Disease Markers 23 (2007) 197–198
IOS Press

Foreword

Magnus von Knebel Doeberitz* and Nicolas Wentzensen
Guest Editors
University of Heidelberg, Germany

AF854602

The year 2006 was marked by an important event in cancer prevention: 30 years after Harald zur Hausen for the first time hypothesized that human papillomaviruses may be associated with the development of cervical cancer, a prophylactic vaccine against certain types of these viruses was launched to the market in Mexico, the US, Canada, Australia, and several European countries. Initially, the very rare malignant conversion of condylomata accuminata tempted zur Hausen to speculate that infectious genital warts and cervical cancer may have a similar infectious causes. These considerations were strongly supported by observations made by Alexander Meisels in Toronto who found that replicating HPV infections led to the formation of "koilocytes" that are found in condylomata but also in early cervical intraepithelial lesions (CIN 1), the early precursors of invasive cervical cancer. Shortly thereafter, the papillomavirus genotypes 6 and 11 were isolated from condylomata and were used as molecular probes to identify related viral genomes in cell lines and biopsies of cervical cancers. These experiments led to the successful detection of HPV 16 and 18 in the early 1980ies. Subsequent research revealed that oncogenic HPV genes are present in almost all cervical cancers, that the viral genes E6 and E7 are continuously expressed in all cancer cells, that these genes confer transforming activities once they are expressed in cultured human epithelial cells *in vitro* and, importantly, that the inhibition of the expression of these genes results in loss of the neoplastic growth of cervical cancer cells. Since then a tremendous amount of knowledge has been gathered by many scientists, including epidemiologists, pathologists, clinicians and public health physicians on the global distribution of oncogenic papillomaviruses and their disease causing role. It turned out that these viruses are abundant agents infecting the majority of all humans at least once in their lifetime. They use an elegant replication strategy that permits high level expression of viral genes and multiplication of the viral genome with capsid formation only in terminally differentiated epithelial cells at the very surface of the epithelium that are going to be exfoliated as cellular debris anyhow. Thus, they cause little or almost no damage within the infected tissues and replicate usually unrecognized by the host. Danger occurs only when after a rather prolonged period of latent infection some basal cells lose molecular control mechanisms that restrain the virus and usually prevent active expression of viral genes in the basal cells. Uncontrolled expression of the viral oncogenes may then induce chromosomal instability and initiate a dangerous cascade of events that drive the cells through a series of pre-neoplastic lesions into invasive cancer cells.

All this knowledge was combined to design a plan to defeat this cancer-causing virus: Empty viral capsids that resemble normal virus particles, but lacking their dangerous genetic information, have been produced and were injected subcutaneously to stimulate the immune system of vaccinees to produce neutralizing antibodies that prevent the entry of infectious virus particles in the basal cells at risk of being infected by oncogenic papillomaviruses. Initial animal experiments and later large worldwide clinical trials showed excellent protection of the vaccinated individuals in almost 100 % against infectious papillomavirus particles. Thus, the development of these vaccines crowns the 30 year long discovery of human papillomaviruses as cancer causing agents that are responsible for at least the second most frequent cancer in women world wide and thus represent after smoking the second most important carcinogen on earth.

Despite all this success a word of caution: we have not yet reached all the goals. Cervical cancer still is an

*Corresponding author. E-mail: knebel@med.uni-heidelberg.de.

ISSN 0278-0240/07/$17.00

important and costly issue and the prevention approach will only work if at least most women in the world will have access to these vaccines. To achieve this, we will certainly need a lot of time, effort and money. The worst thing to do now would be to neglect the very successful screening programs for cervical cancer that made cervical cancer the prime paradigm for successful cancer prevention strategies. About 60 years ago George Papanicolaou developed a simple cytological staining technique that allowed to identify preneoplastic cells in cytological specimens taken by a little swab, brush or broom from the uterine cervix. Because of its simplicity this method became the most wide spread diagnostic test in oncology and led to reduction of the incidence of cervical cancer by about 70%. The vaccine has to compete with this success and there clearly will be a time period in that we will not be willing to abandon the one or the other.

For the time being, vaccination and screening have to go hand in hand. It is clear that screening needs to be adapted to the new demands. There is a lot of room for improvement in cervical cancer screening and a lot of opportunities to render it more cost-effective. The introduction of costly vaccines together with a costly and ineffective screening program is surely not acceptable. In this issue we have addressed these problems from many points of view covering all timely issues of HPV-related disease, screening techniques, molecular biomarkers as well as therapeutic and prophylactic vaccination approaches.

Jenkins summarizes the various histo- und cytopathological features associated with acute and persistent HPV-infections and provides the reader with the essential knowledge to understand how HPV gene products alter shape and function of normal epithelial cells.

Bosch and de Sanjose present a current and extensive survey of HPV and cervical cancer epidemiology. Moscicki gives an overview of HPV infections, screening, triage, and treatment in adolescents that is highly relevant for vaccination programs, since adolescents represent the primary target population and HPV infection in young girls emerges as a new problem. Shah and Westra provide an up-to-date review of HPV associated disease in the aerodigestive tract, including the benign recurrent respiratory papillomatosis as well as head and neck cancers. Nindl and colleagues have summarized biological and clinical data on the role of human papillomviruses in non-melanoma skin cancer. Palefsky contributes a comprehensive overview of HPV infections in men with respect to disease patterns observed in men, transmission of the virus to women and the related issues concerning the possible vaccination of women and men. Moving towards new approaches in screening, Meijer and colleagues present an extensive survey of different HPV detection methods including genotyping and mRNA detection together with different possible scenarios of their application. Pagliusi contributes an important article on the international standardization of HPV testing.

Further articles address the emerging research on new biomarkers for cervical cancer screening that appear to help to overcome several of the important limitations of the current cancer early detection strategies. Doorbar extensively reviews molecular processes in transition from viral infection to the development of high grade disease and cervical cancer. A special focus is put on the changes of the viral life cycle with effects on cellular genes and proteins. Wentzensen and von Knebel Doeberitz summarize the current state of the most promising biomarkers that have been identified so far for revised cervical cancer screening and triage programs and potential clinical applications. The last two articles finally deal with the exciting topic of prophylactic and therapeutic vaccines. Müller and Gissmann contribute an exciting historical essay of the discovery of HPV and the highly interesting process of development of therapeutic and prophylactic vaccines. Kast and colleagues present an excellent and very timely survey on therapeutic vaccines against HPV and associated disease with a detailed description of the lessons learned from the limitations of previous vaccination trials and of novel promising approaches.

We like to express our sincere thanks to all colleagues and scientists who took the effort to contribute to this selection of papers and very much hope that this issue will be an informative source of valuable information particularly for the growing group of people joining the field now and decided to help for their part to defeat human papillomavirus infections and associated cancers.

Disease Markers 23 (2007) 199–212
IOS Press

Histopathology and cytopathology of cervical cancer

David Jenkins
Glaxo Smith Kline Biologicals, Rixensart, Belgium
University of Nottingham, Nottingham, UK
E-mail: David.D.Jenkins@gskbio.com

1. Introduction

Histopathology and cytopathology form the scientific and clinical basis for current prevention and treatment of cervical cancer. Histopathology determines treatment of cancer and precancer through classifying into a diagnosis the patterns of microscopic organization of cells in tissue sections from biopsy or surgical specimens. Although morphological concepts of cervical cancer and precancer evolution are giving way to viral and molecular knowledge, histopathology also remains important as the most widely used clinical endpoints by which the performance of new techniques for cervical cancer prevention are currently evaluated. Cervical cytopathology studies exfoliated cells taken from the surface of the cervix and is the main method of cervical screening in successful cervical cancer prevention programmes.

These techniques have contributed hugely to reducing the burden of cervical cancer. Countries with successful implementation of cytological screening

have shown a reduction in incidence and mortality by 70% or more [1,2]. These figures are historical comparisons and may underestimate the impact as they do not take account of observed increased rates in young women for whom screening provides little protection, and the impact of increasing exposure to oncogenic HPV and other risk factors in some countries as a consequence of major behavioural changes. On this basis, in the UK, the national programme started in 1988 has been estimated to prevent 4,500–6,000 deaths per year, with a very marked decline in [3] rates in women aged 30–34 y. Despite this, because of the difficulties and costs of this approach, globally, there are almost half a million cases of cervical cancer each year.

Concurrently with the enormous success of cytological screening, there has been increasing knowledge of the challenges of the limited reproducibility of the diagnoses, of the complex relationships between cytological and histological diagnosis and the natural history of cervical precancer, particularly the driving role of infection with genital human papillomavirus (HPV).

This review focuses on the concepts and terminology used in classifying morphological changes of cervical precancer and HPV infection, how this links to natural history through information from cervical screening and more recent cohort studies of HPV infection. It addresses the issues around the performance characteristics (reproducibility and accuracy) of cytopathology and histopathology as diagnostic tests, and the implications for cervical screening practice. Finally it discusses the use of cytopathology and histopathology as reference standards and endpoints in clinical research and biomarker development.

2. Historical background

Histopathology has defined historically the concepts of development and progression of cervical precancer to cancer. The idea of carcinoma-in-situ as a cancer precursor dates back to the early cellular pathology of Rudolf Virchow during the nineteenth century. The concept of cervical precancer has been refined

ISSN 0278-0240/07/$17.00

over more than a century to include less severe, dysplastic, changes, and then unified into cervical intraepithelial neoplasia of three grades by Richart [4–6]. Histopathology continues to drive key decisions on treatment of precancer and invasive cancer; and for this reason has been used to define clinical endpoints for research into cervical screening, HPV vaccines and biomarkers.

Cytopathology forms the basis of cervical screening. The proposal can be traced to the Romanian scientists Aurel Babes and Constantin Daniel in 1927 [7]. In 1941 George Papanicolaou and Herbert Traut created widespread attention with their paper on applying the cervical smear technique to women in the Gynaecology department of New York Hospital in the USA [8].

3. Histopathology and the concepts of cervical precancer and cancer

3.1. Normal cervical histology

The normal cervix has two distinct epithelial zones: the ectocervix covered by squamous epithelium, and the endocervix lined by simple glandular epithelium [6, 9]. As a result of squamous metaplasia during adolescence and early adult life the endocervical epithelium is replaced by immature squamous epithelium which eventually matures. This squamous metaplastic area is called the transformation zone and is by far the most common site for development of cervical cancer. What makes the transformation zone uniquely sensitive to HPV-induced carcinogenesis is not well understood. It may be a consequence of exposure of actively proliferating stem cells or transit amplifying cells in the basal layer to HPV, specific molecular properties of the immature metaplastic epithelial cells or the local immune system [10,11].

Underneath the epithelium is a layer of connective tissue and beneath this smooth muscle. There is a local cervical immune system in the epithelium and subepithelial tissue, composed of T and B lymphocytes, plasma cells, NK cells and macrophages and specialized antigen-presenting cells – Langerhans' cells. The local immune system is particularly prominent in certain diseases – for example, lymphoid follicles in follicular cervicitis associated with Chlamydia infection, polymorphs during acute inflammation (eg in gonococcal infection), and the rare condition of eosinophilic cervicitis. Oncogenic HPV, specifically HPV 16 can inhibit activation of the local immune system, manifested as a reduction in numbers of epithelial Langerhans' cells [11,12] This may be a key mechanism of viral persistence. All the different immune cells and other specialized cells such as endocervical cells showing tubal metaplasia may express factors considered as potential biomarkers of carcinogenesis and their presence in clinical studies compared to simple laboratory models complicates the application of biomarkers in clinical practice.

4. The CIN classification

Carcinoma-in-situ (CIS) has long been recognized as the immediate precursor of invasive cancer, and both squamous CIS and glandular, adenocarcinoma-in-situ (AIS) are recognised. The majority of cervical precancer, like invasive cancer (ICC), shows a squamous differentiation. The cervical intraepithelial neoplasia (CIN) classification system was developed to embrace all potential squamous precancerous lesions and to classify the lesions into grades CIN 1, CIN 2 and CIN 3 [13]. The system is descriptive, the morphological changes are regarded as a continuum, and the three grades are defined by arbitrary criteria, the most important of which is the proportion of the epithelium occupied by undifferentiated, basal type cells (Fig. 1). CIS was grouped with severe dysplasia as CIN 3, and mild and moderate grades of dysplastic change reclassified as CIN 1 and CIN 2 respectively. The classification predates and takes no direct account of the oncogenic role or cytopathic effects of different types of HPV. Use of the CIN system is deeply entrenched in clinical practice and provides for a level of continuity in terminology for diagnostic records [6,9,14,15].

An important modification was introduced in 1988 and revised in 2001 [16,17]. The Bethesda system was started as an attempt to define morphological correlates for the different effects of oncogenic and low-risk HPV in cervical lesions, unify morphology of cervical HPV infection and precancer and create a single terminology for histopathology and cytopathology of precancer. For histology two grades of cervical lesion, LSIL and HSIL were defined (Fig. 1). Neither category precisely relates to the presence of low-risk or of oncogenic HPV, as there are no consistent morphological differences between oncogenic and non-oncogenic HPV infection apart from those of progressive neoplastic transformation recorded in CIN. Each category includes a huge range of lesions. In practice LSIL has been used to correspond to CIN 1, with, variably, some, more mi-

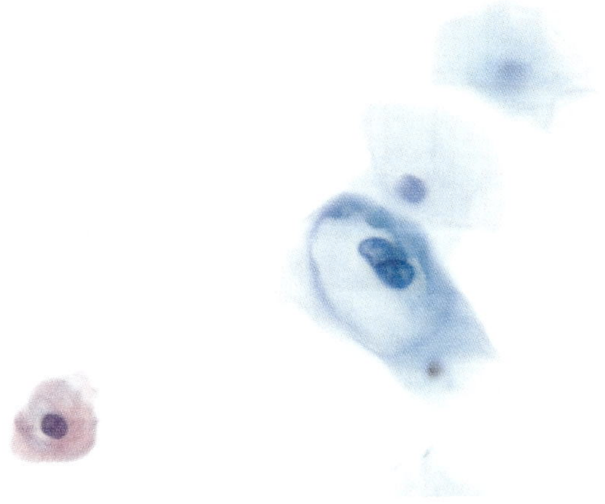

Fig. 1. Schematic representation shows the CIN classification and the Bethesda system, together with the role of HPV infection and persistence. The approximate time to development of lesions estimated from cohort and screening studies is also shown.

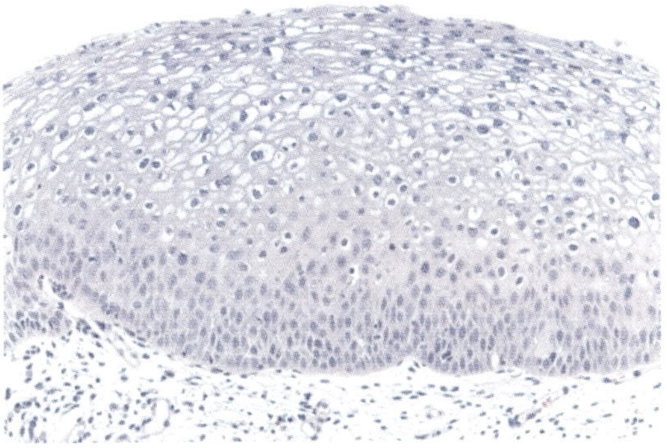

Fig. 2. CIN 1 on cervical biopsy (x20 original magnification) showing hyperplasia of the basal layers (less than one-third of the epithelial thickness) and widespread koilocytosis (vacuolated cells) in the upper layers, together with some binucleate cells. This "typical" case would be accepted by most pathologists as CIN 1, but in other lesions there is widespread variation in the extent and severity of these changes, leading to frequent disagreement on grading.

nor changes of productive HPV infection. HSIL combines CIN2 and CIN 3 into a single category, covering a very wide range of lesions differing widely in morphological, viral and natural history characteristics. The Bethesda system for cytology has, however, proved popular for clinical use [18].

4.1. CIN 1

The characteristics used to define CIN 1 are, firstly, a degree of epithelial hyperplasia, seen as an increase in thickness of the basal and parabasal layers, and secondly, features of HPV replication (productive infection) such as koilocytosis and altered keratinisation, particularly hyperkeratosis and dyskeratosis (Figs 1 and 2). In addition pathologists demand varying degrees of nuclear abnormality for a lesion to qualify as CIN 1 [6,9, 15].

Koilocytosis is the most distinctive feature which is recognized in superficial cells by the wrinkled nuclear outline, with nuclear enlargement and hyperchromasia and a sharply etched perinuclear clearing of the cytoplasm. It is the simplest criterion for productive HPV infection to recognize, but is usually very focal and varies greatly in severity and extent, making it a relatively insensitive criterion for HPV infection. Other changes such as basal cell hyperplasia, multinucleate cells, individual cell keratinisation, parakeratosis and papillomatosis are more widespread and are sensitive but not specific features for HPV infection.

Pathologists have attempted for over twenty years to identify oncogenic changes by conventional morphology from those of a simple productive HPV infection. Progressive and non-progressive infections are not reproducibly distinguishable [19,20] and there is no general agreement about a threshold of histological abnormality distinguishing progressive or persistent precancerous changes within CIN 1 from transient productive infection. The recent suggestion that CIN 1 should be considered to represent simply the morphological manifestations of productive HPV infection is a significant development supported by studies of expression of HPV oncogenes in CIN [21]. However, by convention many pathologists exclude from CIN 1 a whole range of minor morphological features typical of productive HPV infection. This widespread, but unreproducible practice has not been shown to be of predictive value [20,22]. Attempts to include all HPV related changes in a single category of 'low-grade squamous intra-epithelial abnormalities' has led to over-treatment of frequently regressing lesions in very young women [23,24]. Biological markers may represent a solution to this dilemma. Persistence of oncogenic HPV infection over time can distinguish an increased risk of progression to CIN 3 or ICC and the additional expression of the molecular marker p16 can further indicate increased risk of progression [25].

4.2. CIN 2

The diagnosis of CIN 2 is important clinically as it represents what is considered to be a transforming le-

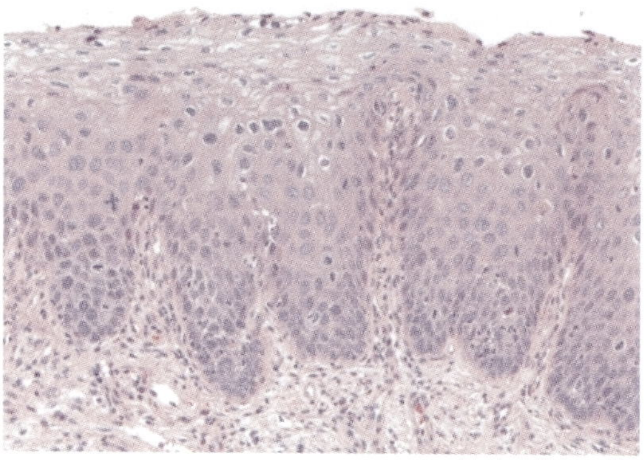

Fig. 3. CIN 2 (x20 original magnification) showing more marked basal hyperplasia (between one- and two-thirds of the epithelial thickness) than CIN 1 with also koilocytosis as in CIN 1. In addition nuclei are enlarged and there are more frequent mitoses and abnormal, multipolar and fragmented mitoses indicating also a high-grade lesion. As in CIN 1 the range of appearances included in CIN 2 leads to disagreement on grading.

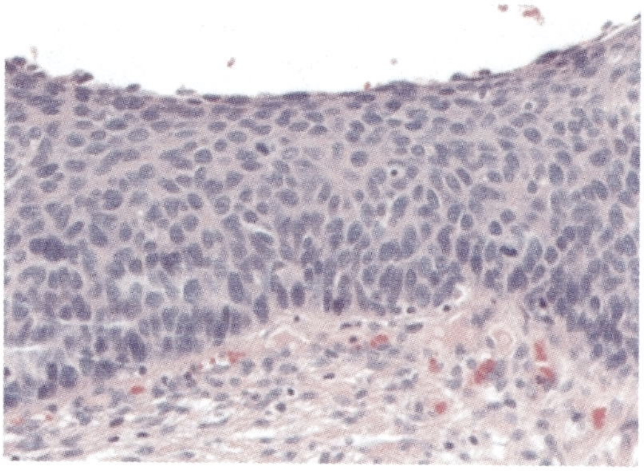

Fig. 4. CIN 3 (x20 original magnification) shows abnormal cells with hyperchromatic (dark) nuclei almost filling the cells occupying almost the entire epithelium. When the entire epithelium is replaced by uniform immature cells it is called carcinoma-in-situ, but in this example there is some flattening and differentiation of cells at the surface.

sion and the threshold for treatment in most cervical screening programmes. The distinction of CIN 2 from CIN 1 is based on a number of different criteria. The nuclear atypia is more severe than CIN 1; immature proliferating cells persist up to the middle third of the epithelium where cytoplasmic maturation commences. Aneuploidy – and related histological features important in discrimination of CIN1 from CIN 2+, particularly abnormal mitoses and mitoses at a high level in the epithelium, koilocytosis and other changes of productive HPV infection remain a common feature, with frequent bizarre koilocytes and apoptotic or dyskeratotic cells (Fig. 3). The limitations of this category in relation to reproducibility and natural history are discussed below.

4.3. CIN 3

CIN 3 is characterized by major loss of orderly maturation of the epithelium with the deepest two-thirds or more of the epithelium replaced by immature abnormal cells with abnormal nuclei and atypical mitoses (Figs 1 and 4). In contrast to the strict definition of carcinoma-in-situ in which the entire epithelium is replaced by such cells, in CIN 3 there may be some flattening and cytoplasmic maturation of surface squamous cells in the upper third of the epithelium, although these cells are abnormal. CIN 3 is considered the HPV-related, immediate intraepithelial precursor of invasive cervical cancer. Lesions with CIN 3 may have a complex architecture, with both high-grade and low-grade components. These have a definite arrangement with a centripetal structure in which CIN 3 is a central core at the inner part of the transformation zone and is surrounded by CIN 1. This complex architecture may affect the expression of molecular markers eg HPV viral load detection in cervical samples.

There is important heterogeneity within CIN 3, especially in lesion size which is not always routinely recorded. This varies widely in extent of involvement of surface epithelium by at least two orders of magnitude and also in depth of extension into cervical crypts [26–29]. Large lesion size has been correlated with cytological grade of abnormality detected in cytological screening, with poor response to local treatment, and very importantly with early invasive or micro-invasive cancer [26,29,30]. As such it may be a reflection of duration and growth of the lesion over many years and may be associated with molecular evidence of accumulating genetic abnormality leading to development of invasive cancer. Other phenotypic changes such as central dyskeratotic necrosis and intralesional squamous maturation are also seen in CIN 3 associated with early invasive cancer [30]. The size of a CIN 3 lesion should be considered in the evaluation of molecular markers for evolution of cervical precancer to cancer.

4.4. Precursors of adenocarcinoma

Adenocarcinoma is thought to arise also through a parallel pathway of cervical glandular intraepithelial neoplasia which is closely associated with squamous CIN [15,31]. The association of adenocarcinoma and oncogenic HPV is as strong as that of squamous carcinoma, although HPV 18 plays a major role and HPV 16 and 18 together are found in more than 80% of cervical adenocarcinoma [10].

The natural history of cervical glandular intraepithelial neoplasia is less well understood than that of squamous intraepithelial neoplasia, with which it is frequently associated. It generally affects the transformation zone, but can also involve endocervical crypts and may be discontinuous and multifocal. It is recognized by a combination of architectural changes in glandular organization and cytological abnormalities including cellular stratification, large and irregular nuclei, prominent nucleoli and mitoses. High-grade glandular precancer (adenocarcinoma-*in-situ*, sometimes called CGIN 3) is relatively well-defined, although it may sometimes be difficult to distinguish from early invasive adenocarcinoma. Low-grade changes (glandular atypia) are more difficult to define, and their outcomes are difficult to predict. These changes are sampled less effectively by conventional cervical cytology, and screening has had less impact on adenocarcinoma than on squamous carcinoma [32] .

4.5. Invasive cervical cancer

The morphology, spread and classification of invasive cervical cancer, stage and grade is described well in standard texts of gynaecological pathology and oncology [31,33,34]. Over 70% of invasive cervical cancer is squamous cell carcinoma with adenocarcinoma and adenosquamous carcinomas making up the majority of the rest, together with infrequent small-cell undifferentiated carcinomas and clear cell carcinomas. The last is associated with vaginal adenosis and prenatal exposure to diethylstilboestrol, but, otherwise, all or almost all cervical cancer is considered as due to oncogenic HPV [35]. The rare verrucous carcinoma may be associated with HPV 6 & 11 [36].

The histological types of squamous carcinoma provide little prognostic information. Small-cell undifferentiated carcinoma shows features of neuro-endocrine epithelial differentiation, and has a less favorable prognosis with surgery. Adenocarcinomas have more positive lymph nodes than squamous carcinomas. The International Federation of Gynecology and Obstetrics (FIGO) staging, based on pathological examination of resected tissue is the basis of determining which approach is used in individual patients in current therapy.

One important category is micro-invasive carcinoma [37–39]. This group of cancers is well defined for squamous carcinoma, but less clear for adenocarcinoma. It constitutes a precisely defined group within the FIGO staging that is usually detected through screening and has very limited superficial invasion only. By setting very precise histological definitions it is possible to identify a group of women with invasive cancer who can be safely managed by local excision.

4.6. Areas of diagnostic difficulty

There are some lesions which are unrelated to HPV or neoplasia in both squamous and glandular epithelium that can cause difficulties and errors in pathological diagnosis. These are problems where biomarkers could be of great value in diagnosis, but also create issues for assessment of biomarkers, as expression of biomarkers may differ physiologically from that of the normal squamous or glandular epithelium in these states. In squamous epithelium some of these changes are: basal cell hyperplasia, immature squamous metaplasia, low-oestrogen states and transitional cell metaplasia. In diagnosing glandular precancer there can be problems with lesions of endometriosis and tubo-endometrioid metaplasia, progestogen-associated changes, inflammatory changes in glandular epithelium, Gartner's duct remnants, endocervical polyps, Arias Stella change and microglandular hyperplasia [40–42].

5. Cytopathology of cervical precancer and cancer

A number of systems have been employed to attempt to classify the visible changes in cervical smears in a way that is reliable and clinically relevant to the management of screen-detected abnormalities. All systems are based on detection in cervical smears of relatively small numbers of cells showing cytological features of productive HPV infection and of the different grades of histological precancer. How these changes are grouped has been the subject of much controversy, reflecting the difficulty of matching cellular morphology of the individual cells to histological diagnosis and then to treatment. Some of the major systems are shown in Table 1.

6. Bethesda classification system

The Bethesda classification is the major current system of terminology providing a standardized format for reporting cervical cytology [7,17,18] (see Table).

Table 1
Terminology used in reports for cytological and histological tests (Source: IARC 2005b)

Papanicolaou System		World Health	CIN	Bethesda	UK classification
Grade	Description	Organization		System	system
Cytological test		Cytological and histological test	Histological test	Cytological and histological test	Cytological
I	Absence of atypical or abnormal cells			Within normal limits	Normal
II	Atypical cytology, but no evidence for malignancy			Benign cellular changes ASC-US/ASC-H	Dyskaryosis
III	Cytology suggestive of, but not conclusive for, malignancy	Mild dysplasia Moderate dysplasia Severe dysplasia	CIN1 CIN2 CIN3	Low-grade SIL High-grade SIL	Mild dyskaryosis Moderately dyskaryosis
IV	Cytology strongly suggestive of malignancy	Carcinoma *in situ*	CIN3		Severe dyskaryosis /invasive carcinoma?
V	Cytology conclusive for malignancy	Microinvasive carcinoma Invasive carcinoma	Invasive carcinoma	Invasive carcinoma	Glandular neoplasia

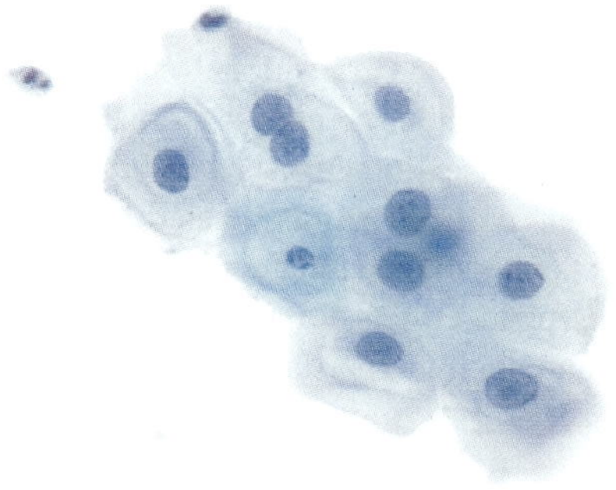

Fig. 5. A group of cells shows changes classified as ASCUS (x60 original magnification). These cells are atypical in terms of nuclear enlargement, a binucleate cell, a "stippled" chromatin, and some vacuolation. These changes can be associated with a wide range of underlying pathology, including CIN2/3 and very occasionally cancer, but often no important pathology.

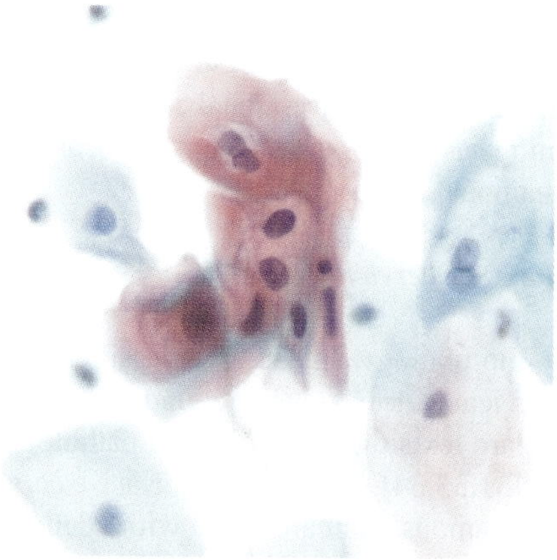

Fig. 6. A group of cells showing changes of LSIL (x60 original magnification). The nuclei are irregular, dark and surrounded by well-defined cytoplasmic vacuolation typical of koilocytes. This picture is relatively reproducible to interpret and associated with productive HPV infection.

It was originally developed at a workshop in Bethesda in 1988, and was widely accepted by the relevant professional societies. In 2001, the American Society for Colposcopy and Cervical Pathology produced a revised consensus statement called "the Bethesda 2001 System" [17]. This can be summarised as:

- Squamous cell abnormalities

  1. Atypical squamous cells of undetermined significance (ASC)
     ASC-US: the commonest abnormality, including a range of minor cellular abnormalities which may or may not be associated with HPV or cervical cancer development (Fig. 5). Women with ASC-US may have findings on cervical examination ranging from negative to invasive cervical cancer.
     ASC-H represents morphological abnormalities where the cytopathologist has difficulty in being confident whether the changes are related to a high-grade precancer or not.
  2. Squamous intraepithelial lesion (SIL) to denote cervical cancer precursors: Low-grade SIL (LSIL) encompassing: productive HPV changes; mild dysplasia or CIN1 (Fig. 6).
     High-grade SIL (HSIL) encompassing: moderate and severe dysplasia CIN2/3 including carcinoma in situ (Fig. 7).

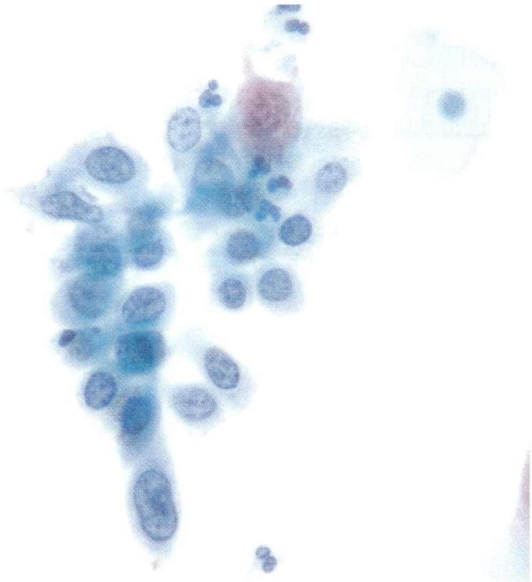

Fig. 7. The changes of HSIL (x60 original magnification) are relatively distinct – a large nucleus with a coarse surrounding membrane and dark blocks of chromatin. They are usually associated with CIN2/3 and cancer.

3. Squamous cell carcinoma (SCC)

- Glandular (columnar) cell abnormalities
  1. Endometrial cells, cytological benign, in a postmenopausal woman
  2. Atypical glandular cells:
     Atypical glandular cells (AGC) which may be endocervical, endometrial, or glandular cells not otherwise specified (AGC NOS)
     Atypical glandular cells, either endocervical or glandular cells favour neoplasia (AGC favour neoplasia)
     Endocervical adenocarcinoma in situ (AIS)
  3. Adenocarcinoma: endocervical; endometrial; extrauterine; no obvious site.

While the Bethesda classification system is used in many countries throughout the world, its use is less common in Europe, where many of the organized screening programmes have their own classification schemes (e.g., Finland, the Netherlands and the UK). The terminology used in these setting generally can be translated into the terms in the Bethesda classification, but there is evidence of country-specific differences in interpretation, which makes precise translation more difficult [43].

Before considering the relationship between cytological findings and underlying cervical disease and how this informs the natural history of the progression from cervical HPV infection to invasive cancer it is necessary to examine the issues around the performance of cytopathology and histopathology as tests.

7. Performance of cytopathology and histopathology as tests

7.1. Reproducibility

Many studies have shown that the reproducibility of cervical cytological and histological interpretations is limited. This has important consequences for clinical practice in cervical screening, especially the requirements for regular repeat testing and follow-up investigations and underlies the importance of training and quality control in cervical cytology and histopathology. It also underlies some of the criticism and litigation aimed at cervical screening despite its success in reducing cervical cancer incidence and deaths. The results of the studies of cytological and histological reproducibility are generally consistent. The largest study of both, the ASCUS-LSIL triage study in the USA showed that, overall, the reproducibility of monolayer cytology was moderate ($K = 0.46$) and equivalent to the reproducibility of punch biopsy and LEEP histopathology. Reproducibility was greatest for high-grade histology, although in this study CIN2 was not separated from CIN 3 and other studies have found CIN 2 to be less reproducible than CIN 3. The lack of reproducibility is generally greatest for less severe interpretations for both cytology and histology, with the interpretation of ASCUS (borderline) cytology and the diagnosis of CIN 1 and CIN 2 histology being the most uncertain diagnoses in most studies [20]. However, the cytological diagnosis of LSIL was found to be reproducible [20]. It is likely that this reproducibility is a consequence of the strict and simple criteria, essentially koilocytosis with nuclear abnormality, required to make the diagnosis.

7.2. Sensitivity and specificity

Cytology shows only a modest overall sensitivity but potential high specificity with regard to detection of CIN lesions with a wide range of performance in different laboratories in different countries, and a trade-off between sensitivity and specificity made differently by different observers. This has been documented in a number of systematic reviews [44,45]. A recent overview of European and North American studies on HPV testing in primary cervical cancer screening showed that the sensitivity of cytology for CIN 2+ was

53% and specificity 96.3%. There was a very wide variation in sensitivity of cytology from 19–77% between different laboratories in different countries, reinforcing the importance of training and quality control. In the same study HPV DNA testing was confirmed as showing better and more consistent sensitivity (96%; range 94–97%) although lower specificity (91%; range 90–91%) [46]. This is similar to other reviews [47,48]. The lower specificity of HPV DNA testing is affected by the age at which screening by HPV DNA is offered and potentially limits this to women over 25–30 y as well as requiring evidence of persistent infection to avoid increasing the cost and inconvenience of referral for colposcopic follow-up.

7.3. *Improving cytological reproducibility and accuracy*

The varied reproducibility of different cyto-histological diagnostic categories suggests that the complexity of the information on which the diagnosis is based, is important in determining agreement. Training in the use of clearly defined criteria is important and requires support by proficiency testing, performance improvement programs or external quality assurance (EQA), and by internal quality assurance using approaches such as rapid re-screening or random re-screening. Such programmes have been introduced into comprehensive training and QC programmes in the USA and in the UK NHS CSP. Automated prescreening and rescreening using image analysis also may assist in standardisation [49].

There is, however, no evidence that expert pathologists perform significantly better, as opposed to differently, compared to other properly trained specialist pathologists. The ALTS study indeed suggests that the correlation for the expert review group of a more strict diagnosis of CIN 1 with HPV DNA positivity was lower than for the clinical centre pathologists, and did not predict outcome [20].

7.4. *Cytohistological relationships*

The overlapping terminology used in cytological and histological classifications of cervical precancer implies a close relationship between the findings of the two methodologies. This is only an approximation. In particular, low-grade cytology (both ASCUS (borderline) and LSIL (mild dyskaryosis)) can be associated with underlying normality, CIN 1, but also CIN2 and CIN 3, and infrequently invasive cancer. The relationship is affected by the subjectivity and limited reproducibility of both tests and colposcopy used to identify lesions for biopsy, and by the sampling process for cytology and biopsy. One important, additional, biological factor that has received only limited attention so far is lesion size, especially for CIN 3 [26–29]. Although there is considerable variation, CIN 1 and CIN 2 lesions are mostly small, with CIN 3 lesions showing a wide range of size. Increasing size of CIN 3 is associated with presence of early invasive cervical cancer and also increases the likelihood of a high-grade cytological abnormality being detected. Small lesions are associated with low-grade cytology and high-grade cytology is associated with large lesions. This is important with regard to the detection of CIN 3 at different ages and to understanding the limitations of knowledge of the natural history of CIN 3.

8. Natural history of cervical precancer and cancer

In an unscreened population it has been estimated from mathematical models that the lifetime risk of cervical cancer is about 3–4%, although the rates up to age 65y in developing countries are about 1.5% [32,50, 51]. Understanding the progression of precancer to invasive cancer is based on analysis of data from cervical screening and from cohort studies. In recent years, this has been supplemented by information on HPV type distribution in cytological abnormality and cohort studies of HPV infection and subsequent cervical precancer or cancer.

8.1. *Screening and cohort studies of women with cytohistological abnormalities*

Data from screening studies was reviewed by Oster (1993). This review found? 3529 cases of CIN 1 of which 57% showed regression, persistence was found in 32%, progression to CIN 3 in 11% and progression to invasive cancer in 1% of cases. The corresponding figures for CIN 2 were 43%, 35%, 22% and 5% respectively. Melnikow [52] demonstrated in a meta-analysis of the published literature similar rates of regression of cytological abnormalities: 68% (95% CI = 58–79%) of ASC-US cases; 47% (95% CI = 36–59%) of LSIL and 35% (95% CI = 17–53%) of HSIL cases. Estimated rates of progression of cytological abnormalities over 24 months range from 7% for ASCUS to about 21% for LSIL. Progression to ICC over 24 months was rare: 1.4% for HSIL and 0.2% for ASC-US [52].

Data from cohort studies indicate that regression of lesions may be very frequent in young women. In one of the few longitudinal studies that included very young women (13–22 y) who were HPV positive at enrolment and had LSIL detected at baseline or during the study 91% (95% CI = 84–99%) regressed by 36 months [23]. Progression to HSIL occurred in 3% at this time. In another study of girls 18 years or younger with LSIL, 28% had regressed by 12 months, 55% by 24 months and 62% by 36 months [53].

8.2. *Distribution of HPV types in precancerous lesions*

The above studies take no account of the impact of HPV type on outcome. Studies of prevalence of different HPV types in cervical precancerous lesions and in cancer have been summarized in a number of systematic reviews [54–56]. The total HPV DNA positivity rose from 71.1% in LSIL to 88.1% in cancer. Such figures are probably substantial underestimates as they are based on a wide range of studies with varying cytology, histology and HPV detection methodology, including sub-optimal studies. The major types of oncogenic HPV are found in all grades of lesions, with HPV 16 predominating. Importantly the distribution of HPV types changes progressively from low-grade to invasive cancer [56,57] with HPV 16 and 18 being the two types which increase in frequency from low-grade to high-grade lesions (2.0 and 1.5 times respectively). There is a decrease in frequency with other oncogenic types ranging from slight (0.85) for HPV 45 to 0.1 for HPV 53. In addition a single cervix may contain multiple lesions which may be of different HPV types. There is a decrease in frequency of multiple type infections from up to 50% in low-grade lesions to about 4% in invasive cancer [54,55,58].

8.3. *Incident and persistent HPV infection and cervical precancer or cancer*

Cohort studies of women uninfected at entry show that incident oncogenic HPV infection is associated with the development of CIN lesions of all grades within 3–24 months. In the case of HPV 16, CIN 1 has been found within 3 months of first detecting infection, and for CIN 2 within 6 months [59,60]. Median time of progression from incident infection to lesions is somewhat longer, around 15-16 months [61,62], although all such estimates are affected by sampling interval and the limited sensitivity of cytology for detecting morphological changes compared to very sensitive viral detection. Many of the issues have been reviewed recently [63,64] Studies also show that the risk of high-grade precancer or invasive cancer is increased with increasing duration of persistence of oncogenic HPV infection especially over 12 months or more [65–69]. Persistent type-specific oncogenic HPV infection has been proposed as a more reliable surrogate indicator of cancer risk for screening and trials than the less reproducible, current, treatment threshold of CIN 2 or worse. The risk for women over 30y with oncogenic HPV of CIN 3 over 10 years of follow-up has been found to be particularly high for certain oncogenic HPVs – 17% for HPV 16 and 14% for HPV 18, compared to 3% for other oncogenic HPV [70] and similar esults have been obtained in other studies [71]. This is consistent with cross-sectional data showing the different distributions of individual oncogenic HPVs between precancers of different grades and cancer.

8.4. *A model of the natural history of cervical carcinogenesis*

Combining information on natural history of cervical precancer from all sources allows proposal of a model going beyond the traditional concept of cervical carcinogenesis proceeding gradually in 10-yearly steps from CIN1 to CIN 2 to CIN 3 over 20–30 years. CIN 1 and CIN 2 can arise within a few months of incident infection and even CIN 3 within 1 year, although the median time for these events is likely to be somewhat longer. Reconciling the cohort studies with the screening data implies there is then likely to be a long period of evolution of high-grade lesions, possibly in transition from CIN 2 to CIN 3, but also probably associated with expansion in size within CIN 3, accompanying multiple genetic and phenotypic changes leading in some women to invasive cancer.

This model leaves open questions which cannot be fully resolved on present evidence. Such uncertainties are important considerations when designing studies of potential biomarkers of precancerous progression, and may be finally resolved by application of markers.

9. Cervical screening

Organised cervical cytological screening has been shown to reduce cervical cancer incidence and mortality by 70–90% [2,72]. Within all major national screening programmes and in the USA where screening practice is recommended by the American Society for Colposcopy and Cervical Pathology on the basis of a National Consensus Conference and by other organisations, cervical screening practice is based on regularly updated guidelines. These are, when possible, informed by critical appraisal of evidence from diagnostic studies, from trials and from mathematical modelling of cost-effectiveness. Current screening is based on regular cervical cytology sampling of adult women at intervals of one to five years. About 1 in 15 women screened have some abnormality requiring further examination or treatment. The management of women with equivocal (ASCUS) smears is an important issue, generating anxiety and cost. About 10% will have CIN2/3 and 1/1000 or less will have cervical cancer. The high sensitivity and hence negative predictive value of HPV DNA testing in the triage situation make this an effective test, and, especially when used as a reflex test on a liquid-based cytology specimen, very efficient. Women who are HPV negative can be reassured and avoid further follow-up. The management of women who are HPV positive is less clear. Immediate colposcopic referral may lead to over-treatment of regressing lesions and will also fail to detect CIN 3 which may develop subsequently [73].

European Union guidelines on cervical screening recommend that cervical cytology should be part of an organised screening programme beginning between 20–30 years and continuing until at least 60 years, with an interval of 3–5 y. In practice there is considerable variation between European countries and even more worldwide. In the USA, although current recommendations support screening at three yearly intervals there is a longstanding, but expensive practice of annual screening starting shortly after commencing sexual activity.

Effectiveness and cost-effectiveness are important issues in screening and very relevant in assessing the likelihood of uptake of a new biomarker. Such issues can be explored by randomised clinical trials (e.g. ALTS) but these use intermediate or surrogate clinical endpoints such as CIN2/3 or CIN3 and any impact on invasive cancer and cost-effectiveness can only be studied prior to widespread clinical implementation by mathematical modelling. Such studies have addressed coverage, interval and age range of screening as well as triage algorithms, HPV DNA testing, liquid-based cytology and, more recently, the potential interaction of cervical screening and prophylactic HPV vaccination. A consistent result of such modelling is that effectiveness of cervical screening is largely driven by coverage of the at-risk population of women and by the frequency of their screening, although increasing this above every three years has little impact. Cost-effectiveness is strongly influenced by the age range over which screening is performed and by the frequency of screening. The performance characteristics of the screening test follow this in importance [74,75]. These characteristics are, however, important in assessing alternative diagnostic tests. One example is that the major limitation of HPV DNA as a screening test is that it does not have high specificity and this is influenced by the frequency of incident and prevalent infection in the population [46, 48]. This varies widely geographically as well as with age. In considering screening tests any impact on frequency of screening could well outweigh other limitations in determining cost-effectiveness. Biomarkers are potentially important as primary screening tests, and, importantly, because of their potential higher specificity for high-grade precancer, as a second stage triage test, preferably as a reflex test which can be performed in the laboratory on a primary liquid-based cytology specimen after cytology or HPV DNA screening.

9.1. Pathology and the assessment of new diagnostic tests for screening and triage

Unlike therapeutics there is no standard regulatory procedure for diagnostic testing. Evaluating a new biomarker often begins with cross-sectional studies in which the potential biomarker is compared for reproducibility, diagnostic sensitivity and specificity on clinical specimens with an established test such as cytology (or even histopathology itself) in predicting a histopathology outcome, usually CIN. CIN 1 is now seen not so much as a precancerous disease entity, but as a histological marker for productive infection. CIN2 & 3, combined with adenocarcinoma-in-situ has been widely used as a combined endpoint of high-grade precancer in clinical trials for the assessment of diagnostic tests or triage algorithms for women with abnormal smears and in primary cervical screening, and also for phase 3 studies of prophylactic HPV vaccines. Making histopathology endpoints reproducible requires the use of a pathology panel through which a review diagnosis based on independent reading and concurrence of at least two expert observers is used to define the endpoints of the study. This approach has been used in clinical trials. When multiple sections are examined from a single block, the grade of a lesion may change through the block. When it is important to link CIN grade to individual HPV types or to markers using extracted DNA or RNA from tissue (as in assessing impact of prophylactic HPV vaccination) it is necessary to link the histology panel diagnosis to a sandwich process of taking sections for DNA or RNA analysis between sections subjected to histological examination.

Demonstration of sensitivity, specificity and reproducibility of a new marker is a basic requirement, but this is not sufficient to ensure uptake and reimbursement as these are also driven by the impact of a new marker on effectiveness and cost-effectiveness. A high sensitivity improves effectiveness and a high specificity improves cost-effectiveness. Neither cervical cytological screening nor HPV DNA testing are perfect by these criteria and programmatic issues such as screening interval and the necessity of triage are heavily influenced by test performance with substantial implications for health care costs and for the women concerned. It is therefore necessary to complement the data on test performance by an exploration in a clinical trial and through mathematical modelling of the true impact of the new test on clinical effectiveness and cost-effectiveness. The endpoint of a trial is usually CIN 2 or CIN 3. CIN 2 is the threshold for surgical treatment of CIN, but some experts have a preference for CIN 3 as the natural history of CIN 2 includes acute and regressing lesions. Studies using CIN3 and ICC as endpoints in the context of screening or other cervical cancer prevention are limited by the requirement for large study populations and/or many years, even decades, of follow-up. Therefore potential impact on invasive cancer is usually assessed by mathematical modelling. Review of the current evaluations of HPV DNA testing and of liquid-based cytology provide a guide as to the approaches needed to assess new biomarkers [46,48, 64].

10. Conclusion

Biomarkers offer exciting opportunities to overcome the limitations of current morphological methods of screening and diagnosis in cervical cancer prevention and cancer management. Understanding the theory and practice of cervical histopathology and cytopathology is important for the assessment of biomarkers. Cytopathology remains the key comparator for evaluating the performance of a biomarker in screening, and histopathology provides the major surrogate endpoints of high-grade precancer – CIN 2 or worse. An important issue for both is standardization of subjective morphological interpretation when used as a comparator or endpoint, requiring careful attention to reproducibility and quality control of the diagnostic processes. Use of multiple readers is essential for key endpoints, and careful attention is also needed to link the histopathology endpoints accurately to their HPV status.

The evaluation of biomarkers for cervical cancer prevention even with standardisation of pathology comparators and endpoints, cannot be considered in isolation from the picture of current clinical and laboratory practices, or from potential future changes in screening practice and other important, new developments such as prophylactic HPV vaccination. Pathology is the key in providing endpoints for assessing diagnostic sensitivity and specificity and for clinical trials. However, in cervical screening and cervical cancer prevention it is effectiveness and cost-effectiveness of cervical cancer prevention that ultimately will determine the use of a new biomarker. The performance data and clinical trial results against surrogate CIN2/3 endpoints are important for providing data for mathematical models to evaluate these rapidly and economically.

A final major issue in planning studies using pathology endpoints is that cervical cancer preventive practice is changing. HPV testing has been introduced widely for triage of ASCUS smears and is under research for primary screening. Most importantly the future impact of prophylactic vaccination against the major types of oncogenic HPV infection, types 16 & 18 needs to be taken into account. Prophylactic HPV vaccination of uninfected women has been shown to prevent abnormal smears and CIN associated with HPV 16 & 18 [60,76–78] and this protection may extend to other HPV types, in particular HPV 45 and 31 [78]. Effective prophylactic vaccination will alter the natural history of the residual precancer when HPV 16/18 driven lesions are removed. The residual disease will be predominantly associated with other oncogenic and non-oncogenic HPV types. The residual oncogenic HPV lesions are probably less aggressive from cohort studies, and the reduction in frequency of high-grade lesions will decrease the predictive value of abnormal screening results [73,79]. This impact on test performance is likely to affect cytology most severely, and, together with the need to identify any true "breakthrough" cases of HPV 16/18 high-grade precancer from other CIN in vaccinated women could drive a change to HPV testing and typing, and the use of biomarkers to improve accuracy. To meet these challenges the assessment of biomarkers against pathology endpoints needs to be done with careful attention to defining pathology endpoints reliably, linking these to HPV status and also with careful consideration of the current and future clinical and epidemiological context in which the biomarker is likely to be used.

Acknowledgments

The author would like to thank Dr. Ron Luff of Quest Diagnostics, Teterboro, NJ, USA, for providing the photomicrographs.

References

[1] M.E. van den Akker-van Marle, M. van Ballegooijen, G.J. van Oortmarssen, R. Boer and J.D. Habbema, Cost-effectiveness of cervical cancer screening: comparison of screening policies, *J Natl Cancer Inst* **94** (2002), 193–204.

[2] A. Anttila, G. Ronco, G. Clifford, F. Bray, M. Hakama, M. Arbyn et al., Cervical cancer screening programmes and policies in 18 European countries, *Br J Cancer* **91** (2004), 935–941.

[3] J. Peto, C. Gilham, O. Fletcher and F.E. Matthews, The cervical cancer epidemic that screening has prevented in the UK, *Lancet* **364** (2004), 249–256.

[4] R.M. Richart, Natural history of cervical intraeithelial neoplasia, *Clin Obstet Gynecol* (1968), 5.

[5] R.M. Richart, Cervical intraepithelial neoplasia, *Pathol Annu* **8** (1973), 301–328.

[6] B. Anderson, Premalignant and malignant squamous lesions of the cervix, in: *Haines and Taylor: Obstetrical and Gynaecological Pathology,* H. Fox, ed., 1995, pp. 273–322.

[7] P. Virtej and C. Vasiliu, Cytodiagnosis in cervical neoplasia: from the Babes/Papanicolaou smear to the actual Bethesda System, *Clin Exp Obstet Gynecol* **30** (2003), 173–177.

[8] G.N. Papanicolaou and H.F. Traut, The diagnostic value of vaginal smears in carcinoma of the uterus. 1941, *Arch Pathol Lab Med* **121** (1997), 211–224.

[9] M.C. Anderson, C.L. Brown, C.H. Buckley, H. Fox, D. Jenkins, D.G. Lowe et al., Current views on cervical intraepithelial neoplasia, *J Clin Pathol* **44** (1991), 969–978.

[10] N. Munoz, X. Castellsague, A.B. de Gonzalez and L. Gissmann, Chapter 1: HPV in the etiology of human cancer, *Vaccine* **24** (2006), S3:S1–S10.

[11] M. Stanley, Immune responses to human papillomavirus, *Vaccine* (2005).

[12] S.K. Tay, D. Jenkins, P. Maddox, M. Campion and A. Singer, Subpopulations of Langerhans' cells in cervical neoplasia, *Br J Obstet Gynaecol* **94** (1987), 10–15.

[13] Histopathology Reporting in Cervical Screening, Ed. Fox H & Buckley CH. NHSCSP Publication 10, 1999, Sheffield ISBN 1 871997 68 2.

[14] D. Jenkins, The pathology of lower genital tract premalignancy, *Clin Pract Gynaecol* (1987).

[15] M. Stoler, *The pathology of cervical neoplasia,* Kluwer Academic Publishers, 2004.

[16] D. Solomon, The 1988 Bethesda system for reporting cervical/vaginal cytological diagnoses, *Acta Cytologica* (1989).

[17] D. Solomon, D. Davey, R. Kurman, A. Moriarty, D. O'Connor, M. Prey et al., The 2001 Bethesda System: terminology for reporting results of cervical cytology, *JAMA* **287** (2002), 2114–2119.

[18] C. Bergeron, The 2001 Bethesda system, *Salud Publica Mex* **45**(Suppl 3) (2003), S340–S344.

[19] D. Jenkins, S.K. Tay, D.J. McCance, M.J. Campion, P.K. Clarkson and A. Singer, Histological and immunocytochemical study of cervical intraepithelial neoplasia (CIN) with associated HPV 6 and HPV 16 infections, *J Clin Pathol* **39** (1986), 1177–1180.

[20] M.H. Stoler and M. Schiffman, Interobserver reproducibility of cervical cytologic and histologic interpretations: realistic estimates from the ASCUS-LSIL Triage Study, *JAMA* **285** (2001), 1500–1505.

[21] K. Middleton, W. Peh, S. Southern, H. Griffin, K. Sotlar, T. Nakahara et al., Organization of human papillomavirus productive cycle during neoplastic progression provides a basis for selection of diagnostic markers, *J Virol* **77** (2003), 10186–10201.

[22] J.T. Cox, M. Schiffman and D. Solomon, Prospective follow-up suggests similar risk of subsequent cervical intraepithelial neoplasia grade 2 or 3 among women with cervical intraepithelial neoplasia grade 1 or negative colposcopy and directed biopsy, *Am J Obstet Gynecol* **188** (2003), 1406–1412.

[23] A.B. Moscicki, S. Shiboski, N.K. Hills, K.J. Powell, N. Jay, E.N. Hanson et al., Regression of low-grade squamous intraepithelial lesions in young women, *Lancet* **364** (2004), 1678–1683.

[24] A. Szarewski and P. Sasieni, Cervical screening in adolescents–at least do no harm, *Lancet* **364** (2004), 1642–1644.

[25] S.S. Wang, M. Trunk, M. Schiffman, R. Herrero, M.E. Sherman, R.D. Burk et al., Validation of p16INK4a as a marker of oncogenic human papillomavirus infection in cervical biopsies from a population-based cohort in Costa Rica, *Cancer Epidemiol Biomarkers Prev* **13** (2004), 1355–1360.

[26] P. Tidbury, A. Singer and D. Jenkins, CIN 3: the role of lesion size in invasion, *Br J Obstet Gynaecol* **99** (1992), 583–586.

[27] M.E. Sherman, S.S. Wang, R. Tarone, L. Rich and M. Schiffman, Histopathologic extent of cervical intraepithelial neoplasia 3 lesions in the atypical squamous cells of undetermined significance low-grade squamous intraepithelial lesion triage study: implications for subject safety and lead-time bias, *Cancer Epidemiol Biomarkers Prev* **12** (2003), 372–379.

[28] M.E. Sherman, S.S. Wang, C.M. Wheeler, L. Rich, P.E. Gravitt, R. Tarone et al., Determinants of human papillomavirus load among women with histological cervical intraepithelial neoplasia 3: dominant impact of surrounding low-grade lesions, *Cancer Epidemiol Biomarkers Prev* **12** (2003), 1038–1044.

[29] M.R. Jarmulowicz, D. Jenkins, S.E. Barton, A.L. Goodall, A. Hollingworth and A. Singer, Cytological status and lesion size: a further dimension in cervical intraepithelial neoplasia, *Br J Obstet Gynaecol* **96** (1989), 1061–1066.

[30] A.I. al Nafussi and D.E. Hughes, Histological features of CIN3 and their value in predicting invasive microinvasive squamous carcinoma, *J Clin Pathol* **47** (1994), 799–804.

[31] N.R. Griffin and M. Wells, *Premalignant and malignant glandular lesions of the cervix,* Edinburgh, Churchill Livingstone, 1995.

[32] D.M. Parkin and F. Bray, Chapter 2: The burden of HPV-related cancers, *Vaccine* **24**(Suppl 3) (2006), S11–S25.

[33] C.H. Buckley, *Tumors of the cervix uteri,* Edinburgh, Churchill Livingstone, 1995.

[34] J.H. Shepherd, Revised FIGO staging for gynaecological cancer, *Br J Obstet Gynaecol* **96** (1989), 889–892.

[35] J.M. Walboomers, M.V. Jacobs, M.M. Manos, F.X. Bosch, J.A. Kummer, K.V. Shah et al., Human papillomavirus is a necessary cause of invasive cervical cancer worldwide, *J Pathol* **189** (1999), 12–19.
[36] C.J. Lacey, C.M. Lowndes and K.V. Shah, Chapter 4: Burden and management of non-cancerous HPV-related conditions: HPV-6/11 disease, *Vaccine* **24**(Suppl 3) (2006), S35–S41.
[37] E. Burghardt, F. Girardi, M. Lahousen, H. Pickel and K. Tamussino, Microinvasive carcinoma of the uterine cervix (International Federation of Gynecology and Obstetrics Stage IA), *Cancer* **67** (1991), 1037–1045.
[38] N. Tsukamoto, T. Kaku, K. Matsukuma, T. Matsuyama, T. Kamura, T. Saito et al., The problem of stage Ia (FIGO, 1985) carcinoma of the uterine cervix, *Gynecol Oncol* **34** (1989), 1–6.
[39] F. Girardi et al., Small FIGO stage Ib cervical cancer, *Gynecologic Oncology* (1994).
[40] S.M. Ismail, Cone biopsy causes cervical endometriosis and tubo-endometrioid metaplasia, *Histopathology* **18** (1991), 107–114.
[41] A. al Nafussi and M. Rahilly, The prevalence of tubo-endometrial metaplasia and adenomatoid proliferation, *Histopathology* **22** (1993), 177–179.
[42] J.A. Ferry and R.E. Scully, Mesonephric remnants, hyperplasia, and neoplasia in the uterine cervix. A study of 49 cases, *Am J Surg Pathol* **14** (1990), 1100–1111.
[43] D.R. Scott, B. Hagmar, P. Maddox, A. Hjerpe, J. Dillner, J. Cuzick et al., Use of human papillomavirus DNA testing to compare equivocal cervical cytologic interpretations in the United States, Scandinavia, and the United Kingdom, *Cancer* **96** (2002), 14–20.
[44] M.T. Fahey, L. Irwig and P. Macaskill, Meta-analysis of Pap test accuracy, *Am J Epidemiol* **141** (1995), 680–689.
[45] K. Nanda, D.C. McCrory, E.R. Myers, L.A. Bastian, V. Hasselblad, J.D. Hickey et al., Accuracy of the Papanicolaou test in screening for and follow-up of cervical cytologic abnormalities: a systematic review, *Ann Intern Med* **132** (2000), 810–819.
[46] J. Cuzick, M.H. Mayrand, G. Ronco, P. Snijders and J. Wardle, Chapter 10: New dimensions in cervical cancer screening, *Vaccine* **24**(Suppl 3) (2006), S90–S97.
[47] M. Arbyn, F. Buntinx, M. Van Ranst, E. Paraskevaidis, P. Martin-Hirsch and J. Dillner, Virologic versus cytologic triage of women with equivocal Pap smears: a meta-analysis of the accuracy to detect high-grade intraepithelial neoplasia, *J Natl Cancer Inst* **96** (2004), 280–293.
[48] M. Arbyn, P. Sasieni, C.J. Meijer, C. Clavel, G. Koliopoulos and J. Dillner, Chapter 9: Clinical applications of HPV testing: A summary of meta-analyses, *Vaccine* **24**(Suppl 3) (2006), S78–S89.
[49] M.E. Sherman, M. Schiffman, R. Herrero, D. Kelly, C. Bratti, L.J. Mango et al., Performance of a semiautomated Papanicolaou smear screening system: results of a population-based study conducted in Guanacaste, Costa Rica, *Cancer* **84** (1998), 273–280.
[50] S.J. Goldie, D. Grima, M. Kohli, T.C. Wright, M. Weinstein and E. Franco, A comprehensive natural history model of HPV infection and cervical cancer to estimate the clinical impact of a prophylactic HPV-16/18 vaccine, *Int J Cancer* **106** (2003), 896–904.
[51] S.J. Goldie, M. Kohli, D. Grima, M.C. Weinstein, T.C. Wright, F.X. Bosch et al., Projected clinical benefits and cost-effectiveness of a human papillomavirus 16/18 vaccine, *J Natl Cancer Inst* **96** (2004), 604–615.
[52] J. Melnikow, J. Nuovo, A.R. Willan, B.K. Chan and L.P. Howell, Natural history of cervical squamous intraepithelial lesions: a meta-analysis, *Obstet Gynecol* **92** (1998), 727–735.
[53] J.D. Wright, R.M. Davila, K.R. Pinto, D.F. Merritt, R.K. Gibb, J.S. Rader et al., Cervical dysplasia in adolescents, *Obstet Gynecol* **106** (2005), 115–120.
[54] G.M. Clifford, J.S. Smith, M. Plummer, N. Muñoz and S. Franceschi, Human papillomavirus types in invasive cervical cancer worldwide: a meta-analysis, *Br J Cancer* **88** (2003), 63–73.
[55] G.M. Clifford, J.S. Smith, T. Aguado and S. Franceschi, Comparison of HPV type distribution in high-grade cervical lesions and cervical cancer: a meta-analysis, *Br J Cancer* **89** (2003), 101–105.
[56] G. Clifford, S. Franceschi, M. Diaz, N. Munoz and L.L. Villa, Chapter 3: HPV type-distribution in women with and without cervical neoplastic diseases, *Vaccine* **24**(Suppl 3) (2006), S26–S34.
[57] S. Franceschi and G.M. Clifford, Re: A study of the impact of adding HPV types to cervical cancer screening and triage tests, *J Natl Cancer Inst* **97** (2005), 938–939.
[58] G.M. Clifford, R.K. Rana, S. Franceschi, J.S. Smith, G. Gough and J.M. Pimenta, Human papillomavirus genotype distribution in low-grade cervical lesions: comparison by geographic region and with cervical cancer, *Cancer Epidemiol Biomarkers Prev* **14** (2005), 1157–1164.
[59] L.A. Koutsky, K.K. Holmes, C.W. Critchlow, C.E. Stevens, J. Paavonen, A.M. Beckmann et al., A cohort study of the risk of cervical intraepithelial neoplasia grade 2 or 3 in relation to papillomavirus infection, *N Engl J Med* **327** (1992), 1272–1278.
[60] D.M. Harper, E.L. Franco, C. Wheeler, D.G. Ferris, D. Jenkins, A. Schuind et al., Efficacy of a bivalent L1 virus-like particle vaccine in prevention of infection with human papillomavirus types 16 and 18 in young women: a randomised controlled trial, *Lancet* **364** (2004), 1757–1765.
[61] R.L. Winer, N.B. Kiviat, J.P. Hughes, D.E. Adam, S.K. Lee, J.M. Kuypers et al., Development and duration of human papillomavirus lesions, after initial infection, *J Infect Dis* **191** (2005), 731–738.
[62] H. Trottier, S. Mahmud, L. Lindsay, D. Jenkins, S. Wieting and E. Franco, Natural history of HPV infection and cervical lesions in women from the placebo arm of an AS04 adjuvanted HPV-16/18 L1 vaccine trial. EUROGIN.
[63] A.B. Moscicki, M. Schiffman, S. Kjaer and L.L. Villa, Chapter 5: Updating the natural history of HPV and anogenital cancer, *Vaccine* **24**(Suppl 3) (2006), S42–S51.
[64] H.C. Kitchener, P.E. Castle and J.T. Cox, Chapter 7: Achievements and limitations of cervical cytology screening, *Vaccine* **24**(Suppl 3) (2006), S63–S70.
[65] J.P. Bory, J. Cucherousset, M. Lorenzato, R. Gabriel, C. Quereux, P. Birembaut et al., Recurrent human papillomavirus infection detected with the hybrid capture II assay selects women with normal cervical smears at risk for developing high grade cervical lesions: a longitudinal study of 3,091 women, *Int J Cancer* **102** (2002), 519–525.
[66] V. Dalstein, D. Riethmuller, J.L. Pretet, C.K. Le Bail, J.L. Sautiere, J.P. Carbillet et al., Persistence and load of high-risk HPV are predictors for development of high-grade cervical lesions: a longitudinal French cohort study, *Int J Cancer* **106** (2003), 396–403.
[67] N.F. Schlecht, S. Kulaga, J. Robitaille, S. Ferreira, M. Santos, R.A. Miyamura et al., Persistent human papillomavirus infec-

tion as a predictor of cervical intraepithelial neoplasia, *JAMA* **286** (2001), 3106–3114.

[68] G.Y. Ho, R.D. Burk, S. Klein, A.S. Kadish, C.J. Chang, P. Palan et al., Persistent genital human papillomavirus infection as a risk factor for persistent cervical dysplasia, *J Natl Cancer Inst* **87** (1995), 1365–1371.

[69] K.L. Wallin, F. Wiklund, T. Angstrom, F. Bergman, U. Stendahl, G. Wadell et al., Type-specific persistence of human papillomavirus DNA before the development of invasive cervical cancer, *N Engl J Med* **341** (1999), 1633–1638.

[70] M.J. Khan, P.E. Castle, A.T. Lorincz, S. Wacholder, M. Sherman, D.R. Scott et al., The elevated 10-year risk of cervical precancer and cancer in women with human papillomavirus (HPV) type 16 or 18 and the possible utility of type-specific HPV testing in clinical practice, *J Natl Cancer Inst* **97** (2005), 1072–1079.

[71] P.E. Castle, D. Solomon, M. Schiffman and C.M. Wheeler, Human papillomavirus type 16 infections and 2-year absolute risk of cervical precancer in women with equivocal or mild cytologic abnormalities, *J Natl Cancer Inst* **97** (2005), 1066–1071.

[72] M. Hicks and M. Piver, How to obtain an accurate pap smear, *Med Asp Human Sexuality* (1991).

[73] D. Jenkins, Public Health issues related to HPV vaccination, in: *Emerging issues on HPV infections from science to practice,* J. Monsonego, ed., Karger, 2006.

[74] S.J. Goldie, J.D. Goldhaber-Fiebert and G.P. Garnett, Chapter 18: Public health policy for cervical cancer prevention: The role of decision science, economic evaluation, and mathematical modeling, *Vaccine* **24**(Suppl 3) (2006), S155–S163.

[75] S.J. Goldie, J.J. Kim and E. Myers, Chapter 19: Cost-effectiveness of cervical cancer screening, *Vaccine* **24**(Suppl 3) (2006), S164–S170.

[76] L.A. Koutsky, K.A. Ault, C.M. Wheeler, D.R. Brown, E. Barr, F.B. Alvarez et al., A controlled trial of a human papillomavirus type 16 vaccine, *N Engl J Med* **347** (2002), 1645–1651.

[77] C. Mao, L.A. Koutsky, K.A. Ault, C.M. Wheeler, D.R. Brown, D.J. Wiley et al., Efficacy of human papillomavirus-16 vaccine to prevent cervical intraepithelial neoplasia: a randomized controlled trial, *Obstet Gynecol* **107** (2006), 18–27.

[78] D.M. Harper, E.L. Franco, C.M. Wheeler, A.B. Moscicki, B. Romanowski, C.M. Roteli-Martins et al., Sustained efficacy up to 4.5 years of a bivalent L1 virus-like particle vaccine against human papillomavirus types 16 and 18: follow-up from a randomised control trial, *Lancet* **367** (2006), 1247–1255.

[79] E.L. Franco, J. Cuzick, A. Hildesheim and S. de Sanjose, Chapter 20: Issues in planning cervical cancer screening in the era of HPV vaccination, *Vaccine* **24**(Suppl 3) (2006), S171–S177.

Disease Markers 23 (2007) 213–227
IOS Press

The epidemiology of human papillomavirus infection and cervical cancer

F. Xavier Bosch and Silvia de Sanjosé
Institut Català d'Oncologia, Epidemiology and Cancer Registration Unit, Av. Gran Via, s/n Km. 2,7, E-08907 L'Hospitalet de Llobregat, Barcelona, Spain
Tel.: +34 93 2607812; Fax: +34 93 2607787; E-mail: x.bosch@ico.scs.es

Abstract. Cervical cancer has been recognized as a rare outcome of a common Sexually Transmitted Infection (STI). The etiologic association is restricted to a limited number of viral types of the family of the Human Papillomaviruses (HPVs). The association is causal in nature and under optimal testing systems, HPV DNA can be identified in all specimens of invasive cervical cancer. As a consequence, it has been claimed that HPV infection is a necessary cause of cervical cancer. The evidence is consistent worldwide and implies both the Squamous Cell Carcinomas (SCC), the adenocarcinomas and the vast majority (i.e. $> 95\%$) of the immediate precursors, namely High Grade Squamous Intraepithelial Lesions (HSIL)/Cervical Intraepithelial Neoplasia 3 (CIN3)/Carcinoma *in situ*. Co-factors that modify the risk among HPV DNA positive women include the use of oral contraceptives (OC) for five or more years, smoking, high parity (five or more full term pregnancies) and previous exposure to other sexually transmitted diseases such as Chlamydia Trachomatis (CT) and Herpes Simplex Virus type 2 (HSV-2). Women exposed to the Human Immunodeficiency Virus (HIV) are at high risk for HPV infection, HPV DNA persistency and progression of HPV lesions to cervical cancer.

Keywords: Cervical cancer, human papillomavirus, HPV, epidemiology

1. Epidemiology of human papillomavirus infections and cervical cancer

HPV infections of the cervix and the epidemiology of cervical cancer in relation to HPV are being investigated using as markers of exposure the presence of viral DNA in cellular scrapes or in biopsy tissue. Early DNA detection methods lead to the hypothesis that there was an association between cervical cancer and HPV exposure, however the development of Polymerase Chain Reaction (PCR) and other amplification techniques allowed an accurate assessment of the presence of viral DNA in cervical specimens as well as a quantification of the strength of the association down to the level of HPV type and of variants of the main types. Serological tests to detect antibodies to HPV antigens following natural infections are still in evaluation phase for large epidemiological studies. Natural HPV infections only trigger a measurable antibody response under special situations, resulting in significant under-detection. In contrast antibody response to current HPV vaccines based on pseudo viral like particles (VLPs) from the L1 genomic region of type specific HPVs is universal and antibody titers are several fold (up to 40-fold) higher that antibody titers following natural infection. Therefore, most of the epidemiology of HPV and cervical cancer is largely based on DNA detection techniques of which most of the studies included in this review have used either the clinically validated Hybrid Capture 2 method (HC2) or some of the internationally validated PCR-based systems [1].

1.1. Prevalence of human papillomavirus DNA. The international perspective

The prevalence of HPV DNA in cervical specimens from the general population and from samples of women with normal cytology has been reported. The variability of results is considerable and relates to the selection of women included in the surveys (i.e. proba-

ISSN 0278-0240/07/$17.00

bilistic samples of the population, women in screening programs and opportunistic series from clinical settings) and to the testing systems employed. Two recent sources have provided estimates that may reflect the global prevalence, the age-specific prevalence and the type-specific prevalence as well as an approximation to describing the international variability. In a multicentric and centrally coordinated international study, the International Agency for Research on Cancer (IARC) provided data from 15 areas in four continents among women 15–74 year old. The point age standardized prevalence was 10.5 (95%CI 9.9–11.0) and ranged from a low end (less than 5%) in Mediterranean countries and in some countries in South East Asia to a high end (greater than 15%) in several countries in Latin America and in a few populations in Africa) [2].

The second source is a comprehensive review of the literature that used standardized criteria for study inclusion and statistical analyses that adjusted the estimates for the variables were influential in the comparability of studies. In this review, the estimates of the population prevalence worldwide (all ages) among women with normal cytology was of 10.41% with a 95%CI 10.2–10.7. The age specific prevalence showed higher proportions among the young age groups, a decline in the young adults and a variable pattern afterwards. In most countries, notably in the Americas, the prevalence increased again in the post-menopausal age groups. In Europe, the same pattern in the 40+ age group is maintained in most surveys whereas in other high prevalence countries in Asia the HPV DNA prevalence remained fairly constant across all age groups [de Sanjose et al. in press]. Figure 1 shows the summary of the age-specific HPV DNA prevalence in women with normal cytology in a model that compiled data from close to 140,000 women reported in 67 studies from Africa (7 studies), America (17 studies), Europe (27 studies) and Asia (16 studies). The reason for the second increase in the HPV detection rate in the old age groups is unclear. The consistency of the finding in many individual studies in countries with substantial variability in sexual behaviour would indicate that the observation translates biological changes related to menopause-hormonal and immunological status that would facilitate HPV DNA detection from exposures earlier in life that remained silent/undetectable for a number of years. However, individual cohort studies and sexual behaviour surveys also indicate that additional number of new sexual partners habits in middle age and above might partially explain the second peak of genuine incident infections [3].

The HPV type-specific prevalence of the five most common HPV types in women with normal cytology is show in Fig. 2. HPV 16 is identified in 2.25% of women (25.5% of positives) followed by HPV 18 (0.8%), 31 (0.8%), 58 (0.7%) and 52 (0.6%). This distribution reflects the biological advantage of HPVs 16 and 18 for persistency. The 33% relative proportion afforded by HPVs 16 and 18 combined in women with normal cytology is in contrast with the 70% relative frequency of these two viral types observed in invasive cervical cancer and translates the biological advantage for progression of HPV 16 and 18 also observed in several natural history studies [4].

1.2. Behavioural determinants of human papillomavirus infection

Several groups of studies have clearly shown that HPV is predominantly and largely transmitted through sexual intercourse. Other forms of transmission have been occasionally described, but its implication in cervical cancer is likely to be marginal, if any.

Epidemiological studies investigating risk factors for HPV infection clearly and consistently have shown that the key determinants among women are the number of sexual partners, the age at which sexual intercourse was initiated and the likelihood that at least one of her sexual partners was an HPV carrier as measured by his sexual behaviour traits [5]. The role of males as possible vectors of HPV was measured in the early epidemiological studies by questionnaires that addressed the sexual behaviour of the husbands or sexual partners of cervical cancer cases and controls. More recent studies had, in addition, the ability to measure HPV DNA in exfoliated cells from the penile shaft, the coronal sulcus and from the distal urethra [6].

Case-control studies have established that the risk of cervical cancer for a given woman is predictable by the sexual behaviour of her husband as much as for her own sexual behaviour. In populations where female monogamy is dominant, the population of female sex workers plays an important role in the maintenance and transmission of HPV infections. Moreover, the probability that a woman is an HPV carrier and her risk of developing cervical cancer have been shown to be related to the presence of HPV DNA in the penis or the urethra of her husband or sexual partner. These observations confirmed in terms of HPV infections a scientific hypothesis formulated almost 30 years ago that male sexual behaviour is a central determinant of the incidence of cervical cancer [7].

Studies on virgins offer a unique opportunity to demonstrate the predominantly sexual nature of HPV

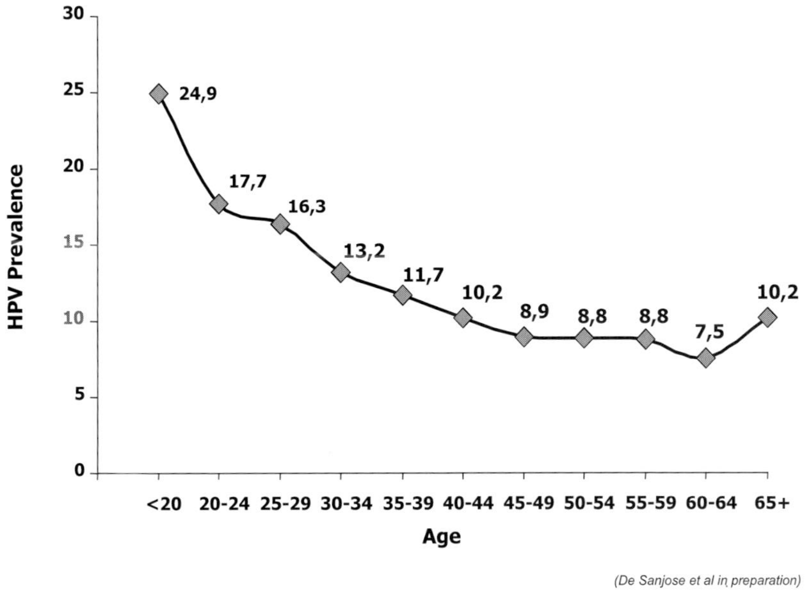

Fig. 1. World-wide age-specific HPV-DNA prevalence among women from the general population.

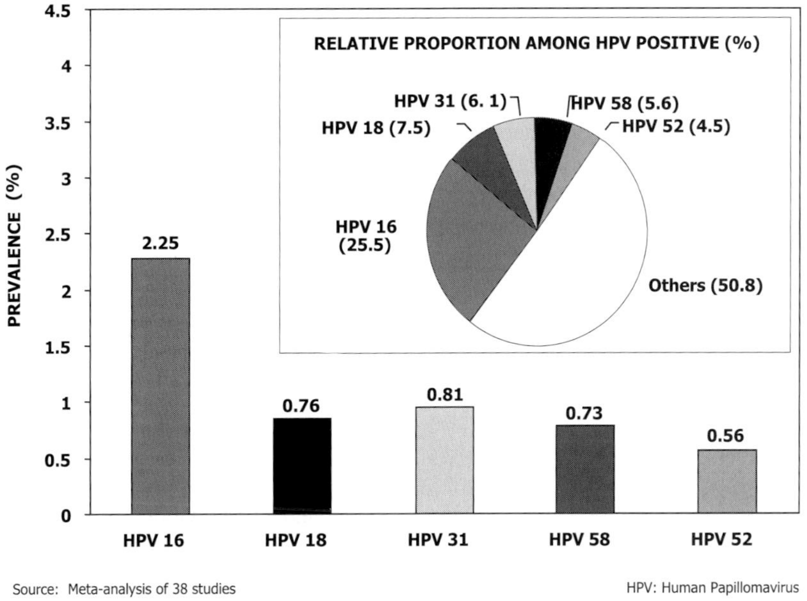

Fig. 2. Overall HPV type specific prevalence & relative proportion of the 5 most common types among HPV positive women with normal cytology.

transmission. Prevalence estimates of high risk HPV DNA infection from early studies in virgins range from 0% to 31%. The wide range of these estimates indicates the influence of methodological issues including the sampling method used (scrapes vs. lavage), the subsite from which the samples were collected (cervical, vaginal or vulvar) and the HPV DNA detection method used. Variables of significant interest include the sensitivity of the test, the number of HPV types used in the testing system and the protocols followed to classify the HPV negative specimens and the HPV of unknown nature usually classed as HPV X. As HPV testing variability was better understood, several studies in which identical sampling methods were taken from all women in a closed cohort and in which HPV DNA was reliably measured, concluded that HPV DNA in cervical specimens is only detected in the sexually experienced women [5,8].

A longitudinal study of virgins who started sexual activity during the study period in a Danish population-based cohort study of 100 virgins and 105 monogamous women showed that all women who stayed virginal throughout follow-up were consistently negative for both HPV DNA and HPV 16 serum antibodies at enrolment and at each follow-up visit. Only a fraction of those virgins who initiated sexual activity became positive for HPV DNA or HPV 16 serum antibodies. The most important determinant of HPV DNA acquisition in this study was the number of sexual partners the woman had had between enrolment and the follow-up visit, both among initially virginal women and among initially monogamous women [5]. In this study, detection of HPV 16 serum antibodies and development of cervical lesions occurred only after HPV transmission, suggesting that sexual intercourse is a necessary step in the acquisition of genital HPVs and in the development of the early stages of cervical neoplasia. A prospective study including 105 HPV-negative women carried out in the San Francisco bay area found that sexual behaviour, specifically exposure to new partners, represented the strongest risk factor for incident HPV infection. The association between sexual behaviour and incident HPV was quite notable, as the risk increased nearly 10-fold for each new partner per month reported.

Many epidemiological studies have consistently shown that sexual behaviour-related characteristics of the individual and his or her partners are the most important risk factors for the acquisition of genital HPV types. The relationship between number of partners and age at first intercourse with the corresponding detection of cervical and penile HPV DNA in adult women and men was examined among the controls (2,225 women and 1,140 men) of a series of 12 case-control studies of cervical cancer carried out by the IARC in 10 countries: Algeria , Brazil, Colombia, India, Morocco, Paraguay, Peru, Spain, Thailand and the Philippines. The study showed that, in both sexes, genital HPV DNA detection increased significantly with increasing lifetime number of sexual partners and with decreasing age at first sexual intercourse [7,8].

HPV data on social groups known to have or have had a high risk sexual behaviour, such as female sex workers and of attendees of STDs clinics have provided further evidence that HPVs are predominantly sexually transmitted. Two studies conducted in Spain and Denmark compared HPV DNA prevalence among women from the general population and women belonging to high-risk groups In all age groups, HPV prevalence was highest among female sex workers, followed by women attending STDs clinics or incarcerated. Women from the general population had much lower age-specific HPV prevalence rates [9,10].

1.3. The role of male in the transmission of human papillomavirus and the risk of cervical cancer

After the identification of HPVs as the sexually transmitted agents etiologically linked to cervical cancer, firm evidence for a role of men as carriers and vectors of oncogenic HPVs resulted from studies that introduced HPV DNA detection in penile samples. However, studies in males are limited because of lack of standardization of the methods to obtain cells from the male external genitalia. The largest study to date exploring the male role in cervical carcinogenesis using PCR technology for the detection of penile HPV is the multicentric case-control study coordinated by the IARC. This large study involved over 1,900 couples that were enrolled in one of seven case-control studies of cervical carcinoma *in situ* and cervical cancer carried out in Brazil, Colombia, The Philippines, Spain and Thailand [7,8,11]. Participating men answered a detailed risk-factor questionnaire and provided a specimen of exfoliated cells from the distal urethra, the glans and the coronal sulcus for HPV DNA detection.

Figure 3 shows the correlation between penile HPV DNA and the sexual behaviour of the couple for subjects enrolled in the studies conducted in Colombia [8] and Spain [7]. Penile HPV prevalence clearly increased with increasing numbers of sexual partners the men reported had had. The increase was observed in male partners of both monogamous and non-monogamous women and penile HPV prevalence was systematically higher in husbands of non-monogamous women than in husbands of monogamous women [6].

Findings from the IARC studies conducted in low- to intermediate-risk countries such as Spain, Thailand and the Philippines, indicate that the men's lifetime number of sexual partners and reporting sex workers as sexual partners are key determinants of cervical cancer risk in their wives. In Spain, the presence of HPV DNA in the husband's penis conveyed a 5-fold increased risk of cervical cancer to their wives. The odds of cervical cancer among monogamous women increased up to 9 to 10 fold in relation to the presence of high-risk HPV types in the penis of their husbands. The ex-

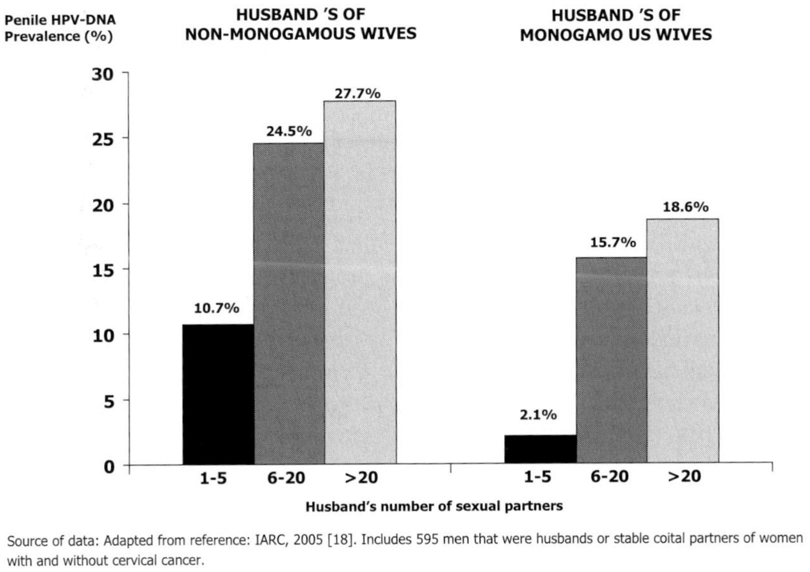

Fig. 3. Penile Human Papillomavirus DNA prevalence by number of sexual partners of husbands of monogamous and non-monogamous women in Spain and Colombia.

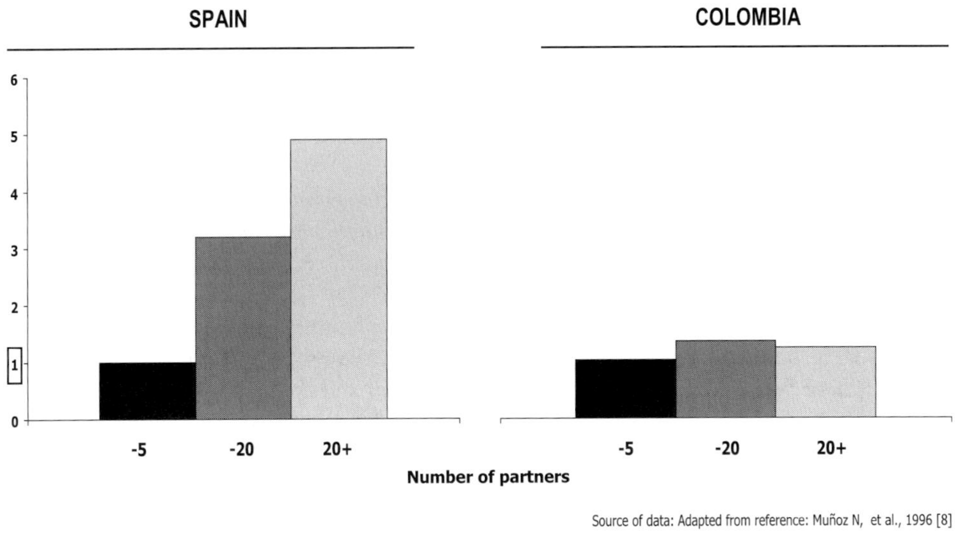

Fig. 4. Husband's lifetime number of partners and risk of cervical cancer among wives in a low risk (Spain) and a high risk country (Colombia).

cess risk associated with HPV type 16 was 6 to 9 fold. Furthermore, the prevalence of penile HPV showed a positive trend with increasing number of sexual partners and with the number of sexual partners who were sex workers [7]. In contrast, in high-risk countries such as Colombia and Brazil, no associations with cervical cancer risk were found with penile HPV DNA or with any other indicators of male sexual behaviour (Fig. 4) [8]. The lack of association between most male sexual behaviour-related variables and cervical cancer risk found in high-risk countries could be explained by the hypothesis that, in these populations, HPV is a widespread infection that it reduces the ability of case-control studies to discriminate subjects at a higher risk. Cross-sectional HPV DNA detection in the penis of adult men, even if high, is still a poor reflection of lifetime exposure to HPV. Other biological markers of lifetime sexual promiscuity in men such as seropositivity to Chlamydia Trachomatis (CT) are more consistent in discriminating women at a high-risk of cervical cancer in relation to the behaviour of their male sexual partners [12].

The clinical implications of recognizing the role of men as occasional carries of HPV DNA and of subclinical lesions that are source and routes of HPV transmission are still under evaluation. In some instances, careful examination of the male external genitalia of sexual partners of women with HPV DNA or CIN lesions unveils minute lesions amenable to treatment. These examinations, usually called penoscopy or genitoscopy, include observations under a colposcopic lens of the external genitalia including the scrotum and perianal regions, with or without acetic acid preparation. It is generally accepted that HPV visible lesions in men should be treated, however the lack of specific antiviral treatment detracts from recommendations of systematic examinations and additional diagnostic procedures and eventual treatments of male partners. Some literature is available indicating that the systematic and regular use of condoms accelerates regression of male and female lesions as well as of HPV DNA clearance [13].

Studies that have addressed concordance of genital HPVs in heterosexual couples found a relatively poor correlation of HPV positivity and HPV type in cervical and penile samples [6]. This is particularly important in the interpretation of case-control studies in which women harbours cervical neoplasia, thus a long-term consistent carrier of type-specific HPV-DNA whereas the husband is, or has been, a transient HPV DNA carrier. Moreover, in some couples, the current partner may not be the relevant one in determining the woman's risk of HPV persistence and progression to cervical neoplasia. Agreement in HPV findings, however, was also modest in couples where both – wife and husband – reported only one lifetime sexual partner [14]. Among women with cervical neoplasia, the relevant infection may have occurred years earlier, and the relatively low prevalence of penile HPV infection in their husbands suggests that viral shedding of advanced cervical lesions is limited. Also cross-sectional detection of penile HPV may measure relatively recent exposures to HPVs that may be unrelated to the initiation of cervical neoplasia in the partner. Finally, the low agreement may be partly due to technical reasons, since a smaller amount of penile exfoliated cells may be obtained in men relative to the cellular yield obtained from the cervix.

The IARC multicentric study on male circumcision and its association with cervical cancer compared penile HPV DNA prevalence in circumcised and uncircumcised men and estimated the woman's risk of cervical cancer according to the husband's circumcision status. The study found that circumcised men were about 3 times less likely to harbour HPV in their penis than uncircumcised men. Male circumcision also reduced the risk of both genital HPV DNA prevalence and cervical cancer in the female partner, particularly and most strongly, in women whose male consorts had had a promiscuous sexual history [11]. Further, the protection afforded by male circumcision also refers to the seroprevalence of CT [15]. These findings, along with the literature on HIV transmission, also indicating a strong protection of circumcised men against HIV carriage and transmission, underline the relevance of circumcision for the prevention of STIs including HPV.

Transmission of genital warts, largely due to HPV 6 and 11 occurs during sexual intercourse with and infected partner. The infection is highly prevalent, with estimates of point prevalence around 1% the sexually active population with cumulative exposure of 17% in the age range 20 of 29% [16]. Risk factors have been clearly linked to the number of sexual partners and infectivity is high with transmission rates estimates of 60% 65% [17]. Genital warts do not convey high-risk of cervical cancer but HPV 6 and 11 have occasionally been related to rare forms of vulvar verrucous carcinomas of the Buschke-Lowestein type.

1.4. Other routes of transmission of human papillomavirus. Recurrent respiratory papillomatosis

Despite the overwhelming evidence that genital HPVs are predominantly sexually transmitted, some clinical and epidemiological observations have documented that genital HPVs can also be transmitted in other ways, especially from mother to child. This is consistent with other microbial and viral infections which are predominantly or exclusively sexually transmitted in adults (e.g., HIV, Hepatitis B Virus (HBV), HSV-2, CT, Treponema Pallidum (TP) and Neisseria Gonorrhoea (NG)) and that may be transmitted to newborns if present in the genital tract of a woman during pregnancy or at the time of delivery. The evidence for the non-sexual transmission of HPVs has been reviewed by several authors concluding that: 1) Genital HPV infections, including genital warts, may occur in sexually naïve populations such as virgins, infants, and children; 2) There is some evidence of horizontal transmission of low-risk HPVs; 3) Vertical and perinatal transmission of HPVs from mother to child, does exist, although rates are small and vary widely; 4) High-risk genital

HPVs have been detected in non-genital mucosa, such as that in the mouth, oropharynx and conjunctiva, and they have been associated with a fraction of cancers of the oral cavity and oropharynx and with conjunctival SCC.

HPV transmission from the genital tract to the upper respiratory was first suggested in 1956, in a case report of a male child who was born to a mother with condyloma that developed symptoms of laryngeal papillomatosis and penile warts at 3 and 6 months after birth. Recurrent laryngeal papillomatosis is a rare, potentially life-threatening condition, associated with HPV types 6 and 11, the HPV types most commonly detected in genital warts. The disease can disseminate through the tracheobronchial tree and progress to pulmonary papillomatosis and subsequent fatal chest infection. Since the disease has a bimodal age distribution with the first peak occurring in infancy, it has been postulated that juvenile papillomatosis may be related to HPV infection acquired from a mother with genital warts or a subclinical HPV infection. A study showed that the risk of the juvenile form of laryngeal papillomatosis appeared to be highest in first-born infants delivered vaginally to an adolescent mother. In contrast, the risk factors identified for the adult onset of the disease included lifetime number of sex partners and high frequency of oral sex, suggesting orogenital transmission [18].

A number of other case report series have indicated the possible non-sexual horizontal transmission of HPVs, particularly of the low-risk HPV types. HPV DNA was detected in finger brush samples of 3 out of 8 women (one with the same types) with cervical HPV, and in 9 out of 13 men (5 with the same types) with penile HPV. In total, 27% of patients had the same HPV types detected in both genital and hand samples. These findings raise the possibility that patients with genital warts may transfer not only genital HPVs to their sexual partners by finger-genital contact but also horizontally to their children. Finger-conjunctiva HPV transmission has been suggested by studies reporting presence of HPV DNA, predominantly type 16, in human ocular surface squamous neoplasias, including conjunctival carcinomas. Indirect transmission via HPV-contaminated fomites (clothing, sheets, towels, objects, and instruments) has also been suggested by some studies, but its impact in passing and inducing active infections is most likely small if any [18]. Although HPV DNA has been occasionally isolated from medical instruments or in the event of medical examinations or treatments (i.e. at the time of laser ablation of CIN lesions in the vaporization fumes), there is at present no evidence that the isolated viral DNA is able to initiate an infection of the patient, her partner or the care taker.

2. Human papillomavirus and cervical neoplastic lesions

The evidence relating HPV infections to cervical cancer includes a large and consistent body of studies indicating a strong and specific role of the viral infection in all settings where investigations have taken place. The association has been recognized as causal in nature by a number of international review parties since the early 90's [19,20].

2.1. Human papillomavirus DNA prevalence in cervical cancer specimens

State-of-the art amplification techniques used in case-control studies, case-series and prevalence surveys have unequivocally shown that, in adequate specimens of cervical cancer, HPV DNA can be detected in 90 to 100% of the cases. Figure 5 shows the prevalence of HPV DNA in specimens of invasive cervical cancer identified in six regions of the world and investigated using PCR technology in a common centralized research laboratory. Allowing for the sampling and testing variability, these results are consistent with a universal presence of these viral markers in established cancerous lesions. The prevalence applies equally to the most common SCC and to the rarer adenocarcinoma, although the HPV type distribution in these two histological forms varies slightly. Further, detailed investigations of the few cervical cancer specimens that appear as HPV DNA negatives in most series has been occasionally conducted and the results strongly suggest that these are largely false negatives. As a consequence, the claim has been made that this is the first necessary cause of a human cancer ever identified, providing a strong rationale for the use of HPV tests in screening programs and for the development of HPV vaccines [21,22].

2.2. Human papillomavirus types involved in cervical cancer and pre-cancerous lesions

Of the more than 35 HPV types found in the genital tract, HPV 16 accounts for some 50% to 60% of the cervical cancer cases in most countries, followed by HPV 18: 10–20%, HPV 45: 4–8% and HPV 31:

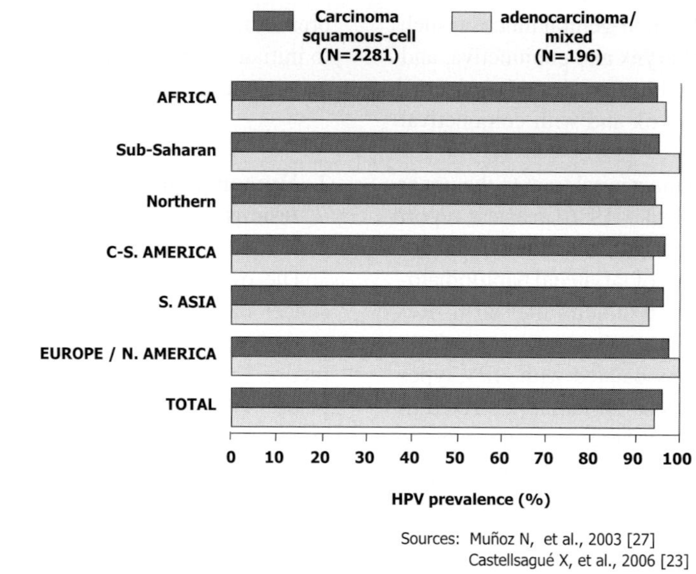

Fig. 5. HVP DNA prevalence in cervical cancer by study region and histology.

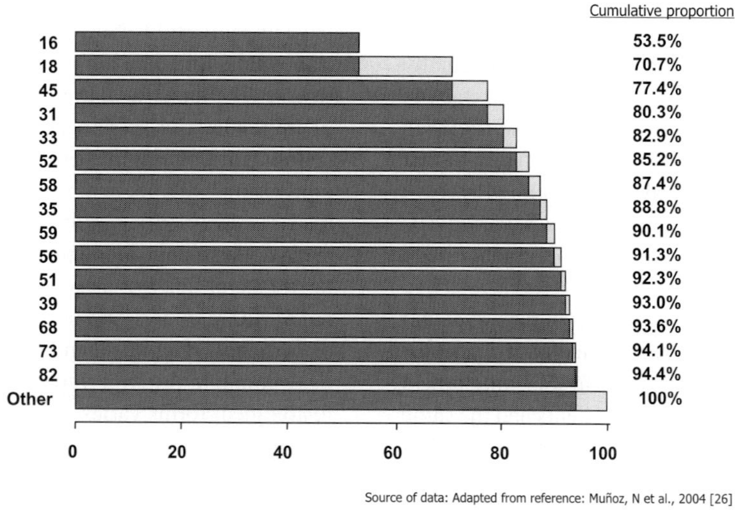

Fig. 6. Relative contribution of HPV types to cervical cancer: All world regions combined.

1–5%. Figure 6 [23] shows the cumulative distribution of 15 HPV types in a series of close to 3,000 cervical cancer cases. Of these, the 5 most common (HPVs 16, 18, 45, 31 and 33) account for 80% of the distribution in squamous cell cancers and of 94% in adenocarcinomas. In most studies, HPV 18 predominates in adenocarcinomas in absolute or relative terms. The reasons for such specificity are unknown.

The positive selection of HPV 16 in cervical cancer cases across the cervical neoplastic spectrum translates the biological advantage of this type in fully expressing its oncogenic capacity. A study among women with different degrees of HIV induced immunosuppression pointed at the likely increased ability of HPV 16 to escape immunesurveillance as compared to other HPV types as one possible mechanism of such advantage [24].

Table 1 compares the HPV type distribution in cervical cancer in the pre-neoplastic precursor lesions HSIL/CIN 2/3 and in women with normal cytology in the published meta-analyses of the literature. The table shows that HPVs 16, 18 and 45 are the only viral types that are more frequently found in the invasive form of neoplasia than in the precursor lesions. These

Table 1
Comparison of overall and type-specific HPV prevalence between Squamous Cell Carcinoma (SCC), High Squamous Intraepithelial Lesion (HSIL) cases and women with normal cytology

A summary of literature reviews						
HPV	SCC (1)		HSIL (1)		NORMAL CYTOLOGY (2)	
TYPE	n	HPV (%)	n	HPV (%)	n women tested	HPV+%
ALL	8550	87.6	4338	84.2	5.764	10.41
16	8594	54.3	4338	45.0	4.385	2.25
18	8502	12.6	4338	7.1	4.286	0.76
33	8449	4.3	4302	7.2	4.136	0.52
45	5174	4.2	2214	2.3	3.554	0.42
31	7204	4.2	4036	8.8	4.157	0.81
58	5646	3.0	2175	6.9	4.155	0.73
52	5304	2.5	2153	5.2	3.927	0.56

HPV: Human Papillomavirus.
SCC: Squamous Cell Carcinoma.
HSIL: High Squamous Intraepithelial Lesion.
Sources of data: Adapted from reference: (1) G.M. Clifford et al. [25]; (2) S. de Sanjose et al. (in press).

findings are interpreted as if the ability to progress was increased in HSIL lesions due to these three HPV types than the corresponding lesions attributed to other HPV types [25]. These results are consistent with some observations from cohort studies indicating that the probability or progression given persistence is significantly higher in women exposed to HPVs 16 or 18 that to any other viral types [4].

The distribution of HPV types in cervical cancer in five different regions in the world is described in Table 2 [26]. It is clear that HPVs 16 and 18 are consistently the first two types involved in all regions explored so far. HPV 45 seems to be a natural candidate for the third ranking place and some additional variability exists thereafter for the relatively rarer HPV types.

2.3. *Risk estimates from case control studies*

Observations on pre-invasive disease and cohort studies on the HPV natural history have intrinsic limitations for making inferences on cervical cancer causality. This is because in controlled settings, biological progression is not allowed to continue beyond the stage of high-grade squamous intraepithelial lesions (HSIL/CIN 3) or carcinoma *in situ*. It is thus of importance to notice that the information applicable to cervical cancer would primarily come from case control studies in which the target disease is directly investigated.

In an effort to simplify the vast literature of case control studies, the results of the IARC multicenter case control study on invasive cervical cancer will be used as example. In brief, this project included nine case-control studies in different parts of the world, mostly in high-risk countries. A common protocol and questionnaire were used, and HPV DNA testing was done in two central research laboratories using the MYO9/11 and the General Primer (GP) GP5+/6+ PCR testing systems. Figure 7 shows the summary results on the HPV DNA prevalence in case and control specimens, the risk estimates and their confidence intervals for SCC. The figure shows very high Odds Ratios (ORs) with estimates in the range of 50 to 150 with several estimates in the several hundred range. These risk estimates lead to calculations of attributable fractions in the range of 90 to 95% [27].

The results are strikingly consistent in the literature for pre-invasive lesions, for SCC and adenocarcinomas and for studies that tested for HPV DNA as a group or studies that restricted the analyses to HR HPV types. Studies that have compared risk factors for CIN 3 and invasive cancer have not reported any significant differences in their associations with HPV or with their epidemiological profile (reviewed in [19]).

The pool of IARC studies was large enough to provide type-specific risk estimates for 18 types. Restricting the analyses to the studies that used the GP5+/6+ HPV detection system and to SCCs, the adjusted OR for HPV DNA detection (the factor by which the reference risk of cervical cancer is multiplied if HPV DNA is detected) was OR = 158.2 (95% Confidence Interval (CI) = 113.2–220.6). The risk estimates for adenocarcinomas was OR = 81.3 (95% CI = 42.0–157.1) [23]. Type specific risk estimates for squamous cell cancer are shown in Fig. 8 and were as follows: HPV 16: OR = 435; HPV 18: OR = 248; HPV 45: OR = 198;

Table 2
Prevalence of the most common HPV types in cervical cancer by region

Sub-Saharan Africa		Northern Africa		Central-South America		South Asia		Europe & North America	
HPV type	%	HPV type	%	HPV type	%	HPV type	%	HPV type	%
HPV 16	47.7	HPV 16	67.6	HPV 16	57.0	HPV 16	52.5	HPV 16	69.7
HPV 18	19.1	HPV 18	17.0	HPV 18	12.6	HPV 18	25.7	HPV 18	14.6
HPV 45	15.0	HPV 45	5.6	HPV 31	7.4	HPV 45	7.9	HPV 45	9.0
HPV 33	3.2	HPV 33	4.0	HPV 45	6.8	HPV 52	3.1	HPV 31	4.5
HPV 58	3.2	HPV 31	3.4	HPV 33	4.3	HPV 58	3.0	HPV 56	2.2

HPV: Human Papillomavirus.
Source of data: [Adapted from reference: N. Muñoz et al. [26].

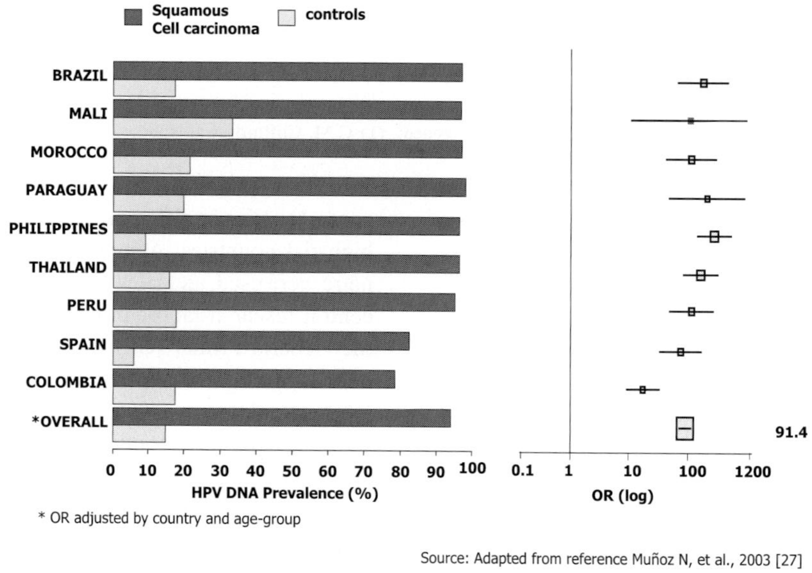

Fig. 7. HPV-DNA prevalence and odds ratios for squamous carcinoma of cervix by country.

HPV 31: OR = 124; HPV 52: OR = 200; HPV 33: OR = 374; HPV 58: OR = 115; HPV 35: OR = 74; HPV 59: OR = 419; HPV 51: OR = 67; HPV 56: OR = 45; HPV 39: infinity; HPV 68: OR = 54. The risk for any given high-risk type was not statistically different from the risk reported for HPV 16. Likewise, the proportion of multiple types in a given specimen varies across studies and particularly in relation to the HPV detection method used. However, in all studies of invasive carcinoma the risk linked to multiple HPV types does not vary significantly from the risk linked to single HPV types.

These studies and a recent International review done at IARC concluded that the evidence is now sufficient to consider as high-risk carcinogenic types HPVs 16, 18, 31, 33, 35, 39, 45, 51, 52, 56, 58, 59, 68, 73 and 82 [IARC, in press]. A second group of HPV types are rarely found in cases and have been classified as Low-risk types and these include HPVs 6, 11, 40, 42, 43, 44, 54, 61, 70, 72, 81 and CP6108. From IARC's and other studies, a small group of HPV types remains in the category of uncertain risk currently including HPVs 26, 53, 66 and perhaps others.

2.4. Cohort studies

Repeated sampling of women being followed for viral persistence and cervical abnormalities has shown that the median duration of the infections is around 8 months for high risk HPV types as compared to 4.8 months for the low-risk HPV types. In unrelated studies, the time estimates were fairly consistent. In one study in a high-risk population in Brazil, the mean duration of HPV detection was 13.5 months for high-risk HPV types and 8.2 months for the non-oncogenic types. HPV 16 tended to persist longer than the average for high-risk types other than HPV 16. The results were remarkably similar in a student population in the Unit-

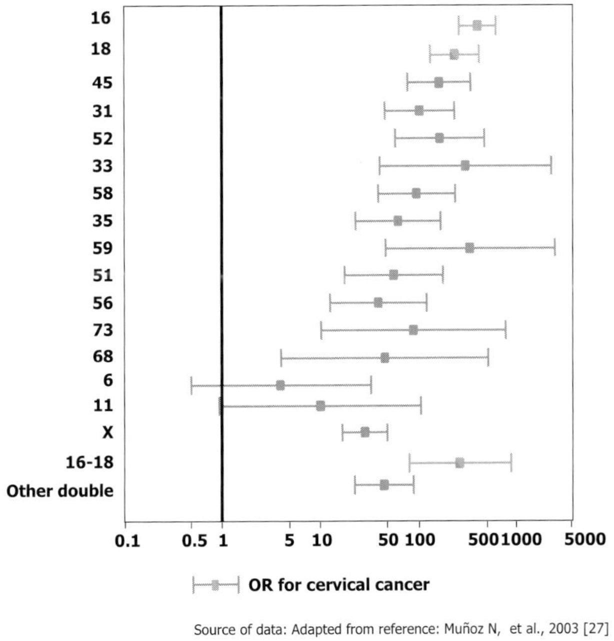

Fig. 8. HPV type-specific risk estimate for cervical cancer.

ed States and in the United Kingdom. However, the currently observed time intervals may still suffer from imprecision in the estimates of time at first exposure, from the variability in the end-point definition and from censoring due to treatment of the early lesions.

Follow-up studies of women with and without cervical abnormalities have indicated that the continuous presence of high risk HPV is necessary for the development, maintenance and progression to CIN 3 and above. A substantial fraction (i.e. 15–30%) of women with high risk HPV DNA who are cytomorphologically normal at recruitment will develop CIN 2/3 within the subsequent 4-year interval. Conversely, among women found to be high risk HPV DNA negative and cytologically identified as atypical squamous cells of undetermined significance (ASCUS), or borderline or mild dysplasia, CIN 2/3 is unlikely to develop during a follow-up of two years and their cytology is likely to return to normal. Women found positive for-low risk HPVs rarely become persistent carriers and their probability of progression to CIN 2/3 is extremely low (reviewed in [19]).

As on going cohorts expand their follow up time, more precise estimates are being provided on the predictive value of viral persistence as defined by repeated measurements of viral types and variants. One of such cohorts in Sao Paulo has shown that the incidence of cervical lesions in women who were twice HPV-negative was 0.73 per 1,000 women-months. The corresponding incidence among women with repeated HPV-16 or HPV-18 positive results was 8.68, a 12-fold increased incidence. The OR for HPV persistence among women who were twice HPV positive for the same oncogenic types was OR = 41.2 (95% CI = 10.7–158.3).

The follow up studies in Costa Rica are beginning to assess the potential for progression-to-neoplasic lesions of some of the most frequent high-risk HPV types. The study confirms that the risk of progression (given persistence) is significantly higher for HPV 16 and 18 HPV carriers over the risk related to any of the remaining high-risk types included in the cocktail test HC2 [4].

Finally, persistence of HPV DNA detection after treatment for CIN 2/3 is an accurate predictor of relapse, significantly more sensitive than repeated vaginal cytology within the 24 months following surgery [28]. These results are useful in defining the clinical role of HPV testing. In screening, in the management of ASCUS and the follow up of women following treatment for HSIL.

3. Other environmental risk factors for cervical cancer

Most of the sexual behaviour parameters that were linked to cervical cancer in the past are being re-evaluated in studies that considered the strong influence of the presence of HPV. Soon after the introduction of HPV testing in research protocols, it became clear that the key risk factors that reflected sexual behaviour, such as the number of sexual partners, merely reflected the probability of HPV exposure. Because of the growing evidence that HPV is a necessary factor in cervical cancer, it soon became a standard procedure in the reports of case control studies to include analyses restricted to HPV positive cases and controls to properly assess the contribution of additional factors to the risk of cervical cancer. In relation to invasive cervical cancer, the IARC's pooled HPV positive restricted analyses included HPV positive 1,768 cases and 262 HPV positive controls and the key findings concerning environmental risk factors are discussed briefly.

3.1. Long term use of oral contraceptives

Ever use of OC was associated with a significant increase in risk of cervical cancer (OR = 1.47 (95% CI = 1.02–2.12) with a clear dose response relationship with duration. The use of OCs for less than 5 years was not related to the risk of cervical cancer (OR = 0.77 (95% CI = 0.46–1.29)) but it increased significantly for 5–9 years of use (OR = 2.72 (95% CI = 1.36–5.46)) and for 10+ years of use (OR = 4.48 (95% CI = 2.24–9.36)).

The evidence for an association of cervical cancer with the use of oral or other hormonal contraceptives is not entirely consistent. A number of studies that investigated HPV positive women found no associations or only weak associations with HSIL/CIN 3 in subgroup analyses. These apparently conflicting results may reflect the increased cytological surveillance of women that are taking OCs in developed countries and the use of different case definition (ASCUS up to HSIL/CIN3 as opposed to cervical cancer) in cohort studies.

Because of the potential public health importance of an interaction between long-term use of OCs and HPV infections in the development of cervical cancer, efforts are now being devoted to verify the results in different populations. A meta-analyses on the association between hormonal contraceptives and cervical cancer concludes that there is a linear dose response relationship and that the effect tends to return to average within a time interval of 5 to 10 years after OC cessation. The relevant units at the World Health Organization examined the evidence with an international working group that recognized the significance of the association. However, the group also concluded that, in balance, the benefits currently achieved by the use of OCs in developing countries (i.e. unwanted pregnancy avoidance) outbalance the increase in risk and should not require a major change in the current family planning strategies.

3.2. High parity

In the IARC case control studies, HPV positive women who reported seven or more full term pregnancies had a four-fold increased risk of cervical cancer as compared to similar HPV positive women that were nulliparous (OR = 3.8 (95% CI = 2.7–5.5)). There was still a two-fold increased risk when women reporting 7 or more pregnancies were compared to HPV positive women who reported 1–2 full term pregnancies [29]. Similar results were obtained in Costa Rica and Thailand as well as among women with pre-invasive disease in the Portland Cohort Study. In Denmark and in the Manchester cohort study, two populations with low parity, the effects are less visible for pre-neoplastic lesions (reviewed in [30]).

It has been speculated that the general reduction in the average number of births in developed countries over the last decades may have contributed to the reduction in cervical cancer incidence but formal proof of the hypothesis has not yet been produced.

The combined effect in the risk of cervical cancer of parity and exposure to OCs has been examined and shown that at each level of OCs use there is an increased risk with a significant trend with the number of lifetime pregnancies. The trend is more remarkable as women refer use of OCs for extended periods of time. As compared to nulliparous women not having used OCs, use for longer that five years and having had more than five full term pregnancies increases the risk by a significant 11-fold [29]. In many of the studies reported, it was difficult to further analyse the association by type of OC use or by estrogens/progesterone dose levels. It is now recognized that current formulations have significantly reduced the product composition and the observed results might apply differently to current users of OCs. However, these observations underline the need to continue conducting studies on the interaction of steroids with the biology of HPV.

3.3. Cigarette smoking

The pooled results of the IARC's studies found that "ever smoking" was associated with a two-fold, statistically significant, increased risk of cervical cancer with a significant dose response. These findings are consistent with those found for "current vs. never smoking" among HPV positive women for pre-neoplastic cervical lesions in virtually all cohort studies in Costa Rica (OR = 2.3), the US Portland (OR = 2.7 for CIN 2–3), in Copenhagen (OR = 1.9) and a large cohort study in Manchester (OR = 2.2) [30]. These studies are providing growing evidence on the carcinogenic effect of cigarette smoking in women with persistent HPV infection. The monograph program at IARC reviewed the evidence in 2002 and concluded that smoking was an independent risk factor for cervical cancer [31]. However the mechanisms by which cigarette smoking may affect cervical cancer (i.e. a direct effect of the tobacco metabolites, an indirect effect related to tobacco-induced immunosupression or to reduced dietary antioxidants) remain elusive.

3.4. Co-infection with the Human Immunodeficiency Virus

The evidence of a putative interaction between HPV and Human Immunodeficiency Virus (HIV) in the origin of cervical cancer was formally recognized when cervical cancer was included as one of the criteria of acquired immune deficiency syndrome (AIDS) among HIV positive women. The subsequent literature largely confirmed the evidence although some major confounders of the epidemiological association tend to obscure the results notably the powerful impact of screening in some populations, the medical surveillance of HIV carriers in developed countries and the short survival time of HIV/AIDS patients in many populations at high risk of cervical cancer in relation to the time intervals between HPV infection and cervical cancer [32].

3.5. Co-infection with other sexually transmitted infections

Markers of exposure to two other Sexually Transmitted Infections (STIs) have been repeatedly although inconsistentcy found associated to cervical cancer. Results from the IARC's multicenter study found a 2-fold increased risk in cervical cancer for the presence of antibodies to CT (OR = 2.1 (95% CI = 1.1–4.0)) and of antibodies to HSV 2 (OR = 2.19 (95%CI = 1.41–3.40) [33,34]. Non-specific inflammatory changes have also been related to modest increases in risk for pre-neoplastic cervical lesions among HPV positive women. The difficulties with the evaluations of such factors lie in the strong co-linearity observed among all STIs and the limitations of some of the biomarkers currently used to assess ever exposure or persistent exposure. to assess ever exposure or persistent exposure.

4. Conclusion

In the last two decades, the aetiology of cervical cancer has become a coherent description that includes the identification of a limited group of HPV types as the necessary, etiologic agents with a few additional co factors intervening as such in the presence of the viral DNA. The association is universal and the HPV type variability is geographically limited. The clinical implications of these findings have resulted in novel screening and vaccination strategies for the prevention of cervical cancer. Current vaccines may prompt a change in the paradigm of cervical cancer prevention.

Acknowledgments

We acknowledge Meritxell Nomen and Cristina Rajo who were responsible for the secretarial workload. Partial support has been received from the Fondo de Investigaciones Sanitarias, Spain (FIS PI030240 and FIS 01/1237), from the European Commission (QLG4-CT-2000-01238 & QLG4-CT-2001-30142), from the Agència de Gestió d'Ajuts Universitaris I de Recerca (2005SGR00695) and from the Instituto de Salud Carlos III (Red de CÁNCER RCESP C03/09 & Red de Salut Pública RTICCC C03/10).

Partial support has been received from the Marato de TV3 Foundation (051530).

References

[1] T. Iftner and L.L. Villa, Chapter 12: Human papillomavirus technologies, *J Natl Cancer Inst Monogr* (2003), 80–88.

[2] G.M. Clifford, S. Gallus, R. Herrero, N. Munoz, P.J. Snijders, S. Vaccarella, P.T. Anh, C. Ferreccio, N.T. Hieu, E. Matos, M. Molano, R. Rajkumar, G. Ronco, S. de Sanjose, H.R. Shin, S. Sukvirach, J.O. Thomas, S. Tunsakul, C.J. Meijer and S. Franceschi, Worldwide distribution of human papillomavirus types in cytologically normal women in the International Agency for Research on Cancer HPV prevalence surveys: a pooled analysis, *Lancet* **366** (2005), 991–998.

[3] N. Munoz, F. Mendez, H. Posso, M. Molano, A.J. van Den Brule, M. Ronderos, C. Meijer and A. Munoz, Incidence, duration, and determinants of cervical human papillomavirus infection in a cohort of Colombian women with normal cytological results, *J Infect Dis* **190** (2004), 2077–2087.

[4] M.J. Khan, P.E. Castle, A.T. Lorincz, S. Wacholder, M. Sherman, D.R. Scott, B.B. Rush, A.G. Glass and M. Schiffman, The elevated 10-year risk of cervical precancer and cancer in women with human papillomavirus (HPV) type 16 or 18 and the possible utility of type-specific HPV testing in clinical practice, *J Natl Cancer Inst* **97** (2005), 1072–1079.

[5] S.K. Kjaer, B. Chackerian, A.J.C. van der Brule, E.I. Svare, G. Paull, J.M.M. Walboomers, J.T. Schiller, J.E. Bock, M.E. Sherman, D.R. Lowy and C.J.L.M. Meijer, High-Risk Human Papillomavirus Is Sexually Transmitted: Evidence from a Follow-up Study of Virgins Starting Sexual Activity (Intercourse), *Cancer Epidemiol Biomark Prev* **10** (2001), 101–106.

[6] X. Castellsague, A. Ghaffari, R.W. Daniel, F.X. Bosch, N. Munoz and K.V. Shah, Prevalence of penile human papillomavirus DNA in husbands of women with and without cervical neoplasia: a study in Spain and Colombia, *J Infect Dis* **176** (1997), 353–361.

[7] F.X. Bosch, X. Castellsagué, N. Muñoz, S. de Sanjosé, A.M. Ghaffari, L.C. González, M. Gili, I. Izarzugaza, P. Viladiu, C. Navarro, A. Vergara, N. Ascunce, E. Guerrero and K.V. Shah, Male sexual behavior and Human Papillomavirus DNA: key risk factors for cervical cancer in Spain, *J Natl Cancer Inst* **88**(15) (1996), 1060–1067.

[8] N. Muñoz, X. Castellsagué, F.X. Bosch, L. Tafur, S. de Sanjosé, N. Aristizabal, A.M. Ghaffari and K.V. Shah, Difficulty in Elucidating the Male Role in Cervical Cancer in Colombia, a High-Risk Area for the Disease, *J Natl Cancer Inst* **88**(15) (1996), 1068–1075.

[9] S. de Sanjose, F.X. Bosch, I. Valls, M.P. Canadas, X. Castellsague, B. Lloveras and K.V. Shah, Prevalence of HPV cervical infections among imprisoned women in Barcelona, Spain, *Sex Transm Infect* **76** (2000), 58.

[10] S.K. Kjaer, E.I. Svare, A.M. Worm, J.M. Walboomers, C.J. Meijer and A.J. van Den Brule, Human papillomavirus infection in Danish female sex workers. Decreasing prevalence with age despite continuously high sexual activity, *Sex Transm Dis* **27** (2000), 438–445.

[11] X. Castellsague, F.X. Bosch, N. Munoz, C.J. Meijer, K.V. Shah, S. de Sanjose, J. Eluf-Neto, C.A. Ngelangel, S. Chichareon, J.S. Smith, R. Herrero, V. Moreno and S. Franceschi, Male circumcision, penile human papillomavirus infection, and cervical cancer in female partners, *N Engl J Med* **346** (2002), 1105–1112.

[12] J. Smith, R. Herrero, K. Erles, D. Grimm, N. Muñoz, F.X. Bosch, L. Tafur, K.V. Shah and J.R. Schlehofer, Adeno-associated virus seroposivility and HPV-induced cervical cancer in Spain and Colombia, *Int J Cancer* **94** (2001), 520–526.

[13] M.C. Bleeker, C.J. Hogewoning, F.J. Voorhorst, A.J. van Den Brule, P.J. Snijders, T.M. Starink, J. Berkhof and C.J. Meijer, Condom use promotes regression of human papillomavirus-associated penile lesions in male sexual partners of women with cervical intraepithelial neoplasia, *Int J Cancer* **107** (2003), 804–810.

[14] S. Franceschi, X. Castellsague, L. dal Maso, J.S. Smith, M. Plummer, C. Ngelangel, S. Chichareon, J. Eluf-Neto, K.V. Shah, P.J. Snijders, C.J. Meijer, F.X. Bosch and N. Munoz, Prevalence and determinants of human papillomavirus genital infection in men, *Br J Cancer* **86** (2002), 705–711.

[15] X. Castellsague, R.W. Peeling, S. Franceschi, S. de Sanjose, J.S. Smith, G. Albero, M. Diaz, R. Herrero, N. Munoz and F.X. Bosch, Chlamydia trachomatis infection in female partners of circumcised and uncircumcised adult men, *Am J Epidemiol* **162** (2005), 907–916.

[16] C. Munk, E.I. Svare, P. Poll, J.E. Bock and S. Krüger Kjaer, History of Genital Warts in 10,838 Women 20 to 29 Years of Age From the General Population, *Sex Transm Dis* **24**(10) (1997), 567–572.

[17] C.J. Lacey, Therapy for genital human papillomavirus-related disease, *J Clin Virol* **32**(Suppl 1) (2005), S82–S90.

[18] F.X. Bosch and T. Iftner, *The Aetiology of Cervical Cancer,* Sheffield, UK: NHS Cervical Screening Programme, 2005.

[19] International Agency for Research on Cancer. IARC Handbooks of Cancer Prevention. Cervix Cancer Screening. Lyon: IARC Press, 2005.

[20] F.X. Bosch, A. Lorincz, N. Muñoz, C.J.L.M. Meijer and K.V. Shah, The causal relation between human papillomavirus and cervical cancer, *J Clin Pathol* **55** (2002), 244–265.

[21] F.X. Bosch, M.M. Manos, N. Munoz, M. Sherman, A.M. Jansen, J. Peto, M.H. Schiffman, V. Moreno, R. Kurman and K.V. Shah, Prevalence of human papillomavirus in cervical cancer: a worldwide perspective. International biological study on cervical cancer (IBSCC) Study Group, *J Natl Cancer Inst* **87** (1995), 796–802.

[22] J.M. Walboomers, M.V. Jacobs, M.M. Manos, F.X. Bosch, J.A. Kummer, K.V. Shah, P.J. Snijders, J. Peto, C.J. Meijer and N. Munoz, Human papillomavirus is a necessary cause of invasive cervical cancer worldwide, *J Pathol* **189** (1999), 12–19.

[23] X. Castellsague, M. Diaz, S. de Sanjose, N. Munoz, R. Herrero, S. Franceschi, R.W. Peeling, R. Ashley, J.S. Smith, P.J. Snijders, C.J. Meijer and F.X. Bosch, Worldwide human papillomavirus etiology of cervical adenocarcinoma and its cofactors: implications for screening and prevention, *J Natl Cancer Inst* **98** (2006), 303–315.

[24] H.D. Strickler, J.M. Palefsky, K.V. Shah, K. Anastos, R.S. Klein, H. Minkoff, A. Duerr, L.S. Massad, D.D. Celentano, C. Hall, M. Fazzari, S. Cu-Uvin, M. Bacon, P. Schuman, A.M. Levine, A.J. Durante, S. Gange, S. Melnick and R.D. Burk, Human papillomavirus type 16 and immune status in human immunodeficiency virus-seropositive women, *J Natl Cancer Inst* **95** (2003), 1062–1071.

[25] G.M. Clifford, J.S. Smith, M. Plummer, N. Muñoz and S. Franceschi, Human papillomavirus types in invasive cervical cancer worldwide: a meta-analysis, *Br J Cancer* **88** (2003), 63–73.

[26] N. Munoz, F.X. Bosch, X. Castellsague, M. Diaz, S. de Sanjose, D. Hammouda, K.V. Shah and C.J. Meijer, Against which human papillomavirus types shall we vaccinate and screen? The international perspective, *Int J Cancer* **111** (2004), 278–285.

[27] N. Munoz, F.X. Bosch, S. de Sanjose, R. Herrero, X. Castellsague, K.V. Shah, P.J. Snijders and C.J. Meijer, Epidemiologic classification of human papillomavirus types associated with cervical cancer, *N Engl J Med* **348** (2003), 518–527.

[28] M. Kyrgiou, G. Koliopoulos, P. Martin-Hirsch, M. Arbyn, W. Prendiville and E. Paraskevaidis, Obstetric outcomes after conservative treatment for intraepithelial or early invasive cervical lesions: systematic review and meta-analysis, *Lancet* **367** (2006), 489–498.

[29] N. Munoz, S. Franceschi, C. Bosetti, V. Moreno, R. Herrero, J.S. Smith, K.V. Shah, C.J. Meijer and F.X. Bosch, Role of parity and human papillomavirus in cervical cancer: the IARC multicentric case-control study, *Lancet* **359** (2002), 1093–1101.

[30] X. Castellsague and N. Munoz, Chapter 3: Cofactors in human papillomavirus carcinogenesis – role of parity, oral contraceptives, and tobacco smoking, *J Natl Cancer Inst Monogr* (2003), 20–28.

[31] IARC. IARC Monographs. Vol. 38. Tobacco Smoking and Tobacco Smoke. 2002.

[32] J.M. Palefsky and E.A. Holly, Chapter 6: Immunosuppression and co-infection with HIV, *J Natl Cancer Inst Monogr* (2003), 41–46.

[33] J.S. Smith, R. Herrero, C. Bosetti, N. Munoz, F.X. Bosch, J. Eluf-Neto, X. Castellsague, C.J. Meijer, A.J. van Den Brule, S. Franceschi and R. Ashley, Herpes simplex virus-2 as a human papillomavirus cofactor in the etiology of invasive cervical cancer, *J Natl Cancer Inst* **94** (2002), 1604–1613.

[34] J.S. Smith, N. Munoz, R. Herrero, J. Eluf-Neto, C. Ngelangel, S. Franceschi, F.X. Bosch, J.M. Walboomers and R.W. Peeling, Evidence for Chlamydia trachomatis as a human papillomavirus cofactor in the etiology of invasive cervical cancer in Brazil and the Philippines, *J Infect Dis* **185** (2002), 324–331.

Disease Markers 23 (2007) 229–234
IOS Press

HPV infections in adolescents

Anna-Barbara Moscicki*
Division of Adolescent Medicine, University of California, San Francisco, CA, USA

Abstract. Adolescents who are sexually active have the highest rates of prevalent and incident HPV infection rates with over 50–80% having infections within 2–3 years of initiating intercourse. These high rates reflect sexual behavior and biologic vulnerability. Most infections are transient in nature and cause no cytologic abnormality. However, a small number of adolescents will not clear the infection. Persistence of HPV is strongly linked to the development of high-grade squamous intra-epithelial lesions (HSIL) and invasive cancer. The HSIL detected, however, does not appear to progress rapidly to invasive cancer. Understanding the natural history of HPV in adolescents has shed light into optional treatment strategies which include watchful observation of atypical squamous cells of undetermined significance (ASCUS) and low grade (LSIL). The association between age of first intercourse and invasive cancer cannot be ignored. Consequently, initiating screening at appropriate times in this vulnerable group is essential. In addition, with the advent of the HPV vaccine, vaccination prior to the onset of sexual activity is critical since most infections occur within a short time frame post initiation.

Keywords: Natural history, HPV, SIL, adolescents

1. Introduction

One of the primary interests in human papillomavirus (HPV) is tied to its unique oncogenic properties. Virtually all squamous cell invasive cancers of the cervix are due to HPV infections. This striking finding is overshadowed by the commonness of this virus. HPV is the most common sexually transmitted infection with over 80% of sexually active women having been exposed to the virus; most within 3–4 years after sexual debut [1,2]. What still intrigues scientists is the long gap between first infection (usually under 21 years of age) and development of invasive cancer in women several decades later. The high prevalence of HPV in young women underscore the vulnerability of adolescents to HPV but the low prevalence of cervical cancer in this age group underscore the benign nature of initial HPV infections. The high incidence of HPV in young women plus the risk of invasive cancer and young age at first intercourse suggests that there are behavioral and/or biologic risks that place the adolescent vulnerable to not only HPV but persistent HPV infection. This Chapter will discuss rates of acquisition in adolescents, the natural history of infections and dysplasia, biologic changes unique to adolescents and preferred treatment recommendations for HPV in adolescents.

2. Incidence of HPV infection in adolescents

Most prevalence studies have demonstrated a 6–8 fold difference in HPV in younger women compared to older. Rates have ranged from 12% to 56% in women under 21 years compared to 2–7% in women over 35 years of age [3–6]. Although this trend has been relatively consistent in studies from developed countries, some countries show no increase across ages or a second increase in older women. A study from Costa Rica suggested that a second rise occurs after the age of 50 years; however, those rates still do not reach those found in adolescents [7].

In a study reported in 2001, approximately 55% of adolescents and young women acquired a cervical HPV infection within 36 months after joining the study [8]. This was approximately within 5–7 years after initiating sexual intercourse. The greatest risk factor for hav-

*Address for correspondence: Anna-Barbara Moscicki, MD, University of California San Francisco, 3333 California Street, Suite 245, San Francisco, CA 94118, USA. Tel.: +1 415 476 5139; Fax: +1 415 476 6106; E-mail: moscickia@peds.ucsf.edu.

ISSN 0278-0240/07/$17.00

ing an incident infection was reporting a new sexual partner. The risk was over 10 fold for each new partner reported per month since the last visit 4 months ago. A recent analysis of a similar cohort showed that of 620 adolescent and young women entered into the study, 37% had a prevalent cervical infection at baseline and 63.3% had an incident infection with a cumulative rate of 75% within approximately 5–6 years after sexual debut (unpublished; personal communication Moscicki).

Another recent study examined 60 adolescents who were asked to obtain weekly vaginal samples and had cervical samples obtained at 3-month intervals [2]. Seventy seven percent were found to have a positive sample for high risk HPV by 2.2 years of follow-up. The most common type in this study was HPV 52; 38.3% had this type detected followed by HPV 16 with a cumulative prevalence of 31.3%. If only cervical infections were considered, 36% had a HR HPV type detected within follow-up showing that half of the detected HPV infections were from vaginal swabs only. This is not surprising since many more samples from the vagina were obtained in this study than from the cervix. On the other hand, this finding also suggests that many of the vaginal infections do not cause cervical infections and are not at risk for causing invasive cervical cancer.

Age related incidence rates, however, have not been consistent across all HPV types. In a recent study in Costa Rica, women under 25 years of age were also more likely to have infection with certain HPV types but not all. It was noted that the alpha nine HPV types (16 and 16 related types) were 2–3 times more common in women under 25 years than women over 35 years [9]. However other types, such as type 61 or 71 increased with increasing age. Of note, these HPV types (61 and 71) are not high-risk types suggesting their presence is unimportant.

3. Vulnerability

The high incidence of HPV in adolescents has been frequently blamed on sexual behavior. Adolescents are much more likely than older women to have had multiple partners within a shorter time frame, such as 6–12 months, than older women. The ease of HPV transmission during sexual activity has been demonstrated in numerous studies [8,10]. But in addition, to high incidence rates, studies have shown that young age at first intercourse is a risk for the development of cancer in later life with a 3–4 fold increased risk of developing invasive cancer if a women initiated intercourse under the age of 18 years of age compared to 20 or older [11, 12]. These studies imply that there may be a biologic vulnerability related to the cervix of young women. Certainly, the adolescent cervix in general is structurally different than the adult women's cervix [13]. Embryologically, the cervix is initially lined by columnar epithelium in utero. Urogenital squamous epithelium replaces the columnar epithelium; however the replacement is incomplete with an abrupt squamous-columnar junction occurring on the ectocervix. The adolescent enters puberty with relatively large areas of columnar epithelium (Fig. 1) compared to the adult women. Due to increased estrogenic activity and resulting acidity of the vagina, uncommitted generative cells of the columnar epithelium begin to transform themselves into squamous epithelium. Eventually, columnar epithelium transforms into squamous epithelium with a new columnar junction occurring well into the os. The predominant cell type in adults is the mature squamous cell (Fig. 2). Both columnar and metaplastic squamous cells are vulnerable to HPV probably for a variety of reasons of which thinness of the epithelium may be one factor (i.e. easy access to basal epithelial cells).

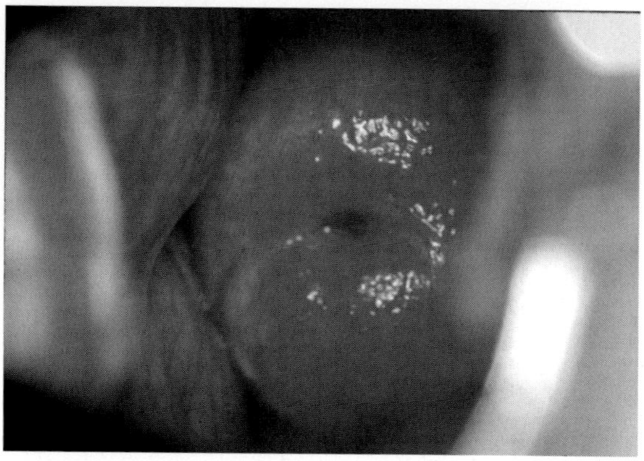

Fig. 1. Colpophotograph of a 16 year old. Note the large area of columnar epithelium in comparison to mature squamous epithelium and abrupt squamo-columanr junction seen well onto the ectocervix.

The transformation process is referred to as squamous metaplasia. The importance of the transformation zone is known since all squamous cell cancers of the cervix appear to arise within the transformation zone. Hence its vulnerability has been well established. Since the process of squamous metaplasia appears to be most active during adolescence, it may represent a vulnerability to the establishment of HPV infections. Triggers of squamous metaplasia include sexual activity. Adolescents with exposure to multiple sexual partners have cervixes that appear more adult

Table 1
Cytologic categories using Bethesda

Bethesda Classification	W.H.O. Classification
ASCUS (ASC)	Atypia
undetermined significance (ASC-US)	
cannot exclude HSIL (ASC-H)	
LSIL (low-grade squamous intra-epithelial lesions)	Condyloma
	CIN 1
HSIL (high-grade squamous intra-epithelial lesions)	CIN 2, CIN 3. Carcinoma *in situ*

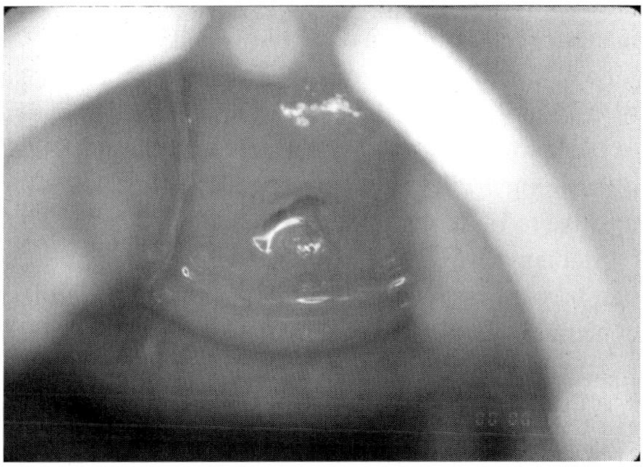

Fig. 2. Colpophotograph of a 20 year old. Note the entire cervix is covered by mature squamous epithelium with the squamo columnar junction not visible.

like with small areas of ectopy [14,15]. It may be women with multiple partners are exposed to sexually transmitted infections, which induce inflammation, repair and metaplasia or semen itself may induce metaplasia. Whatever the reason, rapidly proliferating cellular populations of squamous metaplasia is presumably vulnerable to HPV infection. HPV replication and patterns of transcription are highly dependent on the differentiation program of keratinocytes in the cervical squamous epithelium. Therefore, it is somewhat intuitive that squamous metaplasia is particularly favorable to HPV survival. The environment is conducive to viral replication, and possibly persistence. The high rates of LSIL (see Table 1 for definition of LSIL) in adolescent populations described below support this premise. The protective barrier reflected by the mature squamous epithelium may be an important factor why adult women have lower rates of infection. Rates of LSIL range from 2 to 14% [16–19] in adolescents while in older women ($>$ 30 years) the rates range from 0.6 to 1%. It is important to emphasize, however, that HPV detection in adolescents is most commonly associated with normal cytology. Over three-quarters of HPV-infected adolescents have normal cytology [8]. Whether microscopic abnormalities that remain undetected occur in this group is still controversial. But either way, LSIL, particularly in adolescents appear as benign as HPV infections with normal cytology (see Natural histories of HPV, LSIL, and HSIL in adolescents below).

The expression of viral proteins result in basal cell proliferation, nuclear enlargment and abnormal mitotic figures; all features of SIL [20]. A study of adolescent women showed that those large amounts of metaplastic change visible on colpopophotographs were more likely to develop LSIL if infected with HPV than adolescents with a relatively quiescent cervixes [21].

Few studies have attempted to examine biologic vulnerability to HPV infection. Castle et al. [22] found that the alpha nine types (16, 31, 33, 35, 52, 58, and 67) were detected more commonly among women with greater areas of ectopy. However, the opposite was true of the 3 α 15 α types (61, 71, 72, 81, 83, 84, 89) where prevalence increased with increasing maturity. These authors suggested that the epithelial type helped explain their findings.

4. Natural histories of HPV, LSIL and HSIL in adolescents

Numerous studies have documented the transient nature of HPV infection in adolescents and young women with 50% of women clearing an initially detected infection within 6 months, and 90% clearing within 24 months [1,23,24]. It appears that certain HPV types, such as HPV 16, clear more slowly than other high or low risk types. Certainly, new infections of the same type may occur blurring the true regression rates. There is also evidence that having multiple types of HPVs also slows clearance in adolescents [25,26]. Whether this reflects a global defect in the immune response or whether multiple HPV types act synergistically is unclear. These studies are also difficult to interpret since the reproducabilty between laboratories of detecting multiple types is low. *C. trachomatis*, a common infection in adolescents, has been shown by one study to enhance HPV persistence [27,28]. Since TH1 responses are thought to be responsible for HPV clearance, the authors hypothesized that *C. trachomatis* in some women may be associated with a Th2 type response which in turns results in HPV persistence. This finding with C. trachomatis has not been seen in other studies of HPV persistence [29].

Certainly, many of the HPV infections result in LSIL as mentioned above. The benign nature of LSIL is demonstrated by its high rate of regression that parallels the high rate of regression of HPV. A study of adolescents and young women showed that 92% of LSIL regressed within 36 months of observation [26]. Only 3 % of the adolescent women went onto develop HSIL. Rates of regression of both HPV and LSIL among older women appear to be less frequent; hence detection of HPV or LSIL in older women (defined as > 30 years) most likely reflects an already persistent infection and an increased risk for HSIL.

The role of HPV persistence in the development of HSIL has been established. However, how long persistence is required for HSIL development remains controversial. One of the problems in defining such risks is that CIN 2 and 3 make up the term HSIL (see Table 1) and the natural history of CIN 2 and 3 are likely different. So studies using HSIL have found different rates than those using CIN 2 or 3. Several countries that have collected rates for CIN 3 show that rates of CIN 3 appear to peak in women aged 27–30 years; 7–10 years after peak rate for HPV infections [30]. In comparison, the risk of developing cytologic "HSIL" in adolescents is probably equal that of women aged 20–30 years of age. Mount and colleagues [19] review of cytology found 0.7% of 15–19 year olds had HSIL compared to 0.8% of women aged 20-29 years and 0.7% in 30–39 year-olds. In a nationwide organized cervical screening program in Norway, 0.2% of 20,000 smears from adolescents aged 15–19 years were reported as having HSIL [17]. The reason for these differences is that the rates of CIN 2 most likely out number the rates of CIN 3 in adolescents whereas in older women CIN 3 predominates. So these studies that detect HSIL cytology in adolescents most likely reflect CIN 2 cases.

Given these limitations, it appears that CIN 1 and 2 develop shortly after infection in some women with others taking up to 1–3 years before detection. Moscicki et al. [8] found that 25% of women developed LSIL within 3 years with the risk of of developing cytology diminishing after 3 years. Woodman et al. [31] noted that 3% of HPV negative and 7% of HPV positive adolescents developed HSIL within 19 months of acquiring HPV.

In general, the natural history of LSIL in adolescents parallels that of HPV with few progressing to HSIL. In a longitudinal study of LSIL, only 3% of adolescents went onto HSIL within 3 years [26]. In contrast, a retrospective chart review of adolescents < 19 years of age with cytologic LSIL reported that 31% progressed to HSIL by 36 months [32]. Since this study involved chart reviews, it is not clear if the HSIL reflected new lesions or actual progression of LSIL. In addition, only a third of the original cohort was followed for 36 months. These differences between studies may be a matter of interpretation of cytology and histology or a reflection of different population characteristics. None of the studies found invasive cancer. In comparison to older women, Cox et al. [33] showed that 12.8% of older women will progress from LSIL or ASCUS/HPV positive to HSIL within 2 years.

Studies of HSIL are few since carcinoma-in-situ is part of what is now termed HSIL and there are ethical concerns in monitoring these lesions without treatment. In addition,

CIN 2 is not a very reproducible diagnosis by pathologists and there is considerable debate as to whether CIN 2 behaves more like CIN 1 or more like CIN 3 [34]. The importance of these differences for adolescents is that CIN 2 lesions make up the majority of HSIL while CIN 3 is less common [16,19]. No studies to date are available for progression of CIN 2 or 3 in adolescents. However, prevalence studies in US adolescents have consistently shown that adolescents rarely have invasive cancer [16,19]. According to the most recent US SEER statistics (1995–1999), the incidence of invasive cancer in women under among 20 years of age is 0–3 per million [35]. Little information is available on the rare cases of invasive cancer such as presence of immunodeficiency disorders.

5. Cervical cancer screening

The high rates of regression in adolescents of HPV and LSIL have spurred a movement in the US to push back the age when to initiate screening. Older guidelines included all adolescents once sexually active [36, 37]. Recently, guidelines were constructed on risk behaviors (i.e. initiating sexual activity) and a time frame [38]. Through cost effective modeling, it was shown that initiating screening 3 years after the onset of sexual activity or 21 years of age, whichever comes first, would be cost-effective. In addition, these guidelines were felt to encompass screening in high-risk groups (i.e. those initiating sexual activity at early ages) [36,37].

Although cervical cancer screening in adolescents yield low benefits, the age limit to begin screening remains controversial. As mentioned, US guidelines base risk of cancer on sexual behavior. This type of screening is strategic in identifying the highest risk youth. Although the recommendations were based on sexual behavior reporting, most agree that a cap is needed for women who are unwilling or unable to report sexual activity. The upper age limit of 21 years used by the American Cancer society was primarily based on expert opinion. In the US, this age was considered a realistic age for compliance and access to patients, particularly that the US has no organized screening program. In countries with organized screening such as the United Kingdom, new recommendations start screening at 25 years [39]. In contrast, Australia has new guidelines that recommend screening begin at the ages of 18 years, or one to two years after first sexual intercourse, whichever is later [40]. Data show that some rare cases of invasive cancer will occur in the 20–24 year old group; hence precancers in this group would be missed if screening begins after 20 years of age.

6. ASCUS and LSIL triage

The high rates of LSIL and HPV regression have led to more reasonable guidelines for adolescents [41]. ASCUS triage with HPV testing has been incorporated into many triage schemes. However, recent study of population performances show that up to 77% of adolescents with ASCUS will be positive for high-risk HPV types. This has called into question the use of HPV triage in adolescent populations [42]. Repeat cytology 6 to 12 months is now often favored over HPV triage. Similar conservative observation of LSIL by cytology is also recommended with repeat cytology 6 to 12 months later rather than immediate referral to colposcopy [43]. Since ASCUS-HR HPV type has a similar history as LSIL, similar strategies can be given to these lesions if HPV testing is performed on the ASCUS smear. At first repeat cytology, HSIL or higher should be referred for colposcopy. At second repeat cytology, any abnormality on repeat cytology for ASCUS, ASCUS HR, and LSIL follow-up leads to referral to colposcopy. Because of the high rates of HPV infection in adolescents, follow-up with HPV testing for any of these lesions is of questionable value. No cost-effective analysis for this age group has been performed.

Appearance of HSIL on cytology at any follow-up visit should be referred to colposcopy.

Because of the frequency of HPV infections in adolescents, HPV testing for primary screening is not recommended.

7. Treatment of SIL

Treatment of LSIL among adolescents is considered unwarranted. Recommendation for treatment of HSIL for adolescents is similar to that of adults. Some have recommended cryotherapy over LEEP for suitable cases (small accessible lesions) in adolescents because of the lower rate of complication associated with cryotherapy. A recent meta-analysis of LEEP procedures showed increased risk of preterm delivery, low birth weight, and premature rupture of membranes [44].

In summary, HPV is undoubtedly the cause of cervical cancer. However, HPV detection, specifically in adolescents, is not an absolute marker of cervical cancer risk. Adolescents are at high risk of acquiring HPV infection with over 50–80% having infections within 2–3 years of initiating intercourse. These high rates are due either to sexual behavior, biologic vulnerability or a combination of both. Most infections are transient in nature and cause no cytologic abnormality. However, a small number of adolescents will not clear the infection and develop HSIL. The HSIL detected, however, does not appear to progress rapidly to invasive cancer since cancers in this age group remain rare. Understanding the natural history of HPV in adolescents has shed light into optional treatment strategies which include watchful observation of ASCUS and LSIL. The association between age of first intercourse and invasive cancer cannot be ignored. Consequently, initiating screening at appropriate times in this vulnerable group is essential. With the HPV vaccine on the horizon, it will be essential to vaccinate children prior to the onset of sexual activity; prior to acquisition of HPV. Accordingly, adolescents who initiate sexual activity may not have yet developed an HPV infection and should receive vaccination as well. All adolescents vaccinated must be counseled about the important of continued cancer screening.

References

[1] A.B. Moscicki, S. Shiboski, J. Broering, K. Powell, L. Clayton, N. Jay, T.M. Darragh, R. Brescia, S. Kanowitz, S.B. Miller, J. Stone, E. Hanson and J. Palefsky, *J Pediatr* **132** (1998), 277.

[2] F.M. Brown, W.C. Faquin, D. Sun, C.P. Crum and E.S. Cibas, *Am J Clin Pathol* **112** (1999), 765.

[3] A.B. Moscicki, J. Palefsky, J. Gonzales and G. Schoolnik, *Pediatr Res* **28** (1990), 507.
[4] A.B. Moscicki, J.H. Ellenberg, S.H. Vermund, C.A. Holland, T. Darragh, P.A. Crowley-Nowick, L. Levin and C.M. Wilson, *Arch Ped Adolesc Med* **154** (2000), 127.
[5] C. Ferreccio, R.B. Prado, A.V. Luzoro, S.L. Ampuero, P.J. Snijders, C.J. Meijer, S.V. Vaccarella, A.T. Jara, K.I. Puschel, S.C. Robles, R. Herrero, S.F. Franceschi and J.M. Ojeda, *Cancer Epidemiol Biomarkers Prev* **13** (2004), 2271.
[6] W.D. Rosenfeld, S.H. Vermund, S.J. Wentz et al., *Am J Dis Child* **143** (1989), 1443.
[7] R. Herrero, A. Hildesheim, C. Bratti, M.E. Sherman, M. Hutchinson, J. Morales, I. Balmaceda, M.D. Greenberg, M. Alfaro, R.D. Burk, S. Wacholder, M. Plummer and M. Schiffman, *J Natl Cancer Inst* **92** (2000), 464.
[8] A.B. Moscicki, N. Hills, S. Shiboski, K. Powell, N. Jay, E. Hanson, S. Miller, L. Clayton, S. Farhat, J. Broering, T. Darragh and J. Palefsky, *JAMA* **285** (2001), 2995.
[9] P.E. Castle, A.C. Rodriguez, F.P. Bowman, R. Herrero, M. Schiffman, M.C. Bratti, L.A. Morera, D. Schust, P. Crowley-Nowick and A. Hildesheim, *Clin Diagn Lab Immunol* **11** (2004), 399.
[10] A. Burchell, R. Winer, S. de Sanjose and E. Franco, *Vaccine Monographs* (2006), in press.
[11] J. Green, A. Berrington de Gonzalez, S. Sweetland, V. Beral, C. Chilvers, B. Crossley, J. Deacon, C. Hermon, P. Jha, D. Mant, J. Peto, M. Pike and M.P. Vessey, *Br J Cancer* **89** (2003), 2078.
[12] C.H. Sierra-Torres, S.K. Tyring and W.W. Au, *Int J Gynecol Cancer* **13** (2003), 617.
[13] A. Singer, in: *The Cervix,* J.A. Gordon and A. Singer, eds, WB Saunders, Philadelphia, 1978, p. 87.
[14] A. Singer, *Br J Obstet Gynaecol* **82** (1975), 81.
[15] A.B. Moscicki, Y. Ma, C. Holland and S.H. Vermund, *J Infect Dis* **183** (2001), 865.
[16] S.B. Sadeghi, E.W. Hsieh and S.W. Gunn, *Am J Obstet Gynecol* **148** (1984), 726.
[17] T. Bjorge, A.B. Gunbjorud, F. Langmark, G.B. Skare and S.O. Thoresen, *Cancer Detection and Prevention* **18** (1994), 463.
[18] L.T.M. Schydlower, M.H. Greenberg and C.P.H. Patterson, *Clinical Pediatrics* **20** (1981), 723.
[19] S.L. Mount and J.L. Papillo, *Pediatrics* **103** (1999), 539.
[20] D. Solomon, D. Davey, R. Kurman, A. Moriarty, D. O'Connor, M. Prey, S. Raab, M. Sherman, D. Wilbur, T.J. Wright and N. Young, *JAMA* **287** (2002), 2114.
[21] A.B. Moscicki, V. Grubbs-Burt, S. Kanowitz, T. Darragh and S. Shiboski, *Cancer* **85** (1999), 1139.
[22] P.E. Castle, J. Jeronimo, M. Schiffman, R. Herrero, A.C. Rodriguez, M.C. Bratti, A. Hildesheim, S. Wacholder, L.R. Long, L. Neve, R. Pfeiffer and R.D. Burk, *Cancer Res* **66** (2006), 1218.
[23] G.Y. Ho, R. Bierman, L. Beardsley, C.J. Chang and R.D. Burk, *NEJM* **338** (1998), 423.
[24] M. Evander, K. Edlund, A. Gustaffson, M. Jonsson, R. Karrlson, E. Rylander and G. Wadell, *The Journal of Infectious Diseases* **171** (1995), 1026.
[25] A.B. Moscicki, J.H. Ellenberg, S. Farhat and J. Xu, *J Infect Dis* **190** (2004), 37.
[26] A.B. Moscicki, S. Shiboski, N.K. Hills, K.J. Powell, N. Jay, E.N. Hanson, S. Miller, L. Canjura-Clayton, S. Farhat, J.M. Broering and T.M. Darragh, *Lancet* **364** (2004), 1678.
[27] I. Silins, W. Ryd, A. Strand, G. Wadell, S. Tornberg, B.G. Hansson, X. Wang, L. Arnheim, V. Dahl, D. Bremell, K. Persson, J. Dillner and E. Rylander, *Int J Cancer* **116** (2005), 110.
[28] E. Samoff, E.H. Koumans, L.E. Markowitz, M. Sternberg, M.K. Sawyer, D. Swan, J.R. Papp, C.M. Black and E.R. Unger, *Am J Epidemiol* **162** (2005), 668.
[29] A.B. Moscicki, J.H. Ellenberg, S. Fahrat and J. Xu, *Journal of Infectious Diseases* **190** (2004), 37.
[30] M. Schiffman and S.K. Kjaer, *J Natl Cancer Inst Monogr* **31** (2003), 14.
[31] C.B. Woodman, S. Collins, H. Winter, A. Bailey, J. Ellis, P. P., M. Yates, R.T. P. and L.S. Young, *Lancet* **357** (2001), 1831.
[32] J.D. Wright, R.M. Davila, K.R. Pinto, D.F. Merritt, R.K. Gibb, J.S. Rader, D.G. Mutch, F. Gao and M.A. Powell, *Obstet Gynecol* **106** (2005), 115.
[33] J.T. Cox, M. Schiffman and D. Solomon, ASCUS-LSIL Triage Study (ALTS) Group, *Am J Obstet Gynecol* **188** (2003), 1406.
[34] K. Syrjanen, V. Kataja, Yliskoski, F. Chang and S. Syrjanen, *Obstet Gynecol* **79** (1992), 675.
[35] P.G. Chan, H.Y. Sung and G.F. Sawaya, *Obstet Gynecol* **102** (2003), 765.
[36] American College of Obstetricians and Gynecologists, **152** (1995).
[37] American Medical Association, in, American Medical Association, Chicago, IL, 1992.
[38] D. Saslow, C.D. Runowicz, D. Solomon, A.B. Moscicki, R.A. Smith, H.J. Eyre and C. Cohen, *CA Cancer J Clin* **52** (2002), 342.
[39] NHS Cancer Screening Programmes, in, NHS Cervical Screening Programme, http://www.cancerscreening.nhs.uk/cervical/index.html#invited, 2006.
[40] National Health and Medical Research Council, in, 2005.
[41] T.C.J. Wright, J.T. Cox, L.S. Massad, L.B. Twiggs, E.J. Wilkinson, *JAMA* **287** (2002), 2120.
[42] G. Sawaya, *JAMA* **294** (2005), 2210.
[43] American Society for Colposcopy and Cervical Pathology, in, 2006.
[44] M. Kyrgiou, G. Koliopoulos, P. Martin-Hirsch, M. Arbyn, W. Prendiville and E. Paraskevaidis, *Lancet* **367** (2006), 489.

Disease Markers 23 (2007) 235–245
IOS Press

Genital HPVs in the aerodigestive tract: Etiologic association with a subset of oropharyngeal/tonsillar cancers and with recurrent respiratory papillomatosis[1]

Keerti V. Shah[a,*] and William H. Westra[b]
[a]*Department of Molecular Microbiology and Immunology, Bloomberg School of Public Health, Johns Hopkins University, Baltimore, MD, USA*
[b]*Department of Pathology, School of Medicine, Johns Hopkins University, Baltimore, MD, USA*

1. Introduction

The mucosal human papillomaviruses (HPVs) primarily infect the genital tract, but they also infect the mucosa lining the aerodigestive tract where they are etiologically linked to two clinical entities. The high-risk HPV type 16, which is responsible for about 50% of cervical cancers, is linked to a subset of oropharyngeal/ tonsillar cancers. Low-risk HPV types 6 and 11, which cause a large majority of genital warts, are also responsible for juvenile-onset as well as adult-onset recurrent respiratory papillomatosis (RRP).

2. HPVs and Head and Neck Squamous Cell Carcinomas (HNSCC)

Each year there are more than 550,000 newly diagnosed cases of HNSCC world wide, and these contribute to 300,000 annual cancer-related deaths [1]. Often considered a single and uniform tumor type, HNSCC in reality is a heterogeneous mix of cancers that differ in many ways including site of origin, causation, and behavior. Anatomically, HNSCCs originate from the mucosa lining the sinonasal tract, oral cavity, larynx and pharynx (inclusive of the nasopharynx, oropharynx and hypopharynx). The contribution of various risk factors is strongly influenced by social and ethnic factors. Cigarette smoking and alcohol consumption are by far the most widely recognized risk factors for HNSCC as a whole, but they are not the only ones. For example, oral cancers linked to betel quid chewing predominate in parts of India, and nasopharyngeal cancers associated with Epstein-Barr virus are common in China.

Infection with high-risk genital tract HPVs has long been established as the etiology of cancers of the female and male genital tracts, but its contribution to tumorigenesis of the head and neck has been an unsettled topic under intense investigation since the 1980s. Early studies reporting on the prevalence of HPV sequences in cancers and non-neoplastic tissues of the head and neck were marred by widely disparate results [2]. In one of the first studies to provide compelling evidence for the etiological role of HPV in HNSCC, Steenbergen et al. [3] observed the presence of integrated HPV-16 genome, HPV-16 transcripts and specific chromosomal alterations in both a primary oral squamous cell carci-

[1]This study was supported in part by grant number P50 CA96784 from the National Cancer Institute, NIH, Bethesda MD, USA.
*Corresponding author: 615 N. Wolfe Street, Baltimore, MD 21205, USA. Tel.: +1 410 955 3189; Fax: +1 443 287 4563; E-mail: kvshah@jhsph.edu.

ISSN 0278-0240/07/$17.00

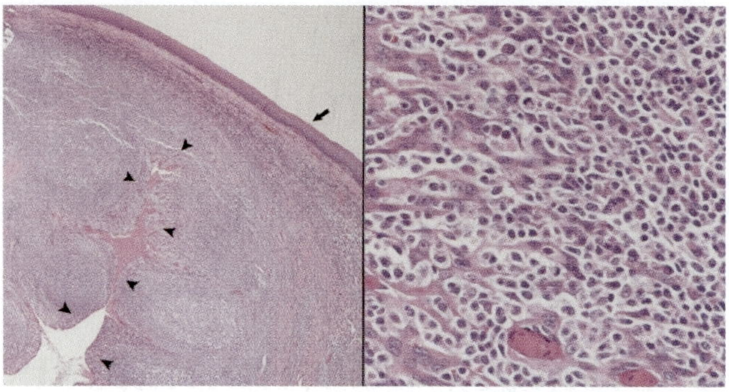

Fig. 1. Histology of the normal tonsil. The surface of the tonsil is lined by a layer of stratified squamous epithelium (left panel, arrows). Deep invaginations of the epithelium into the underlying lymphoid tissue are known as tonsillar crypts (left panel, arrowheads). The epithelium lining these crypts is disrupted by numerous permeating lymphocytes that separates the epithelium into cords of basaloid cells (right panel).

noma and in the cell line derived from the cancer. In the early 1990s, reports from Europe began to more clearly pinpoint the tonsil as an anatomic site targeted by HPV-16. Using an in-situ hybridization approach, Niedobitek et al. [4] frequently detected HPV-16 hybridization signals in HNSCC arising from the palatine tonsils. Using a PCR-based approach, Snidjers et al. [5,6] reported HPV-16 viral transcripts and evidence of HPV-16 integration in a high percentage of oropharyngeal carcinomas compared to HNSCCs arising in non-oropharyngeal sites.

As the role of HPV-16 in head and neck tumorigenesis becomes better understood, these HPV-16-related cancers are becoming increasingly recognized as a biologically distinct subgroup of HNSCCs with a characteristic pathological and clinical profile [7,8]. Compared to their non-HPV counterparts, HPV-16-related HNSCCs less frequently harbor inactivating mutations targeting the p53 and retinoblastoma (Rb) tumor suppressor genes. Under the microscope, HPV-16-related HNSCCs consistently demonstrate a "basaloid" appearance in contrast to the conventional keratinizing morphology of most non-HPV-16-related HNSCCs. Patients with HPV-16-related HNSCCs are less likely to use alcohol or tobacco, and they are more likely to experience favorable outcomes. As first suggested by Niedobitek and others [4], another distinctive feature of HPV-16-related HNSCC is its strong tendency to localize to the oropharynx – an anatomic site that includes the base of the tongue, lingual and palatine tonsils, soft palate and uvula. Within the oropharynx, HPV-16 appears to target the specialized reticulated epithelium that lines the tonsillar crypts (Fig. 1).

Several recent reviews have discussed different aspects of the role of HPVs in tumors of the aerodigestive tract [8–10]. This review will summarize the characteristics of HNSCC etiologically linked to HPV infections.

2.1. Virologic characteristics

Kreimer et al. [9] systematically reviewed 60 PCR-based studies to describe the prevalence, viral genotypes, and anatomic distribution of HPVs in over 5000 HNSCCs. In the combined results of the studies, the prevalence of HPV DNA in squamous cell carcinomas of the oropharynx (36%) was significantly higher than that in squamous cell carcinomas of the oral cavity (24%) and larynx (24%). For all three groups, HPV-16 was by far the most common HPV type detected in the HPV-positive carcinomas. The predominance of HPV-16 type in HNSCC is a common finding in the PCR-based studies.

These PCR-based studies reported the presence of HPV-16 in HNSCCs across various anatomic sites, but were unable to describe the distribution of the viral genome in tumor tissues. Unlike PCR-based detection methods, current *in situ* hybridization methods permit direct visualization of HPV-16 in tumor cells. Moreover, the *in situ* methods are highly sensitive and are able to detect a single HPV DNA copy per cell and they are applicable to formalin-fixed paraffin-embedded clinical samples. Punctate staining in the nucleus of the tumor cell is suggestive of an integrated state of the viral genome. Begum et al. [11] performed *in situ* hybridization for HPV-16 DNA on a tissue array assembled from HNSCCs representing all anatomic subsites of the head and neck. They detected HPV-16 in 82% of the oropharyngeal cancers but in only one of 131 cancers (0.8%) arising from non-oropharyngeal sites. All 115 cancers from the oral cavity and the larynx were HPV-16 negative. The HPV prevalence data comparing

Table 1
HPV prevalence in tumor biopsies from different HNSCC sites by PCR and by *in situ* hybridization

Study	Assay	Oropharynx		Oral Cavity		Larynx	
		No.	(% prev)	No.	(% prev)	No.	(% prev)
Kreimer et al. [9]	PCR for all HPVs	969	(35.6)	2642	(23.5)	1435	(24.0)
Kreimer et al. [9]	PCR for HPV-16	969	(30.9)	2642	(16.0)	1535	(16.6)
Begum et al. [11]	ISH for HPV-16 in tumor cell nuclei	45	(82)	61	(0)	54	(0)

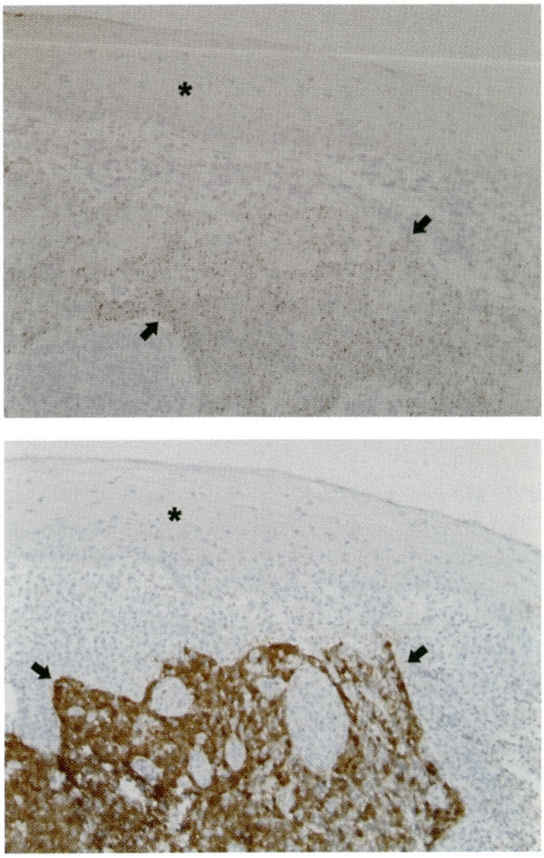

Fig. 2. HPV16 in-situ hybridization and p16 immunohistochemistry of a tonsillar carcinoma. Distinct dot-like hybridization signals are localized to the tumor nuclei involving a tonsillar crypt (outlined by arrows), but they are not present in the overlying surface epithelium (asterisk) (A, HPV in-situ hybridization). The pattern of high p16 expression reflects the distribution of HPV virus (B, p16 immunohistochemistry).

PCR-based detection and *in situ* hybridization detection across three anatomic sites [11] are shown in Table 1. They show that although cancers at all three HNSCC sites are HPV-positive by PCR, only the oropharyngeal cancers demonstrate the presence of HPV as visualized by hybridization signals within the tumor nuclei (Fig. 2A). The same conclusion was reached in a study of paraffin sections of metastatic lymph nodes from 68 HNSCC patients by *in situ* hybridization [12]. HPV-16 DNA was found in the tumor nuclei of 22 of 31 patients (71%) whose primary tumor was in the oropharynx, but in none of 37 patients with primary tumors at other sites (21 in oral cavity, 11 in larynx and 5 in hypopharynx). *In situ* hybridization was performed only with HPV-16 probe; thus these studies likely underestimate the true prevalence of HPV-associated cancers by missing the few oropharyngeal cancers associated with some other HPV type. In confirmation of the *in situ* hybridization studies, high copy number of HPV DNA and the presence of HPV E6 and E7 transcripts strongly correlate with tumor origin from the oropharynx [6,13–16]. Gillison et al. [13] tested HPV PCR-positive HNSCC biopsies by *in situ* hybridization and/or Southern hybridization of tissue DNAs. They found that PCR-positive oropharyngeal cancers were much more likely to be positive by either or both of these assays (17 of 24 (71%)) than PCR-positive biopsies from non-oropharyngeal HNSCC sites (one of 13 (8%)).

With respect to the physical state of HPV-16 DNA in HPV-positive oropharyngeal/tonsillar cancers, evidence has been presented for the viral genome being predominantly episomal [14] as well as for its being integrated [6,8,15].

In summary, the majority of squamous cell carcinomas arising from the oropharynx have a transcriptionally active HPV genome localized to the tumor cells, suggesting that they are a result of a clonal expansion of HPV-transformed cells. Tumors with these characteristics appear to be virtually absent from other HNSCC anatomic sites such as the oral cavity and the larynx. Although squamous cell carcinomas of the larynx can arise from malignant transformation of recurrent respiratory papillomas caused by the non-oncogenic HPV types 6 and 11, this is an exceedingly rare phenomenon [17]. HNSCCs which have small copy numbers of HPV DNA by quantitative PCR assays, or HNSCCs that are HPV-negative by *in situ* hybridization, are very likely not etiologically linked to HPV infection.

2.2. *Pathogenesis*

2.2.1. *Pathological aspects*

The HPV-associated HNSCCs have a characteristic appearance under the microscope that is distinct

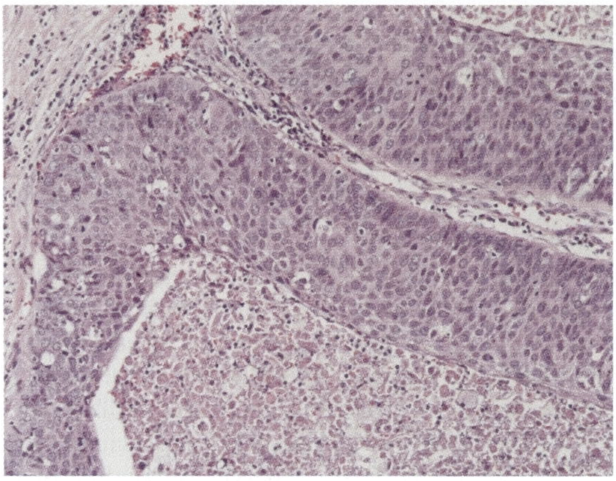

Fig. 3. Characteristic basaloid appearance of an HPV16-related oropharyngeal carcinoma. The carcinoma grows as expanding cellular lobules with central cystic necrosis. The tumor cells are non-keratinizing and have a high nuclear to cytoplasmic (N:C) ratio.

from their non-HPV-related counterparts. In contrast to the keratinizing morphology of conventional HNSCC, these HPV-related tumors tend to be seen as expanding lobules of poorly differentiated and non-keratinizing squamous cells, imparting a "basaloid" appearance [15] (Fig. 3). Of note, this same basaloid morphology has also been observed in the HPV-related squamous carcinomas of the vulva and penis [18].

The consistent localization of HPV-related HNSCC to the oropharynx may reflect viral targeting of the epithelium lining the tonsillar crypts [16]. This specialized lymphoepithelium has a distinctly "basaloid" appearance, is involved in the capture and processing of antigens, and serves as a replication site for important pathogenic viruses (e.g., Epstein-Barr virus, adenoviruses, and herpes simplex virus) and perhaps may serve as a reservoir for HPV following exposure [19]. In their description of the HPV-16 distribution in oropharyngeal carcinomas as visualized by *in situ* hybridization, Begum et al. [11] found that all of the 37 HPV-positive oropharyngeal carcinomas arose either from the lingual ($n = 17$) or palatine ($n = 20$) tonsils, whereas four of the eight HPV-negative oropharyngeal cancers arose from the soft palate, a site unassociated with crypt epithelium. In those HPV-positive cases where all histologic stages of tumor progression were present from epithelial dysplasia to invasive carcinoma, the premalignant changes localized to the tonsillar crypts and were HPV-16 positive. These observations suggest that HPV-16 targets the tonsillar crypt epithelium for the initiation and maintenance of the malignant phenotype.

The propensity of HPV-16 to initiate tumorigenesis from deep within the tonsillar crypts may help account for certain well recognized but poorly understood clinical characteristics of tonsillar carcinoma. First, premalignant changes of the tonsils are rarely clinically evident. This inability to visualize tonsillar dysplasia diminishes the opportunity to remove the tonsils during the early stages of tumor development. Second, tonsillar carcinomas are prone to metastatic spread to regional lymph nodes even when the surface of the tonsils appears visibly unremarkable [20]. Indeed, a significant number of metastatic carcinomas from occult primary tumors are HPV-16 positive (Westra, unpublished results), likely reflecting origin from the deep recesses of the tonsillar crypts. It is not known if this location of HPV infection to the tonsillar crypts will adversely affect the ability to detect HPV as part of screening protocols for early cancer detection. Of note, HPV is readily recovered from exfoliated cervical cells, but it is not consistently recovered in oral rinses obtained from patients with HPV-positive HNSCCs [21].

2.2.2. *Molecular aspects*

Tumorigenesis of the head and neck almost always involves inactivation of the p53 and Rb pathways – two pathways that are intimately involved in regulation of the cell cycle [22]. In non-HPV-related HNSCCs, disruption of the p53 pathways occurs via genetic alterations targeting the p53 gene; and disruption of the Rb pathway predominantly occurs via genetic and/or epigenetic silencing of the p16(INK4A) tumor suppressor gene. In HPV-related HNSCCs, genetic alterations targeting p53 and p16(INK4A) are much less common. Instead, the viral oncoproteins E6 and E7 are expressed and they physically bind and functionally inactivate the p53 and pRb proteins, respectively. Andl et al. [7] were among the first to note the disparity between Rb protein expression and Rb mutational status as a function of HPV infection. Compared to other HNSCCs, Rb protein expression was disproportionately reduced in the tonsillar carcinoma, even though these carcinomas lacked Rb mutations. HPV DNA was identified in 11 of 12 tonsillar carcinomas with reduced Rb expression, but in none of nine tonsillar carcinomas with normal levels of Rb protein. A growing number of studies have also consistently shown that HPV-associated oropharyngeal carcinomas are much less likely to harbor p53 mutations than oropharyngeal carcinomas that are not HPV related [13].

In HPV-positive cervical carcinomas, transcription of the viral oncoprotein E7 physically binds and functionally inactivates the Retinoblastoma (Rb) gene product, causing a perturbation of other key components of the Rb pathway. As one example, functional inactivation of Rb by E7 is known to induce an upregulation of p16 expression [23], reaching levels that can be readily detected by routine immunohistochemistry (IHC) [24]. In effect, immunohistochemical detection of high p16 expression serves as a surrogate marker of infection with high-risk HPVs and, in turn, a marker for neoplastic transformation of the cervix [25]. Immunohistochemical detection of high p16 expression is also an effective ancillary tool for identifying HPV-associated HNSCC. Presence of p16 by IHC correlates very well with the presence of HPV genome by *in situ* hybridization [26] (Fig. 2B). Testing of paraffin-embedded tissue sections for both HPV-16 *in situ* hybridization and p16 IHC is an effective way to screen for HPV-associated HNSCC; positive results in both assays would be expected for most of the HPV-associated HNSCC, and positive results only for p16 IHC may indicate HNSCC associated with HPVs other than HPV-16.

Other differences between HPV-associated and HPV-unassociated HNSCC have been described. Compared with their non-HPV-related counterparts, HPV-related HNSCC are less likely to be associated with inactivation of the tumor suppressor RASSFIA [27], less likely to be associated with inactivation of 14-3-3 sigma, a regulator of senescence in keratinocytes [28]; and less likely to exhibit gross chromosomal changes [29].

2.3. Serologic correlates

Mork et al. [30] conducted a case-control study nested in a large Nordic cohort to examine if the presence of antibodies to HPV-16 and some other HPV types in pre-diagnostic sera (a measure of previous HPV infection) was a risk factor for subsequent HNSCC. They found that antibodies reactive with HPV-16 VLPs in pre-diagnostic sera (on average 9.4 years before diagnosis) conferred a high14-fold risk for oropharyngeal cancers and a lower risk for HNSCC at other anatomic sites. They also examined 160 archived HNSCC tumors for HPV DNA and found HPV-16 DNA in 15 tumors. Detection of HPV-16 DNA in the tumors correlated with pre-diagnostic seropositivity to HPV-16 VLPs.

Antibodies to HPV oncoproteins E6 and E7 are markers of HPV-associated invasive cancer. In a case-control study of women with invasive cervical cancer, Sun et al. [31] found that 63% of cases and 10% of controls had HPV-16 E6 and/or E7 antibodies, and that 21% of cases and 0.5% of controls had antibodies for both HPV-16 E6 and E7. Similar patterns of E6/E7 antibody prevalence are seen with HNSCC. Zumbach et al. [32] reported the presence of HPV-16 E6/E7 antibodies in 7 of 19 (37%) HNSCC patients who had HPV-16 DNA in their tumors and lower prevalences in other groups. In the large international multicenter study [21], the seroprevalence of HPV-16 E6/E7 antibodies was high (65.4%) in patients with HPV DNA-positive oropharyngeal cancers, and low (3.2–4.2%) in patients with HPV DNA-negative oropharyngeal cancers, in patients with oral cancers and in individuals without cancer.

In summary, serologic studies have established that HPV-16 infection precedes the development of HPV-16 DNA-positive HNSCC and that patients with HPV-16-positive oropharyngeal cancer develop antibodies which are markers of HPV-caused cancers.

2.4. Clinical features

Several studies have shown that patients with HPV-positive HNSCCs have a better prognosis than patients with HPV-negative HNSCCs [13]. Mellin et al. [33] compared the clinical outcomes of patients with HPV-16-positive ($n = 23$) and HPV-negative ($n = 29$) tonsillar carcinomas, and found that the risk of cancer-related death was reduced by one-half in the HPV-positive group. In the group of patients with oropharyngeal carcinoma reported by Gillison et al. [13], HPV-positivity was associated with fewer cancer related deaths (3 of 24 HPV-positive cases vs. 10 of 26 HPV-negative cases) and significantly improved disease specific survival. Of the 99 cases of oropharyngeal carcinomas reported by Lindel et al. [34], the 14 HPV-positive cases were associated with a lower recurrence rate and longer patient survival. Li et al. [35] studied 67 patients with tonsillar cancer, 31 of whom had HPV-positive tumors. They found that patients with HPV-positive tumors were 3 times less likely to have recurrence and 5 times less likely to die of the disease than patients with HPV-negative tumors. Weinberger et al. [36] divided 77 patients with oropharyngeal cancers into three groups based on the HPV-16 and p16 status of their tumors. Patients who had HPV-16-positive tumors with high p16 expression (18 cases, group 3) had a better prognosis (five year survival 79%) than patients with HPV-16-negative tumors with low p16 expression (30 cases, group 1, five year survival 20%) or patients with HPV-16-positive tumors with low p16 expression (29 cases, group 2, five year survival, 18%). The HPV-16 viral load was ten-fold

Table 2
Characteristics of HPV-associated HNSCC

Defined by: Transcriptionally active HPV genome localized to tumor cell nuclei
Tumor
– Located almost exclusively in the oropharynx, constituting a significant subset of oropharyngeal carcinomas arising from the lingual and palatine tonsils
– Basaloid histology
– High expression of cellular p16
– Mostly with wildtype p53 and pRb
Patient – compared to other HNSCC patients
– Less likely to have a history of alcohol and tobacco exposure
– More likely to have a history of multiple sexual partners
– More likely to have improved clinical outcomes
– More likely to have antibodies to HPV16 E6 and E7 proteins

higher in group 3 tumors (median, 46 copies per cell) as compared to group 2 tumors (median 3.6 copies per cell). It is possible that the group 3 patients in this study had tumors etiologically linked to HPV-16 and that patients in group 2, with low copy numbers of HPV-16, had tumors not etiologically linked to HPV-16.

The biology underlying the clinical observation of improved prognosis for patients with HPV-associated HNSCC remains to be clarified. Improved outcomes associated with HPV infection is thought to be related to any combination of multiple factors including immune modulation, increased tumor sensitivity to chemoradiation, and a less complex profile of genetic alterations.

2.5. Epidemiologic findings

Patients with HPV-associated oropharyngeal carcinomas are less likely to have a history of exposure to alcohol and tobacco than patients with non-HPV-associated HNSCCs [8].

Risk factors for oral HPV infections are related to sexual behavior and include orogenital contact, multiple sexual partners and HIV infection [37]. In healthy individuals, the prevalence of HPV DNA sequences in tonsillar epithelium is quite low and estimated to be 1% by Kreimer et al. [38] and 0.64% by Hansson et al. [39]. HPV is more prevalent in tonsillar epithelium and in oral rinse specimens in HIV-infected individuals compared to the general population [38]. Further, HPV-associated carcinomas are more likely to occur in HIV-infected individuals than in the general population [40].

2.6. Magnitude of the problem

In his estimates of the global burden of infection-related cancers in 2002, Parkin [41] used a combination of HPV PCR and E6/E7 serology data from cases and controls in the international study of HNSCCs [21] to suggest that, worldwide, 3% of oral cancers (8,200 cases) and 12% of oropharyngeal cancers (6,300 cases) were attributable to HPV infections. By the criteria described earlier in this review (transcriptionally active HPV genome or HPV genome localized to tumor cells), at least one half of all oropharyngeal cancers and practically no oral cavity cancers in the USA and Europe are HPV-associated. If the contribution of HPVs to oropharyngeal cancers is similar elsewhere in the world, about 25,000 of the 51,200 oropharynx cases worldwide might be HPV-related. However, the contribution of HPV infections to these cancers may be geographically variable. Li et al. [35] have reported that 31 of 67 (46%) tonsillar cancers from Australia, but none of 16 tonsillar cancers from China, were HPV-positive by PCR. Also, the incidence of tonsillar cancers has been increasing over the past few decades [42] and it has been suggested that this may be, in part, because of the increasing contribution of HPVs to tonsillar cancer over time [43]. Thus, a crude estimate of HPV-associated cancers worldwide may be in the range of 15,000–25,000 per year.

2.7. Prevention and control

Both of the recently introduced Merck and Glaxo Smith Kline (GSK) HPV-based prophylactic vaccines against cervical cancer include HPV-16 and HPV-18 VLPs. In clinical trials in young women, both vaccines have been shown to be nearly 100% effective in preventing incident HPV-16 and HPV-18 infections and cervical intraepithelial neoplasia (CIN) associated with these types. Trials of the effectiveness of the vaccines in men are in progress. Because the vaccines prevent incident infections, it is very likely that wide-spread

Table 3
Comparison of HPV-associated oropharyngeal squamous cell carcinoma with squamous cell carcinoma of the cervix

	HPV-associated squamous cell carcinoma of the oropharynx	HPV-associated squamous cell carcinoma of cervix
Attributed to HPVs	At least 50% of oropharyngeal cancers	100%
Attributed to HPV-16	90+% of HPV-positive	50% of HPV-positive
Site of precursor lesion	tonsillar crypt	transformation zone
Gender	male predominance	Females

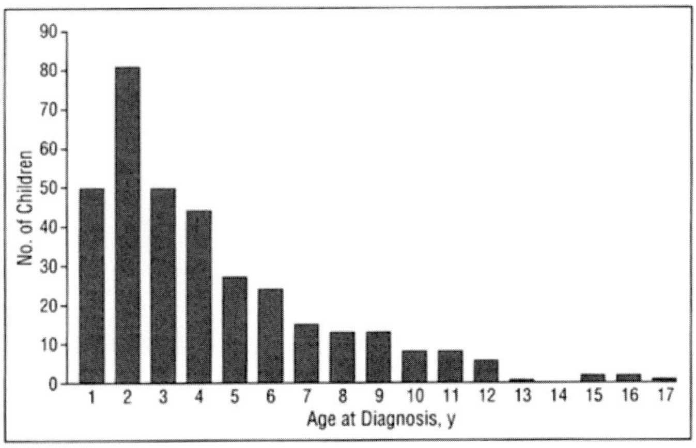

Distribution of age at diagnosis for children enrolled in the recurrent respiratory papillomatosis registry.

Fig. 4. Distribution of age at diagnosis for children enrolled in the recurrent respiratory papillomavirus registry (from [54]).

utilization of these vaccines will reduce the burden of HPV-associated HNSCC.

A number of HPV-16 E6- and E7-based therapeutic vaccines have shown promise in animal models where they protect mice against challenge with HPV-16-transformed tumor cells [44]. Some of these vaccines are in trials in patients with HPV-16-associated oropharyngeal cancers.

2.8. *Summary*

The characteristics of HPV-associated HNSCC are summarized in Table 2. A comparison of some aspects of HPV-associated squamous cell carcinomas of the oropharynx and the cervix is shown in Table 3.

3. HPVs and Recurrent Respiratory Papillomatosis (RRP)

Genital HPVs are also etiologically linked to the benign condition, recurrent respiratory papillomatosis, in the aerodigestive tract. RRP may have onset in childhood (juvenile-onset RRP (JORRP)) with most of the cases occurring in the first 4 years of life (Fig. 4), or in adult life (adult-onset-RRP (AORRP)) with a small peak at 21–30 years.

3.1. *Virologic characteristics*

The non-oncogenic HPV types 6 and 11 that commonly infect the genital tract and are responsible for a large majority of genital warts (condylomas) also account for almost all cases of JORRP and AORRP.

3.2. *Pathogenesis*

For JORRP, the transmission of HPV-6 or HPV-11 most likely occurs intra-partum from mother to child when the fetus is passing through an infected birth canal. This mode of transmission is similar to that of neonatal transmission of herpes simplex virus 2. The manner of transmission in AORRP is not known but it is unlikely that the infection is acquired at birth.

In a child with JORRP, latent HPV infection is apparently widespread throughout the respiratory tract [45]. Papillomas are most frequently found on the vocal cords in the larynx, but may occur at any other site in the respiratory tract. In the genital tract, infection with HPV-6 is more frequent than with HPV-11, but HPV-11 is responsible for a majority of JORRP cases, suggesting that HPV-11 is transmitted more readily than HPV-6 from mother to child. HPV-11 is associated with a more severe clinical course of JORRP [46], as well as with a greater likelihood of malignant transformation of the papilloma [47].

3.3. Clinical features

The course of the disease is highly variable. Although the papillomas are benign and malignant conversion is rare, the recurrent nature of the disease, and the need for repeated surgical interventions to keep the airways open, often impose an enormous burden on the patients and their families (Fig. 5). The number of surgeries required is highest in children with an early onset of disease (Fig. 6), and in severe cases, may exceed 100 [48]. Extension of the disease to the trachea and lungs is a serious complication and it sometimes results from the seeding of infected cells at these sites by the repeated surgical procedures.

3.4. Epidemiologic findings

Maternal condyloma during pregnancy is the overwhelming risk factor for JORRP. About 50% of the mothers of JORRP cases give a history of genital warts during pregnancy [49]. In a population-based study in Denmark [50], maternal condyloma during pregnancy was estimated to increase the risk of JORRP in the child by more than 200 fold. However, the risk of JORRP in a child born to a mother who had condyloma in pregnancy was not large and was estimated to be less than 1%, and a majority of JORRP cases were born to mothers who did not have a history of condyloma during pregnancy.

3.5. Magnitude of the problem

The estimates of the number of JORRP cases in the USA, based on extrapolations from questionnaire data and from a small population-based study are imprecise and have varied from a low of 80 to a high of 2340 [51]. The number of reported cases of JORRP in one survey, without extrapolations, was 840 for the year 1976 [52].

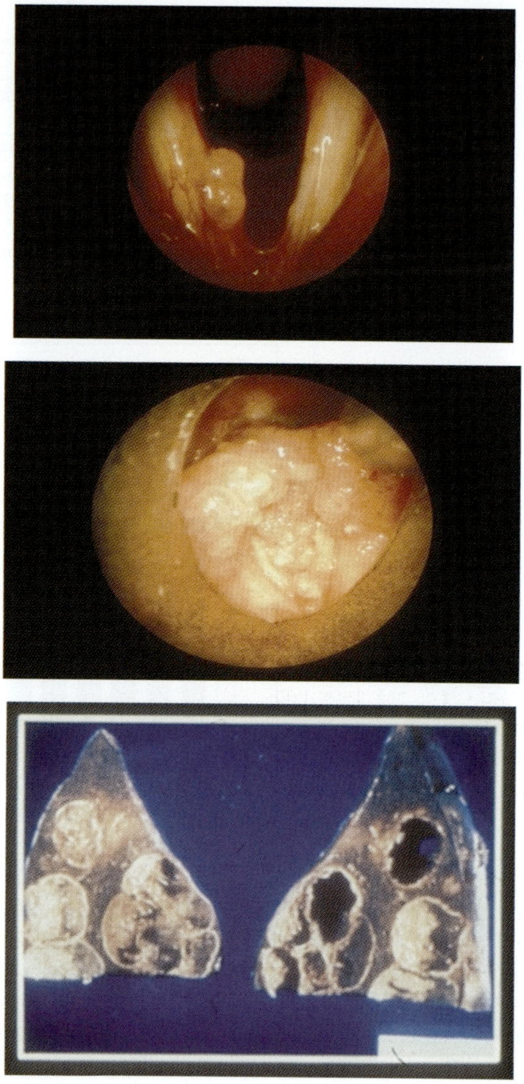

Fig. 5. Clinical presentations of RRP: (a) papilloma on the vocal cord; (b) papilloma obstructing the airway; and (c) papilloma spreading into lungs.

3.6. Prevention and control

Cesarean delivery of the at-risk child might be helpful in preventing JORRP, but it has not been possible to directly evaluate this possibility, because the disease is rare, and the frequency of JORRP even in the high-risk group is low. Indirect evidence for the effectiveness of cesarean delivery has been sought by comparing the cesarean delivery rate in mothers of JORRP cases with national rates [51]. While the data were not consistent across different studies, they suggest that cesarean delivery may afford some protection.

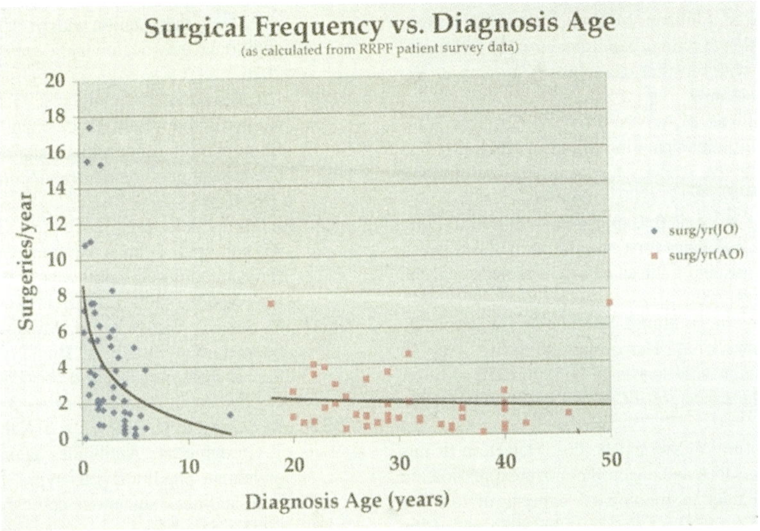

Fig. 6. Number of annual surgeries by age of patient in the Recurrent Respiratory Papillomavirus Foundation Registry (courtesy of Bill Stern).

Prophylactic HPV VLP-based vaccines which include HPV-6 and HPV-11 VLPs, such as Merck's Gardasil®, are anticipated to completely change the landscape for prevention of both JORRP and AORRP. In clinical trials, Gardasil® has been shown to be very effective in protecting young previously uninfected women against incident HPV-6 and HPV-11 infections and against genital warts associated with these two HPV types [53]. Women immunized with Gardasil® are likely to be fully protected against having a child with JORRP. Currently, the Merck Gardasil® vaccine approved by the US FDA is recommended for pre-teen and young women. But older women, pregnant women who have condyloma during pregnancy and even infants born to women who had condyloma during pregnancy could conceivably benefit from the vaccine [51]. Surveillance for JORRP after the introduction of the vaccine will be necessary to evaluate the effectiveness of the vaccine in preventing JORRP.

3.7. Summary

JORRP and AORRP are significant public health problems which at present are difficult to prevent or treat. The HPV VLP-based prophylactic vaccines which include HPV-6 and HPV-11 VLPs have great promise for the reduction of the burden of these diseases.

References

[1] D.M. Parkin, F. Bray, J. Ferlay and P. Pisani, Global cancer statistics, 2002, *CA Cancer J Clin* **55**(2) (2005), 74–108.

[2] S. Franceschi, N. Muñoz, F.X. Bosch, P.J.F. Snijders and J.M.M. Walboomers, Human papillomavirus and cancers of the upper aerodigestive tract: A review of epidemiological and experimental evidence, *Cancer Epidemiol Biomarkers Prev* **5** (1996), 567–575.

[3] R.D.M. Steenbergen, A.J.A. Hermsen, J.M.M. Walboomers, H. Joenje, F. Arwert, C.J.L.M. Meijer et al., Integrated human papillomavirus type 16 and loss of heterozygosity at 11q22 and 18q21 in an oral carcinoma and its derivative cell line, *Cancer Res* **55** (1995), 5465–5471.

[4] G. Niedobitek, S. Pitteroff, H. Herbst, P. Shepherd, T. Finn, I. Anagnostopoulos et al., Detection of human papillomavirus type 16 DNA in carcinomas of the palatine tonsil, *J Clin Pathol* **43** (1990), 918–921.

[5] P.J.F. Snijders, F.V. Cromme, A. van den Brule, H.F.J. Schrijnemakers, G.B. Snow and C.J.L.M. Meijer, Prevalence and expression of human papillomavirus in tonsillar carcinomas, indicating a possible viral etiology, *Int J Cancer* **51** (1992), 845–850.

[6] P.J.F. Snijders, C.J.L.M. Meijer, A. van den Brule, H.F.J. Schrijnemakers, G.B. Snow and J.M.M. Walboomers, Human papillomavirus (HPV) type 16 and 33 E6/E7 region transcripts in tonsillar carcinomas can originate from integrated and episomal HPV DNA, *J Gen Virol* **73** (1992), 2059–2066.

[7] T. Andl, T. Kahn, A. Pfuhl, T. Nicola, R. Erber, C. Conradt et al., Etiological involvement of oncogenic human papillomavirus in tonsillar squamous cell carcinomas lacking retinoblastoma cell cycle control, *Cancer Res* **58** (1998), 5–13.

[8] M.L. Gillison, Human papillomavirus-associated head and neck cancer is a distinct epidemiologic, clinical, and molecular entity, *Semin Oncol* **31**(6) (2004), 744–754.

[9] A.R. Kreimer, G.M. Clifford, P. Boyle and S. Franceschi, Human papillomavirus types in head and neck squamous cell carcinomas worldwide: a systematic review, *Cancer Epidemiol Biomarkers Prev* **14**(2) (2005), 467–475.

[10] P.J.F. Snijders, A. van den Brule, C. Meijer and J. Walboomers, HPV and cancer of the aerodigestive tract, *Papillomavirus Rep* **6** (1995), 157–162.

[11] S. Begum, D. Cao, M. Gillison, M. Zahurak and W.H. Westra, Tissue distribution of human papillomavirus 16 DNA integration in patients with tonsillar carcinoma, *Clin Cancer Res* **11**(16) (2005), 5694–5699.

[12] S. Begum, M.L. Gillison, M.A. Ansari-Lari, K. Shah and W.H. Westra, Detection of human papillomavirus in cervical lymph nodes: a highly effective strategy for localizing site of tumor origin, *Clin Cancer Res* **9**(17) (2003), 6469–6475.

[13] M.L. Gillison, W.M. Koch, R.B. Capone, M.D. Spafford, W.H. Westra, L. Wu et al., Evidence for a causal association between human papillomavirus and a subset of head and neck cancers, *JNCI* **92** (2000), 709–720.

[14] H. Mellin, L. Dahlgren, E. Munck-Wikland, J. Lindholm, H. Rabbani, M. Kalantari et al., Human papillomavirus type 16 is episomal and a high viral load may be correlated to better prognosis in tonsillar cancer, *Int J Cancer* **102**(2) (2002), 152–158.

[15] S. Wilczynski, B. Lin, Y. Xie and B. Paz, Detection of human papillomavirus DNA and oncoprotein overexpression are associated with distinct morphological patterns of tonsillar squamous cell carcinoma, *Am J Pathol* **152** (1998), 145–156.

[16] I. Paz, N. Cook, T. Odom-Maryon et al., Human papillomavirus (HPV) in head and neck cancer. An association of HPV 16 with squamous cell carcinoma of Waldeyer's tonsillar ring, *Cancer* **79** (1997), 595–604.

[17] C.G. Hobbs and M.A. Birchall, Human papillomavirus infection in the etiology of laryngeal carcinoma, *Curr Opin Otolaryngol Head Neck Surg* **12**(2) (2004), 88–92.

[18] M. Sideri, R.W. Jones, E.J. Wilkinson, M. Preti, D.S. Heller, J. Scurry et al., Squamous vulvar intraepithelial neoplasia: 2004 modified terminology, ISSVD Vulvar Oncology Subcommittee, *J Reprod Med* **50**(11) (2005), 807–810.

[19] I. Brook, The clinical microbiology of Waldeyer's ring, *Otolaryngol Clin North Am* **20**(2) (1987), 259–272.

[20] I. Haas, T.K. Hoffmann, R. Engers and U. Ganzer, Diagnostic strategies in cervical carcinoma of an unknown primary (CUP), *Eur Arch Otorhinolaryngol* **259**(6) (2002), 325–333.

[21] R. Herrero, X. Castellsague, M. Pawlita, J. Lissowska, F. Kee, P. Balaram et al., Human papillomavirus and oral cancer: the International Agency for Research on Cancer multicenter study, *J Natl Cancer Inst* **95**(23) (2003), 1772–1783.

[22] A. Forastiere, W. Koch, A. Trotti and D. Sidransky, Head and neck cancer, *N Engl J Med* **345**(26) (2001), 1890–1900.

[23] M. Serrano, G.J. Hannon and D. Beach, A new regulatory motif in cell-cycle control causing specific inhibition of cyclin D/CDK4, *Nature* **366**(6456) (1993), 704–707.

[24] J.P. Klussmann, E. Gultekin, S.J. Weissenborn, U. Wieland, V. Dries, H.P. Dienes et al., Expression of p16 protein identifies a distinct entity of tonsillar carcinomas associated with human papillomavirus, *Am J Pathol* **162**(3) (2003), 747–753.

[25] R. Klaes, T. Friedrich, D. Spitkovsky, R. Ridder, W. Rudy, U. Petry et al., Overexpression of p16(INK4A) as a specific marker for dysplastic and neoplastic epithelial cells of the cervix uteri, *Int J Cancer* **92**(2) (2001), 276–284.

[26] J.P. Klussmann, S.J. Weissenborn, U. Wieland, V. Dries, J. Kolligs, M. Jungehuelsing et al., Prevalence, distribution, and viral load of human papillomavirus 16 DNA in tonsillar carcinomas, *Cancer* **92**(11) (2001), 2875–2884.

[27] S.M. Dong, D.I. Sun, N.E. Benoit, I. Kuzmin, M.I. Lerman and D. Sidransky, Epigenetic inactivation of RASSF1A in head and neck cancer, *Clin Cancer Res* **9**(10 Pt 1) (2003), 3635–3640.

[28] M. Gasco, A.K. Bell, V. Heath, A. Sullivan, P. Smith, L. Hiller et al., Epigenetic inactivation of 14-3-3 sigma in oral carcinoma: association with p16(INK4a) silencing and human papillomavirus negativity, *Cancer Res* **62**(7) (2002), 2072–2076.

[29] B.J. Braakhuis, P.J. Snijders, W.J. Keune, C.J. Meijer, H.J. Ruijter-Schippers, C.R. Leemans et al., Genetic patterns in head and neck cancers that contain or lack transcriptionally active human papillomavirus, *J Natl Cancer Inst* **96**(13) (2004), 998–1006.

[30] J. Mork, A.K. Lie, E. Glattre, G. Hallmans, E. Jellum, P. Koskela et al., Human papillomavirus infection as a risk factor for squamous-cell carcinoma of the head and neck, *N Engl J Med* **344**(15) (2001), 1125–1131.

[31] Y. Sun, J. Eluf-Neto, N. Muñoz, M. Booth, J.M.M. Walboomers, K.V. Shah et al., Human papillomavirus-related serological marker of invasive cervical carcinoma in Brazil, *Cancer Epidemiol Biomarkers Prev* **3** (1994), 341–347.

[32] K. Zumbach, M. Hoffmann, T. Kahn, F. Bosch, S. Gottschlich, T. Gorogh et al., Antibodies against oncoproteins E6 and E7 of human papillomavirus types 16 and 18 in patients with head-and-neck squamous-cell carcinoma, *Int J Cancer* **18**(6) (2000), 815–816.

[33] H. Mellin, S. Friesland, R. Lewensohn, T. Dalianis and E. Munck-Wikland, Human papillomavirus (HPV) DNA in tonsillar cancer: clinical correlates, risk of relapse, and survival, *Int J Cancer* **89**(3) (2000), 300–304.

[34] K. Lindel, K.T. Beer, J. Laissue, R.H. Greiner and D.M. Aebersold, Human papillomavirus positive squamous cell carcinoma of the oropharynx: a radiosensitive subgroup of head and neck carcinoma, *Cancer* **92**(4) (2001), 805–813.

[35] W. Li, C.H. Thompson, C.J. O'Brien, E.B. McNeil, R.A. Scolyer, Y.E. Cossart et al., Human papillomavirus positivity predicts favourable outcome for squamous carcinoma of the tonsil, *Int J Cancer* **106**(4) (2003), 553–558.

[36] P.M. Weinberger, Z. Yu, B.G. Haffty, D. Kowalski, M. Harigopal, J. Brandsma et al., Molecular classification identifies a subset of human papillomavirus – associated oropharyngeal cancers with favorable prognosis, *J Clin Oncol* **24**(5) (2006), 736–747.

[37] F. Coutlee, A.M. Trottier, G. Ghattas, R. Leduc, E. Toma, G. Sanche et al., Risk factors for oral human papillomavirus in adults infected and not infected with human immunodeficiency virus, *Sex Transm Dis* **24**(1) (1997), 23–31.

[38] A.R. Kreimer, A.J. Alberg, R. Daniel, P.E. Gravitt, R. Viscidi, E.S. Garrett et al., Oral human papillomavirus infection in adults is associated with sexual behavior and HIV serostatus, *J Infect Dis* **189**(4) (2004), 686–698.

[39] B.G. Hansson, K. Rosenquist, A. Antonsson, J. Wennerberg, E.B. Schildt, A. Bladstrom et al., Strong association between infection with human papillomavirus and oral and oropharyngeal squamous cell carcinoma: a population-based case-control study in southern Sweden, *Acta Otolaryngol* **125**(12) (2005), 1337–1344.

[40] M. Frisch, R.J. Biggar and J.J. Goedert, Human papillomavirus-associated cancers in patients with human immunodeficiency virus infection and acquired immunodeficiency syndrome, *J Natl Cancer Inst* **92**(18) (2000), 1500–1510.

[41] D.M. Parkin, The global health burden of infection-associated cancers in the year 2002, *Int J Cancer* **118**(12) (2006), 3030–3044.

[42] M. Frisch, H. Hjalgrim, A.B. Jaeger and R.J. Biggar, Changing patterns of tonsillar squamous cell carcinoma in the United States, *Cancer Causes Control* **11**(6) (2000), 489–495.

[43] L. Hammarstedt, D. Lindquist, H.M. Dahlstrand, M. Romanitan, L. Dahlgren, J. Joneberg et al., Human papillomavirus as

a risk factor for the increase in incidence of tonsillar cancer, *Int J Cancer* **119**(11) (2006), 2620–2623.

[44] K. Devaraj, M.L. Gillison and T.C. Wu, Development of HPV vaccines for HPV-associated head and neck squamous cell carcinoma, *Crit Rev Oral Biol Med* **14**(5) (2003), 345–362.

[45] B.M. Steinberg, W.C. Topp, P.S. Schneider and A.L. Abramson, Laryngeal papillomavirus infection during clinical remission, *N Engl J Med* **308** (1983), 1261–1264.

[46] B.J. Wiatrak, D.W. Wiatrak, T.R. Broker and L. Lewis, Recurrent respiratory papillomatosis: a longitudinal study comparing severity associated with human papilloma viral types 6 and 11 and other risk factors in a large pediatric population, *Laryngoscope* **114**(11 Pt 2 Suppl 104) (2004), 1–23.

[47] P.M. Reidy, H.H. Dedo, R. Rabah, J.B. Field, R.H. Mathog, L. Gregoire et al., Integration of human papillomavirus type 11 in recurrent respiratory papilloma-associated cancer, *Laryngoscope* **114**(11) (2004), 1906–1909.

[48] C.S. Derkay, Task force on recurrent respiratory papillomas: a preliminary report, *Arch Otolaryngol Head Neck Surg* **121** (1995), 1386–1391.

[49] T.A. Cook, A.M. Cohn, J.P. Brunschwig et al., Laryngeal papilloma: etiologic and therapeutic considerations, *Ann Otol, Rhinol, Laryngol* **82** (1973), 649.

[50] M.J. Silverberg, P. Thorsen, H. Lindeberg, L.A. Grant and K.V. Shah, Condyloma in pregnancy is strongly predictive of juvenile-onset recurrent respiratory papillomatosis, *Obstet Gynecol* **101**(4) (2003), 645–652.

[51] K.V. Shah, E.R. Unger, C.S. Derkay and B.M. Steinberg, Recurrent respiratory papillomatosis: bright prospects for vaccine-based prevention, *Papillomavirus Rep* **16**(6) (2005), 333–338.

[52] M.S. Strong, C.W. Vaughan and G.B. Healy, Recurrent respiratory papillomatosis, in: *Laryngo-Tracheal Problems in the Pediatric Patient*, M. Healy, ed., Springfield: Thomas, 1979, pp. 88–98.

[53] L.L. Villa, R.L. Costa, C.A. Petta, R.P. Andrade, K.A. Ault, A.R. Giuliano et al., Prophylactic quadrivalent human papillomavirus (types 6, 11, 16, and 18) L1 virus-like particle vaccine in young women: a randomised double-blind placebo-controlled multicentre phase II efficacy trial, *Lancet Oncol* **6**(5) (2005), 271–278.

[54] L.R. Armstrong, C.S. Derkay and W.C. Reeves, Initial results from the national registry for juvenile-onset recurrent respiratory papillomatosis. RRP Task Force, *Arch Otolaryngol Head Neck Surg* **125**(7) (1999), 743–748.

Human papillomaviruses and non-melanoma skin cancer: Basic virology and clinical manifestations

Ingo Nindl*, Marc Gottschling and Eggert Stockfleth
Department of Dermatology, Charité, Skin Cancer Center Charité, University Hospital of Berlin, Charitéplatz 1, D-10117 Berlin, Germany

Abstract. Human papillomaviruses (HPV) infect cutaneous and mucosal epithelia and induce benign and malignant lesions. Non-melanoma skin cancer (NMSC), encompassing basal cell carcinoma and squamous cell carcinoma (SCC), is the most frequent cancer in the Caucasian population, and the incidence has increased dramatically worldwide. Ultraviolet (UV) radiation is a major risk factor for NMSC, and cutaneous HPV is also considered to play an active role during the pathogenesis of these cancers. The first evidence for the involvement of HPV in NMSC was reported in patients with Epidermodysplasia verruciformis (EV). HPV types detected in skin tumours of these patients are referred to as EV/cutaneous HPV types belonging to the beta- and gamma-papillomaviruses (PV). Epidemiological studies have shown a higher risk of several EV/cutaneous HPV types for NMSC. Furthermore, *in vitro* and animal models show transforming properties of some PV types. The anti-apoptotic activities, and the delay of DNA repair mechanism caused by some EV/cutaneous HPV E6 proteins in response to UV-induced mutations, may lead to the persistence of DNA-damaged keratinocytes. Thus, specific EV/cutaneous HPV types as co-factors in association with UV-radiation and the immune system seem to be involved in the early pathogenesis of cutaneous SCC.

Abbreviations: AK, actinic keratosis; EV, Epidermodysplasia verruciformis; HPV, human papillomavirus; LOH, loss of heterozygosity; NMSC, non-melanoma skin cancer; PV, papillomavirus; SCC, squamous cell carcinoma; OTR, organ transplant recipient; UV, Ultraviolet.

1. NMSC and ultraviolet radiation

Non-melanoma skin cancer (NMSC), comprising basal cell carcinoma (BCC), Bowen's disease, cutaneous squamous cell carcinoma (SCC), and its early stage actinic keratosis (AK), is the most frequent malignancy among populations of European origin [1–5]. The tumours are readily diagnosed on the basis of clinical and histopathological appearance (Fig. 1A–C). BCC rarely metastasises and shows ingrowths of epidermal keratinocytes adjacent to palisades of cells resembling those that constitute the lower basal layer [6,7]. They frequently occur on the face and are characteristically indolent, small, pearly edged lesions with sometimes an ulcerated centre. On the contrary, SCC are invasive tumours, whose cells histologically appear like differentiated suprabasal keratinocytes, and approximately 3% metastasises [7]. They grow faster than BCC and produce a more indurated, hyperkeratotic lesion with ulceration. AK and cutaneous SCC frequently occur as multiple primary tumours in the same skin area ('field') in proximity to each other ('field cancerisation'; Fig. 1) [8].

During the last decade, worldwide incidence of NMSC has epidemically increased and now represents approximately 30% of total cancers [9–12]. Particularly, light-skinned and sun-sensitive individuals are affected, and the highest frequencies of the disease are found on sun-exposed sites of the body (Fig. 1G–J) [13]. Furthermore, skin cancer risk is relatively increased in

*Corresponding author: I. Nindl, PhD. Tel.: +49 30 450 518 269; Fax: +49 30 450 518 969; E-mail: ingo.nindl@charite.de.

ISSN 0278-0240/07/$17.00

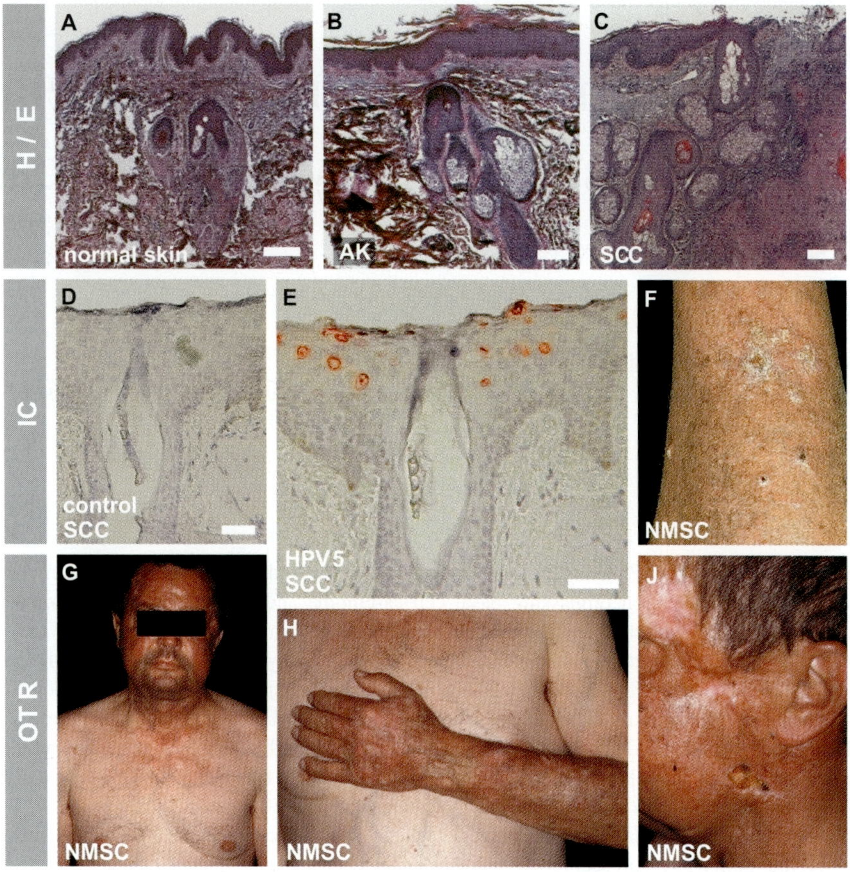

Fig. 1. Non-melanoma skin cancer (NMSC) from an immunocompetent (IC) patient and an immunosuppressed organ transplant recipient (OTR). Sections of paraffin embedded skin tissues stained with haematoxylin and eosin (H / E) for histology (A-C). Normal skin (A), actinic keratosis (AK) (B), and cutaneous squamous cell carcinoma (SCC) (C). Presence of beta-human papillomavirus (HPV) DNA in dysplastic cells of cutaneous SCC (IC patient, 86 years old female) shown by *in situ* hybridisation (ISH) (A. Köhler and I. Nindl, unpublished data) (D,E). Negative control using the HPV 16 genome (D), tyramide signal amplification after ISH, red staining indicate HPV 5 DNA in the nucleus. HPV 5 DNA was not detected in all dysplastic cells, and note the enlarged nuclei in the HPV positive dysplastic cells (E). Field cancerisation with multiple AK and SCC is shown on the forearm of an IC patient (F). Development of multiple AK and SCC exclusively on sun-exposed areas as demonstrated with an immunosuppressed OTR (G-J). Head and chest (G), trunk and left arm (H), left lateral face (J). Originals, magnification scale bars indicate 50 μm.

Caucasians who have been born in countries close to the equator, compared to those who have migrated to them after birth, indicating that the exposure to solar radiation early in life has importance for tumourgenesis [14]. This highlights the role of ultraviolet- (UV) rays as a major environmental risk factor for the development of epithelial skin cancers [15–18]. The major physical adaptation to UV-radiation, which is the most ubiquitous human carcinogen, is pigmentation of the skin, whose degree is largely based on inheritance.

UV-radiation is a component of sunlight and comprises three wavelength classes, UV-C (ranging from 190 to 280 nm), UV-B (280 to 320 nm), and UV-A (320 to 400 nm). The non-ionising radiation cumulatively induces NMSC by at least two interacting rather than separate mechanisms, causing permanent DNA damage and preventing local immunologic recognition of mutant cells [19]. UV-A induces photooxidative stress and secondarily characteristic genome mutations, while UV-B irradiation results directly in the formation of cyclobutane (thymidine) dimers and transitions in DNA. Because of the absence of effective repair mechanisms, such genetic changes lead to permanent mutations in keratinocytes, which subsequently have the potential to progress into epithelial skin cancer [15,18,20,21].

The development of BCC shows a different etiology compared to SCC and is rather marginally subjected to the immune system. It is considered a hair follicle-derived tumour [22] resulting from relatively few genetic alterations that are largely well understood [17].

More than 70% of hereditary and non-hereditary BCC carry a loss of heterozygosity (LOH) at 9q, and loss of 9q22-31 is associated with the Gorlin's syndrome (nevoid BCC syndrome) [23]. In turn, patients suffering from that syndrome exhibit a high risk to develop BCC during the entire lifetime, but are frequently affected by the presence of multiple BCC already at early age [24,25]. The autosomal dominant disorder is based on a germline mutation and persistent inactivation of the tumour suppressor gene *PTCH1* located at chromosome 9q [26–28] that is involved in the sonic hedgehog (SHH) signalling pathway resulting in activation of the transcription factor *Gli1*.

Despite increasing knowledge of BCC development, little is known about the causal alterations of cutaneous SCC. However, the development of SCC clearly results from the mutual interaction of multiple factors that is reflected by, for example, distinct LOH patterns of both various chromosomes and many genes in this disease [29]. LOH has been specifically identified on chromosome 3 (25%), 9 (40%), and 17 (40%), with an overall fractional allelic loss of 30% [30,31]. Recently, 118 differentially expressed genes have been identified by the expression profile of 22,283 genes in normal human skin biopsies compared with AK and cutaneous SCC [32]. Cutaneous SCC is not associated with any hereditary disease, but aneuploidy is frequent occurring in between 20 to 80% of patients [33,34]. UV-B fingerprint type of mutations in NMSC, comprising characteristic C$\rightarrow$T and CC$\rightarrow$TT substitutions, have been particularly identified in the target genes *p53* (chromosome 17p13.1) [35,36], $p16^{\mathrm{INK4a}}$ (chromosome 9p21) [37–40], and *Ha-ras* (chromosome 11p15.5) [17,41,42]. *p53*-mutant cells fail to undergo apoptosis because of UV-induced cellular injury and might also have a selective growth advantage to repopulate injured areas after sunburn events [36,43]. Thus, genomic instability is a driving force in skin cancer development in general, but *p53* mutations rather than $p16^{\mathrm{INK4a}}$ and/or *Ha-ras* mutations seem to be early events during the development of SCC (Nindl et al., unpublished data) [17].

The number of NMSC is remarkably increased in organ transplant recipients (OTR) underscoring the correlation between skin cancer and immune status [44]. Cumulatively, the main risk factors for cutaneous SCC are long-term exposure to UV-radiation, fairly pigmented skin, and immune status. Furthermore, several studies reveal a role of human papillomaviruses (HPV) in the multi-step process of skin carcinogenesis as a co-factor with UV-radiation [45].

2. Human Papillomaviruses

Papillomaviruses (PV) are small DNA viruses with a genome of nearly 8,000 base pairs. They are host specific and have been found in more than 20 different mammalian and avian species. HPV infect keratinocytes of skin and mucosa (Fig. 1D–E), and their lifecycle is adapted to the differentiation of the host cells [46]. Presently, about 100 HPV types have been completely sequenced and are classified into mucosal/genital and cutaneous types based on sequence analyses and clinical manifestation. Phylogenetic analysis of complete L1 gene sequences identify a series of taxonomic units such as alpha-, beta-, and gamma-PV [47]. The human mucosal/genital types belong to the alpha-PV and can be divided into low-risk and high-risk types as inferred from their association with benign and malignant cervical lesions [48–50]. Low-risk types such as HPV 6 and HPV 11 have the potential to induce genital warts (Condylomata acuminata), whereas high-risk types such as HPV 16 and HPV 18 are causally involved in carcinogenesis of the uterine cervix and other mucosae of anogenital and oropharyngeal sites [49,51]. Cutaneous HPV are phylogenetically heterogeneous, and the classical cutaneous warts-associated types (species 2 and 4 of alpha-PV, mu-, and nu-PV) can be distinguished from the Epidermodysplasia verruciformis (EV)-associated or EV/cutaneous types (beta- and gamma-PV) [47,52].

The E5 proteins are considered to access oncogenic potential and are specifically present in alpha- and delta-PV but are absent in EV/cutaneous types. The alpha-PV E5 proteins are classified into four groups based on the clinical manifestations of the corresponding viral infection: the presence of E5-alpha that is found in high-risk types correlates with cervical cancer, E5-gamma and/or E5-delta are associated with mucosal benign lesions, and E5-beta corresponds to benign cutaneous lesions [53,54]. Recent studies reveal a pathogenic role of EV/cutaneous HPV types in the development of NMSC (Fig. 2). In order to prove the causal involvement of HPV in the development of malignancies, specific criteria have to be fulfilled such as the presence and activity of the virus in cells of human skin cancer lesions and evidence on transforming properties of viral genes.

3. HPV and NMSC

3.1. *Epidermodysplasia verruciformis*

The rare heritable disorder EV was initially described in 1922 by the Swiss physician Felix Lewandowsky

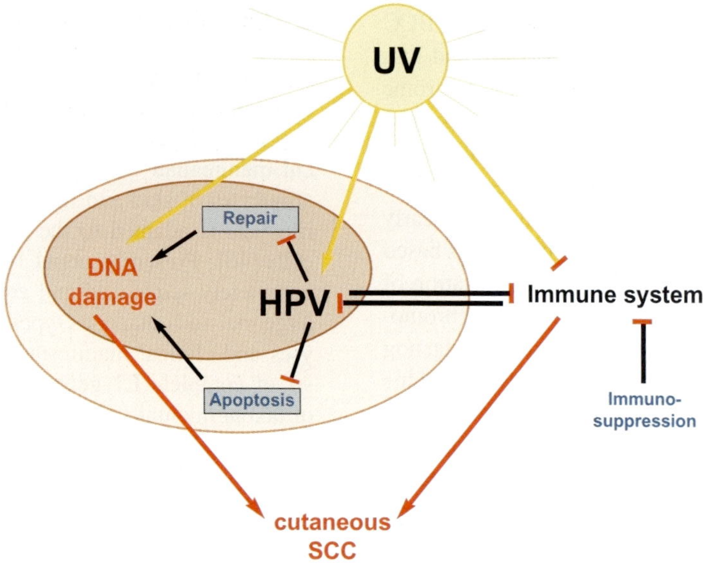

Fig. 2. Multiple risk factors during skin carcinogenesis. Important risk factors for cutaneous squamous cell carcinoma (SCC) are (i) UV-radiation, (ii) EV/cutaneous HPV, and (iii) the immune status. UV-radiation increases the expression of viral genes, induces DNA-damage in keratinocytes, and locally causes immunosuppression. The anti-apoptotic activities, and the delay of DNA repair mechanisms, influenced by HPV in response to UV-induced mutations may lead to the persistence of DNA-damaged keratinocytes and subsequently to skin cancer. Additionally, a low immune status is associated with an increased risk for the development of cutaneous SCC.

under the assistance of Wilhelm Lutz [55]. The disease exhibits extensive polymorphous warts mainly located on sun-exposed sites, which proceed into cutaneous SCC in about 30% of the patients [56,57]. The first evidence for the involvement of HPV in skin cancer was reported from EV patients. The EV types HPV 5 and HPV 8 have been detected in 90% of cutaneous SCC in these patients, whereas HPV 14, HPV 17, HPV 20, and HPV 47 are rarely found in this carcinoma [58].

The genome of EV/cutaneous HPV types is mostly not integrated into the host genome and persists extrachromosomally [59]. This is in contrast to cervical cancer-associated high-risk alpha-HPV, whose viral genome is usually integrated into the host chromosome(s) [60]. HPV DNA persist in high copy numbers in cutaneous SCC (100–300 viral copies per cell equivalent), but not all cancerous cells are HPV-infected [61]. EV/cutaneous HPV types are transcriptionally active in both AK and cutaneous SCC [62,63]. Moreover, persistent HPV infections in cutaneous primary and metastasised SCC from EV patients have been reported [64,65], which may result from a defect of the innate or adaptive immune system by a still unknown mechanism [66].

The eight vertebrate transmembrane cochlear (TMC) expressed genes are evolutionary conserved and encode proteins that constitute three subfamilies. The proteins comprise at least eight membrane-spanning domains, and are located in the endoplasmatic reticulum [67]. The first susceptibility gene locus associated with EV (i.e., EV1) is mapped to chromosome 17q25 [68] and the second locus (EV2) to chromosome 2p21-p24 [69]. Two homologous genes, *TMC6* (*EVER1*) and *TMC8* (*EVER2*), have been identified at the EV1 locus, and nonsense mutations of these genes increase the susceptibility to infection with particular beta-HPV types resulting in a higher risk for cutaneous SCC [70,71]. They appear to be involved in the regulation of the immune system, and additionally in the replication of EV/cutaneous HPV, but the precise function has still to be determined. Moreover, antibodies against beta-HPV types have been found at young ages from EV patients, but age-matched sera from the general population are usually HPV-seronegative (M. Pawlita, personal communication) indicating that viral replication is perturbed in EV patients. Future studies are highly desirable, since knowledge about the mechanism will provide further insights in how EV/cutaneous HPV are controlled at the cellular level and how weak control may contribute to the increased risk for skin cancer.

3.2. General population

Among children from 1 month to 4 years, the prevalence of cutaneous HPV DNA in forehead swabs vary between 50 to 70% [72]. Asymptomatic cutaneous HPV infections of normal skin thus occur very early in infancy caused by a high multiplicity of HPV. Boxman and colleagues [73] firstly detected EV/cutaneous HPV types in hair follicles from eyebrows, arms, and/or legs in 10 of 22 healthy volunteers (45%). Furthermore, cutaneous HPV types have been found in plucked eyebrow hairs in up to 67% of immunocompetent individuals [73–75] and hair follicles are probably a reservoir of EV/cutaneous types. An individual spectrum of EV/cutaneous HPV types is present in plucked hairs from immunocompetent individuals, and similar types are found in different skin areas from both sun-exposed and non sun-exposed sites [76]. Possibly, the skin of each human is infected with an individual pattern of cutaneous HPV types, whose replication is controlled by the immune system. Genital alpha-HPV has been rarely detected in skin samples indicating the high specificity of HPV types to the host tissue.

Over the last two decades, several PCR methods using degenerate, nested and/or type-specific primers followed by sequencing, hybridisation, or cloning and sequencing have been developed to detect a broad range of cutaneous HPV types [73,77–81]. Different prevalence rates of EV/cutaneous HPV types have been reported in NMSC from immunocompetent patients, most likely due to the differences in the detection system used. This assumption has been confirmed by studies reporting increased prevalence rates when a combination of different primer sets have been applied [82, 83]. Recently, two high-throughput PCR-based HPV detection systems have been developed in order to identify EV/cutaneous HPV types with a high sensitivity and both systems are applicable for future large epidemiological studies [84,85].

Overall, the number of EV/cutaneous HPV types in NMSC is higher (27 to 85%) compared to normal skin (15 to 35%) [86–92]. The highest prevalence rate of EV/cutaneous HPV types have been detected in 97 of 114 immunocompetent AK patients (85%) [90]. Moreover, the virus load in skin tumours is low, and a single HPV copy can be detected in only 10 to 1,000 dysplastic cells [88,93,94]. The highest virus load of 6 EV/cutaneous HPV types examined was found in 20 AK, followed by 6 SCC, and has been least in 1 metastasis [95]. Thus, the virus load of EV/cutaneous HPV in cutaneous SCC is very low, and the number of HPV infected cells may decrease during skin carcinogenesis.

An increased risk of SCC, but not BCC, has been associated with EV/cutaneous HPV types in two epidemiological studies investigating viral DNA in eyebrow hairs [75,96]. EV/cutaneous HPV types were detected in hairs from 17 of 25 SCC (68%) *versus* 14 of 25 controls (56%) resulting in a non-significant positive association of HPV with SCC (odds ratio 2.00, 95% confidence interval 0.50–8.0) [75]. In another case-control study, a positive association of EV/cutaneous HPV and SCC was found (odds ratio 1.7, 95% confidence interval 1.1–2.7), with prevalence rates of 75% in SCC (116 of 155) *versus* 58% in controls (216 of 371) [96]. However, an association of a specific HPV type with SCC has not been determined to date. In a few, small epidemiological studies investigating seroreactivity of EV/cutaneous HPV an increased risk of HPV 8 and SCC has been reported [97–99]. A larger study has examined antibody response to six EV/cutaneous types (i.e., HPV types 5, 8, 15, 20, 24, and 38) in 161 SCC, 454 BCC, and 386 control patients [100]. Seroreactivity of HPV 8 and HPV 38 was significantly increased in SCC *versus* controls. In a recent large epidemiological case-control study, antibodies against 16 HPV types (HPV 1, 2, 3, 5, 6, 8, 9, 10, 15, 16, 20, 24, 32, 36, 38, and 57) belonging to beta-, alpha-, and mu-PV have been investigated in 252 SCC, 525 BCC, and 461 control patients using a newly developed multiplex serology [101]. An increased risk of beta-HPV, particularly HPV 5 (odds ratio 1.8, 95% confidence interval 1.0 to 3.1) and SCC, but no association of HPV seropositivity and BCC was found. In conclusion, clinical and epidemiological data support a role of EV/cutaneous HPV in the development of SCC and not BCC.

3.3. Immunosuppressed organ transplant recipients

Persistent HPV-induced warts, AK, and cutaneous SCC, which mainly arise on sun-exposed sites, are the main types of cutaneous tumours in immunosuppressed OTR [4,102,103]. Within 15 years after transplantation, up to 40% of renal transplant recipients have developed NMSC [104]. These cancers predominately represent SCC, but only to a lesser extent BCC. Compared to the general population, the incidence of cutaneous SCC and BCC is approximately 150-fold and 10-fold higher in transplant recipients, respectively, thus leading to a reversal of the SCC to BCC ratio of 1:4 in the general population to 5:1 in transplant recipients [16,44,105,106]. Cutaneous SCC in OTR shows characteristic clinical and morphological features with HPV-induced warts [107]. An important observation is the association and co-localisation of cutaneous SCC with HPV-induced warts in OTR indicating that persistent warts may be progress into skin cancer [108]. Overall, the EV/cutaneous HPV prevalence rate, and the number of multiple types, was higher in cutaneous SCC from immunosuppressed OTR in comparison to the general population. Moreover, OTR have a higher HPV prevalence rate of up to 90% in cutaneous SCC compared to normal skin (11 to 32%) [79,87, 88,92,109–113]. In up to 92% of plucked eyebrow hairs, EV/cutaneous HPV types have been detected [73, 74] leading to low differences in comparison to HPV prevalence of patients with cutaneous SCC. A large European epidemiological study examined the risk of EV/cutaneous HPV types for SCC in 219 OTR with and 550 without a history of cutaneous SCC. An increased risk of one or more EV/cutaneous HPV types in eyebrow hairs for cutaneous SCC have been found in OTR (odds ratio 3.00, 95% confidence interval 1.5–6.2) (J.N. Bouwes Bavinck and the EPI-HPV-UV-CA group, abstract, 4th HPV and Cancer Meeting, November 2006, Turin, Italy). Moreover, a higher prevalence of seroreactivity against beta-HPV was found in OTR with SCC (60%) *versus* in OTR without SCC (55%). Persistent EV/cutaneous HPV infection with the same variant in primary skin SCC, recurrence, and metastases in organ transplant recipients has been reported [94]. Two studies report viral activity of EV/cutaneous HPV types in cutaneous SCC [114,115]. E2 and E4 transcripts have been detected in 20% of warts and 38% of SCC, and E6/E7 transcripts have been found in a single SCC only [114]. Transcriptional activity of the EV/cutaneous HPV types 8, 9, and 15 of E6/E7 has been detected in 4 of 10 viral positive AK and cutaneous SCC from immunosuppressed OTR [115]. Thus, viral activity of early genes seems to be present in at least a subset of AK and cutaneous SCC suggesting a role for HPV during skin carcinogenesis.

4. Molecular mechanisms and transforming properties of EV/cutaneous HPV

4.1. In vitro models

4.1.1. Monolayer

Using monolayer cultures, the E6 gene of HPV 8 shows transforming properties in rodent fibroblast lines (C127, Rat 1), whereas HPV 8 E7 is involved in the replication of the viral DNA [116]. HPV 47 E6 is required and sufficient for the transformation of the rat fibroblastic cell line (3Y1) [117]. The E6 genes of the EV/cutaneous HPV types 5, 8, 14, 20, 21, 25, and 47 induce morphological transformation in 3Y1 cells [118]. The oncogenic potential of HPV types 5, 8, and 47 is higher than those of HPV types 14, 20, 21, and 25. The E7 genes of HPV 8 and HPV 47 fail to induce morphological transformation in rodent fibroblast lines suggesting that E6 rather than E7 is correlated to malignant conversion [116,119]. However, HPV 8 E7 is able to transform rodent cells concertedly with the activated *Ha-ras* oncogene [120]. The first study analysing the ability of cutaneous HPV types to immortalise human foreskin keratinocytes was performed with HPV 1 and HPV 8 [121]. Furthermore, the E6 or E7 gene of HPV 1, showing a transformed phenotype in rodent cells, is not able to immortalise human keratinocytes, and only a weak immortalising potential for HPV 8 E7 has been observed. The E6/E7 protein of EV/cutaneous HPV 38, but not HPV 10 and HPV 20, displays transforming activity by increasing the life span of human primary keratinocytes [122]. Additionally, HPV 38 E7 is able to degrade and inactivate the tumour suppressor gene *pRb*.

Purdie and colleagues [123] were the first to demonstrate UV-induced activation of the viral promotor of the cutaneous type HPV 77 that was identified in cutaneous lesions from OTR. The promotor contains a *p53* binding site, and the response is mediated through the UV-induced expression of *p53*. The influence of UV-radiation varies on viral gene expression of warts-associated types (HPV types 1, 2, 3, 7, 27, 41, and 77) and EV/cutaneous types (HPV types 5, 20, 23, and 38) [124]. The presence or absence of wild-type or mutated *p53* influences the gene expression of HPV types 20, 27, and 77, but not of HPV 41, suggesting that *p53* is not an exclusive factor involved in the interaction between UV-radiation and HPV. UV-induced cytokines activate the promotor of HPV 20, but inhibit the promotor of the warts-associated type HPV 27 [125].

Independently from *p53* degradation, the E6 protein of HPV 5 inhibits apoptosis in response to UV-damage [126] by inactivation of the pro-apoptotic protein *Bak* [127]. Moreover, HPV-negative skin cancers express *Bak* that is in contrast to HPV-positive cancers, in which *Bak* has not been detected. This underscores the importance and clinical relevance of the interaction between the UV-induced *Bak* protein and EV/cutaneous HPV types. E6 of both HPV 1 and HPV 8 binds *XRCC1*, a protein that is required for DNA repair suggesting a link between EV/cutaneous HPV and the according host pathways [128]. The E6 protein of HPV 5 compromises the repair of UV-induced thymine dimers [129], and E6 of HPV 77 additionally forces keratinocytes into the S1-phase by inhibiting *p53*-activated, pro-apoptotic genes [130]. However, the E6 expression of beta-HPV 5 does not interfere with such pro-apoptotic genes indicating that this is probably not the favoured mechanism of EV/cutaneous HPV types in the cell. The anti-apoptotic activity, and the delay of the DNA-repair mechanism, may lead to the persistence of UV-damaged keratinocytes suggesting that cutaneous/EV HPV may be involved in the early stages of skin carcinogenesis.

4.1.2. Organotypic keratinocytes cultures

Functional analyses of EV/cutaneous HPV types have been retarded for a long time because of both the relation between viral development and host cell differentiation, in addition to the lack of a system with continuously differentiating keratinocytes that constitute a stratified epithelium (i.e., the natural target cells of PV). However, the organotypic raft culture partly has such properties and consists of human primary keratinocytes, which stratify and differentiate into a squamous epithelium [131]. Growth and differentiation markers are expressed similarly to the human epithelium making this system a key technology for the investigation of human skin carcinogenesis. The E6/E7 genes of the EV/cutaneous HPV types 5, 12, 15, 17, 20, and 38 have strong effects on the growth and differentiation in organotypic cultures of human primary keratinocytes, but an invasive phenotype have not been observed [132]. HPV 8 E7 promotes invasion of keratinocytes into the dermis [133]. This immortal phenotype was associated with the disruption of the basement membrane and the overexpression of metalloproteinases *MMP-1*, *MMP-8*, and *MT-1-MMP*.

4.2. Animal models

4.2.1. Cattle and horses

Using animal models, the role of PV in skin carcinogenesis has been studied at three different levels, namely in naturally occurring lesions, in colonies of animals that have been collected from the field, and in transgenic animals. Most non-human PV have been isolated and sequenced from severe epithelial diseases of warm-blooded vertebrates including many gregarious animals such as cattle, dog, and rabbit. Bovine papillomavirus type 4 (BPV 4) from the xi-PV is the etiological agent of epithelial papilloma of the upper alimentary canal in cattle [134]. Carcinoma shows characteristic morphological features with papilloma, which can progress into cancer. However, BPV 4 DNA is found in early papilloma of the alimentary tract, but not in advanced papilloma, oesophageal carcinoma, or adenoma and adenocarcinoma of the lower intestine [135,136]. Therefore, the presence of BPV 4 is restricted to the early transformation stages during carcinogenesis ('hit-and-run mechanism'). Decrease of virus load has also been shown in a study investigating AK through SCC developmental stages of human cancers [95]. Thus, the multiple factors including BPV 4 infection that concertedly lead to carcinoma in cattle [137] may serve as animal model for an improved knowledge about the complex role of HPV in human skin cancer.

BPV 1 and BPV 2 belong to the delta-PV exhibiting an E5 open reading frame (ORF), which may have been independently developed from that of the alpha-PV [53]. The virus is able to infect horses and play an important role in the development of equine sarcoids [138–140]. Roughly half of the healthy horses having contact with infected fellows carry BPV 1 in their skin [141]. This indicates that the usually strict specificity of PV to their hosts [142] is occasionally dismantled and that interspecies transmission may rarely occur in PV (although without replicative establishment of the virus). However, the underlying mechanisms and the possible impact on the malignant developments of novel host invasion have not been seriously addressed for PV to date [52]. On the contrary, their presence in humans has exclusively been regarded as old primate inheritance [142].

4.2.2. Cottontail rabbit

Anatomical sites, in which PV cannot complete the productive life cycle, appear particularly involved in the development of skin cancers. This has also been suggested for malignancies caused by cottontail rabbit PV (CRPV) [46] from the kappa-PV. Viral DNA easily induces papillomata making the cottontail rabbit model a powerful system, which identifies the molecular mechanisms that are required for the induction and progression of epithelial neoplasia. Benign papillomata are induced in nearly all rabbits that are infected by CRPV, and 80% of the initially benign epithelial tumours progress into carcinoma within 6 to 14 months [143]. The virus thus plays an active role during skin carcinogenesis of domestic rabbits interacting with chemical carcinogens [144]. Mutation analysis of viral DNA shows that only the E7 gene, but not the E4 gene, is involved in the development of papilloma [145]. However, the E4 gene remains an important factor for viral DNA amplification and expression of the late structural proteins [46]. Mutation of the highly conserved amino acids results in replication-competent but transactivation-deficient E2 proteins [146].

4.2.3. Multimammate mouse

A colony of *Mastomys coucha* (Smith, 1834) [initially determined as *M. natalensis* (Smith, 1834)] has been established from animals collected in South Africa, which spontaneously develop multiple benign skin tumours such as papilloma and keratoacanthoma during aging. The animals are latently infected by the first *Mastomys natalensis* papillomavirus (MnPV 1) [147], which is the etiological agent of the lesions [148–150]. MnPV 1 belongs to the iota-PV and does not contain any E5 ORF. Analogously to HPV 8-induced NMSC in EV patients, MnPV 1 DNA persists episomally, without any evidence of integration [147]. Virus-induced tumours do not regress, but proceed after topical application of carcinogens and tumour promotors of cutaneous SCC [151], which is in contrast to the human keratoacanthoma development. MnPV 1 has a broader tissue specificity than other PV investigated so far, and viral persistence and viral load has been correlated with the development of skin tumors [152]. Thus, *Mastomys coucha* is an excellent animal model for the study of naturally PV-induced skin carcinogenesis.

4.2.4. Transgenic mice

HPV 1 causes hyperproliferation and alterations of skin differentiation in a transgenic mouse model examining benign warts of the animals [153]. The expression of the early genomic region, under the control of the keratin-6 promotor, shows a similar phenotype like human virus-induced warts. Pfister and colleagues have established the first transgenic mouse model for studies on beta-HPV types using the complete early region of HPV 8 under the control of the keratin-14 promotor [154]. The mice have spontaneously developed cutaneous SCC without additional carcinogens, and benign skin tumours have been observed in 91% of the animals. The same research group has generated HPV 8-transgenic mice that affect exclusively the gene(s) E2, E6, E7, or E6/E7. Spontaneously developed skin tumours have been observed in E2-, E6-, and E6/E7-transgenic mice, whereas the exclusive expression of HPV 8 E7 is not sufficient to induce tumour growth (H. Pfister, personal communication). Tommasino and co-workers [155] have established transgenic mice expressing E6/E7 of HPV 38 under the control of the human keratin-10 promoter. The animals have developed skin tumours after a two-stage carcinogen treatment. Cellular proliferation, hyperplasia, and dysplasia in the epidermis have been spontaneously induced by HPV 38 E6/E7. Transforming properties of HPV 8 and HPV 38 have been thus shown in the system of a transgenic mice model.

5. Conclusions

The skin of most humans is infected with an individual spectrum of different cutaneous HPV types, and hair follicles are probably their reservoir. During host-linked evolution, cutaneous HPV types may have established different ecological niches in human skin tissues including a mutualistic cooperation between HPV and their host cells. Specific triggers such as UV-induced DNA-damage in sun-exposed cells, immunosuppression (e.g., locally UV-induced, systemically in OTR), and/or inactivation of host controlled viral life cycle (e.g., in EV patients) lead to increased HPV replication and subsequently to a higher virus load within the cells. The anti-apoptotic effect of cutaneous HPV types in UV-damaged keratinocytes probably results in persistent viral infections and hence the accumulation of further DNA mutations, putatively leading to immortalised cells (Fig. 2). Thus, cutaneous HPV types seem to be involved as a co-factor in the early onset of cutaneous SCC.

Acknowledgements

Our research program is supported by funding from the University Hospital Charité, the Dr. Mildred Scheel Stiftung für Krebsforschung/Deutsche Krebshilfe (grant number 70-2588), the European Community (contract number QLK2-CT-2002-01179), and the Roche Organ Transplantation Research Foundation in Switzerland (grant number 590944305). We acknowledge the native speaker M. Patel for reading the manuscript.

References

[1] R. Marks, G. Rennie and T. Selwood, Malignant transformation of solar keratoses to squamous cell carcinoma, *Lancet* **1** (1988), 795–797.

[2] T. Johnson, D. Rowe, B. Nelson and N. Swanson, Squamous cell carcinoma of the skin (excluding lip and oral mucosa), *J Am Acad Dermatol* **26** (1992), 467–484.

[3] C. Cockerell, Histopathology of incipient intraepidermal squamous cell carcinoma ("actinic keratosis"), *J Am Acad Dermatol* **42** (2000), 11–17.

[4] S. Euvrard, J. Kanitakis and A. Claudy, Skin cancers after organ transplantation, *N Engl J Med* **348** (2003), 1681–1691.

[5] W. Fu and C. Cockerell, The actinic (solar) keratosis: a 21st-century perspective, *Arch Dermatol* **139** (2003), 66–70.

[6] S. Miller, Biology of basal cell carcinoma (Part I), *J Am Acad Dermatol* **24** (1991), 1–13.

[7] G. Bowden, Prevention of non-melanoma skin cancer by targeting ultraviolet-B-light signalling, *Nat Rev Cancer* **4** (2004), 23–35.
[8] D. Slaughter, H. Southwick and W. Smejkal, Field cancerization in oral stratified squamous epithelium; clinical implications of multicentric origin, *Cancer* **6** (1953), 963–968.
[9] D. Miller and M. Weinstock, Nonmelanoma skin cancer in the United States: incidence, *J Am Acad Dermatol* **30** (1994), 774–778.
[10] H. Gloster and D. Brodland, The epidemiology of skin cancer, *Dermatol Surg* **22** (1996), 217–226.
[11] R. DePinho, The age of cancer, *Nature* **408** (2000), 248–254.
[12] T. Diepgen and V. Mahler, The epidemiology of skin cancer, *Br J Dermatol* **146** (Suppl 61) (2002), 1–6.
[13] B. Armstrong and A. Kricker, The epidemiology of UV induced skin cancer, *J Photochem Photobiol* **B63** (2001), 8–18.
[14] M. Staples, M. Elwood, R. Burton, J. Williams, R. Marks and G. Giles, Non-melanoma skin cancer in Australia: the 2002 national survey and trends since 1985, *Med J Aust* **184** (2006), 6–10.
[15] S. Salasche, Epidemiology of actinic keratoses and squamous cell carcinoma, *J Am Acad Dermatol* **42** (2000), 4–7.
[16] E. Stockfleth, C. Ulrich, T. Meyer, R. Arndt and E. Christophers, Skin diseases following organ transplantation-risk factors and new therapeutic approaches, *Transplant Proc* **33** (2001), 1848–1853.
[17] P. Boukamp, Non-melanoma skin cancer: what drives tumor development and progression? *Carcinogenesis* **26** (2005), 1657–1667.
[18] P. Erb, J. Ji, M. Wernli, E. Kump, A. Glaser and S. Büchner, Role of apoptosis in basal cell and squamous cell carcinoma formation, *Immunol Lett* **100** (2005), 68–72.
[19] M. Kripke, Ultraviolet radiation and immunology: something new under the sun-presidential address, *Cancer Res* **54** (1994), 6102–6105.
[20] M. Kripke and M. Fisher, Immunologic parameters of ultraviolet carcinogenesis, *J Natl Cancer Inst* **57** (1976), 211–215.
[21] D. Brash, A. Ziegler, A. Jonason, J. Simon, S. Kunala and D. Leffell, Sunlight and sunburn in human skin cancer: p53, apoptosis, and tumor promotion, *J Investig Dermatol Symp Proc* **1** (1996), 136–142.
[22] D. Jih, S. Lyle, R. Elenitsas, D. Elder and G. Cotsarelis, Cytokeratin 15 expression in trichoepitheliomas and a subset of basal cell carcinomas suggests they originate from hair follicle stem cells, *J Cutan Pathol* **26** (1999), 113–118.
[23] R. Gorlin, Nevoid basal-cell carcinoma syndrome, *Medicine (Baltimore)* **66** (1987), 98–113.
[24] S. Shanley, J. Ratcliffe, A. Hockey, E. Haan, C. Oley, D. Ravine, N. Martin, C. Wicking and G. Chenevix-Trench, Nevoid basal cell carcinoma syndrome: review of 118 affected individuals, *Am J Med Genet* **50** (1994), 282–290.
[25] V. Kimonis, A. Goldstein, B. Pastakia, M. Yang, R. Kase, J. DiGiovanna, A. Bale and S. Bale, Clinical manifestations in 105 persons with nevoid basal cell carcinoma syndrome, *Am J Med Genet* **69** (1997), 299–308.
[26] R. Johnson, A. Rothman, J. Xie, L. Goodrich, J. Bare, J. Bonifas, A. Quinn, R. Myers, D. Cox, E. Epstein Jr. and M. Scott, Human homolog of *patched*, a candidate gene for the basal cell nevus syndrome, *Science* **272** (1996), 1668–1671.
[27] H. Hahn, C. Wicking, P. Zaphiropoulous, M. Gailani, S. Shanley, A. Chidambaram, I. Vorechovsky, E. Holmberg, A. Unden, S. Gillies, K. Negus, I. Smyth, C. Pressman, D. Leffell, B. Gerrard, A. Goldstein, M. Dean, R. Toftgard, G. Chenevix-Trench, B. Wainwright and A. Bale, Mutations of the human homolog of *Drosophila patched* in the nevoid basal cell carcinoma syndrome, *Cell* **85** (1996), 841–851.
[28] A. Chidambaram, A. Goldstein, M. Gailani, B. Gerrard, S. Bale, J. DiGiovanna, A. Bale and M. Dean, Mutations in the human homologue of the *Drosophila patched* gene in Caucasian and African-American nevoid basal cell carcinoma syndrome patients, *Cancer Res* **56** (1996), 4599–4601.
[29] M. Alam and D. Ratner, Cutaneous squamous-cell carcinoma, *N Engl J Med* **344** (2001), 975–983.
[30] A. Quinn, S. Sikkink and J. Rees, Delineation of two distinct deleted regions on chromosome 9 in human non-melanoma skin cancers, Genes Chromosomes, *Cancer* **11** (1994), 222–225.
[31] I. Rehman, M. Takata, Y. Wu and J. Rees, Genetic change in actinic keratoses, *Oncogene* **12** (1996), 2483–2490.
[32] I. Nindl, C. Dang, T. Forschner, R. Kuban, T. Meyer, W. Sterry and E. Stockfleth, Identification of differentially expressed genes in cutaneous squamous cell carcinoma by microarray expression profiling, *Mol Cancer* **5** (2006), 30.
[33] J. Newton, R. Camplejohn and D. McGibbon, A flow cytometric study of the significance of DNA aneuploidy in cutaneous lesions, *Br J Dermatol* **117** (1987), 169–174.
[34] A. Herzberg, B. Kerns, F. Honkanen, J. Pence, J. Iglehart and R. Kinney, DNA ploidy and proliferation index of soft tissue sarcomas determined by image cytometry of fresh frozen tissue, *Am J Clin Pathol* **97** (1992), S29–S37.
[35] N. Dumaz, A. Stary, T. Soussi, L. Daya-Grosjean and A. Sarasin, Can we predict solar ultraviolet radiation as the causal event in human tumours by analysing the mutation spectra of the *p53* gene? *Mutat Res* **307** (1994), 375–386.
[36] A. Ziegler, A. Jonason, D. Leffell, J. Simon, H. Sharma, J. Kimmelman, L. Remington, T. Jacks and D. Brash, Sunburn and *p53* in the onset of skin cancer, *Nature* **372** (1994), 773–776.
[37] N. Soufir, J. Moles, C. Vilmer, C. Moch, O. Verola, J. Rivet, A. Tesniere, L. Dubertret and N. Basset-Seguin, *P16* UV mutations in human skin epithelial tumors, *Oncogene* **18** (1999), 5477–5481.
[38] V. Brown, C. Harwood, T. Crook, J. Cronin, D. Kelsell and C. Proby, $p16^{INK4a}$ and $p14^{ARF}$ Tumor suppressor genes are commonly inactivated in cutaneous squamous cell carcinoma, *J Invest Dermatol* **122** (2004), 1284–1292.
[39] H. Kreimer-Erlacher, H. Seidl, B. Bäck, L. Cerroni, H. Kerl and P. Wolf, High frequency of ultraviolet mutations at the *INK4a-ARF* locus in squamous cell carcinomas from psoralen-plus-ultraviolet-A-treated psoriasis patients, *J Invest Dermatol* **120** (2003), 676–682.
[40] Z. Saridaki, T. Liloglou, A. Zafiropoulos, E. Koumantaki, O. Zoras and D. Spandidos, Mutational analysis of *CDKN2A* genes in patients with squamous cell carcinoma of the skin, *Br J Dermatol* **148** (2003), 638–648.
[41] H. Ananthaswamy and W. Pierceall, Molecular alterations in human skin tumors, *Prog Clin Biol Res* **376** (1992), 61–84.
[42] S. Popp, S. Waltering, C. Herbst, I. Moll and P. Boukamp, UV-B-type mutations and chromosomal imbalances indicate common pathways for the development of Merkel and skin squamous cell carcinomas, *Int J Cancer* **99** (2002), 352–360.
[43] A. Jonason, S. Kunala, G. Price, R. Restifo, H. Spinelli, J. Persing, D. Leffell, R. Tarone and D. Brash, Frequent clones of p53-mutated keratinocytes in normal human skin, *Proc Natl Acad Sci USA* **93** (1996), 14025–14029.
[44] F. Moloney, H. Comber, P. O'Lorcain, P. O'Kelly, P. Conlon and G. Murphy, A population-based study of skin cancer

incidence and prevalence in renal transplant recipients, *Br J Dermatol* **154** (2006), 498–504.
[45] B. Akgül, J. Cooke and A. Storey, HPV-associated skin disease, *J. Pathol* **208** (2006), 165–175.
[46] J. Doorbar, The papillomavirus life cycle, *J Clin Virol* **32** (2005), 7–15.
[47] E.-M. de Villiers, C. Fauquet, T. Broker, H.-U. Bernard and H. zur Hausen, Classification of papillomaviruses, *Virology* **324** (2004), 17–27.
[48] International Agency for Research on Cancer, IARC monographs on the evaluation of carcinogenic risks to humans. Human papillomaviruses, *IARC Lyon France* **64** (1995).
[49] N. Muñoz, F. Bosch, S. de Sanjose, R. Herrero, X. Castellsague, K. Shah, P. Snijders and C. Meijer, Epidemiologic classification of human papillomavirus types associated with cervical cancer, *N Engl J Med* **348** (2003), 518–527.
[50] A. Narechania, Z. Chen, R. DeSalle and R. Burk, Phylogenetic incongruence among oncogenic genital alpha human papillomaviruses, *J Virol* **79** (2005), 15503–15510.
[51] H. zur Hausen, Papillomaviruses and cancer: From basic studies to clinical application, *Nat Rev Cancer* **2** (2002), 342–350.
[52] M. Gottschling, A. Köhler, E. Stockfleth and I. Nindl, Phylogenetic analysis of beta-papillomaviruses as inferred from nucleotide and amino acid sequence data, *Mol Phylogenet Evol* **42** (2007), 213–222.
[53] I. Bravo and A. Alonso, Mucosal human papillomaviruses encode four different E5 proteins whose chemistry and phylogeny correlate with malignant or benign growth, *J Virol* **78** (2004), 13613–13626.
[54] S. Garcia-Vallve, A. Alonso and I. Bravo, Papillomaviruses: different genes have different histories, *Trends Microbiol* **13** (2005), 514–521.
[55] F. Lewandowsky and W. Lutz, Ein Fall einer bisher nicht beschriebenen Hauterkrankung (Epidermodysplasia verruciformis), *Arch Dermatol Syphilol* **141** (1922), 193–203.
[56] S. Jablonska, J. Dabrowski and K. Jakubowicz, Epidermodysplasia verruciformis as a model in studies on the role of papovaviruses in oncogenesis, *Cancer Res* **32** (1972), 583–589.
[57] G. Orth, S. Jablonska, M. Favre, O. Croissant, M. Jarzabek-Chorzelska and G. Rzesa, Characterization of two types of human papillomaviruses in lesions of Epidermodysplasia verruciformis, *Proc Natl Acad Sci USA* **75** (1978), 1537–1541.
[58] S. Majewski and S. Jablonska, Human papillomavirus-associated tumors of the skin and mucosa, *J Am Acad Dermatol* **36** (1997), 659–685.
[59] M. Favre, N. Ramoz and G. Orth, Human papillomaviruses: General features, *Clin Dermatol* **15** (1997), 181–198.
[60] N. Wentzensen, R. Ridder, R. Kläs, S. Vinokurova, U. Schäfer and M. Doeberitz, Characterization of viral-cellular fusion transcripts in a large series of HPV16 and 18 positive anogenital lesions, *Oncogene* **21** (2002), 419–426.
[61] H. Pfister, Chapter 8: Human papillomavirus and skin cancer, *J Natl Cancer Inst Monogr* (2003), 52–56.
[62] M. Yutsudo and A. Hakura, Human papillomavirus type 17 transcripts expressed in skin carcinoma tissue of a patient with Epidermodysplasia verruciformis, *Int J Cancer* **39** (1987), 586–589.
[63] K. Haller, F. Stubenrauch and H. Pfister, Differentiation-dependent transcription of the Epidermodysplasia verruciformis-associated human papillomavirus type 5 in benign lesions, *Virology* **214** (1995), 245–255.
[64] R. Ostrow, M. Bender, M. Niimura, T. Seki, M. Kawashima, F. Pass and A. Faras, Human papillomavirus DNA in cutaneous primary and metastasized squamous cell carcinomas from patients with Epidermodysplasia verruciformis, *Proc Natl Acad Sci USA* **79** (1982), 1634–1638.
[65] H. Pfister and J. Ter Schegget, Role of HPV in cutaneous premalignant and malignant tumors, *Clin Dermatol* **15** (1997), 335–347.
[66] S. Majewski and S. Jablonska, Do Epidermodysplasia verruciformis human papillomaviruses contribute to malignant and benign epidermal proliferations? *Arch Dermatol* **138** (2002), 649–654.
[67] N. Ramoz, L. Rueda, B. Bouadjar, L. Montoya, G. Orth and M. Favre, Mutations in two adjacent novel genes are associated with Epidermodysplasia verruciformis, *Nat Genet* **32** (2002), 579–581.
[68] N. Ramoz, L. Rueda, B. Bouadjar, M. Favre and G. Orth, A susceptibility locus for Epidermodysplasia verruciformis, an abnormal predisposition to infection with the oncogenic human papillomavirus type 5, maps to chromosome 17qter in a region containing a psoriasis locus, *J Invest Dermatol* **112** (1999), 259–263.
[69] N. Ramoz, A. Taieb, L. Rueda, L. Montoya, B. Bouadjar, M. Favre and G. Orth, Evidence for a nonallelic heterogeneity of Epidermodysplasia verruciformis with two susceptibility loci mapped to chromosome regions 2p21-p24 and 17q25, *J Invest Dermatol* **114** (2000), 1148–1153.
[70] G. Keresztes, H. Mutai and S. Heller, *TMC* and *EVER* genes belong to a larger novel family, the *TMC* gene family encoding transmembrane proteins, BMC *Genomics* **4** (2003), 24.
[71] K. Kurima, Y. Yang, K. Sorber and A. Griffith, Characterization of the transmembrane channel-like (TMC) gene family: functional clues from hearing loss and Epidermodysplasia verruciformis, *Genomics* **82** (2003), 300–308.
[72] A. Antonsson, S. Karanfilovska, P. Lindqvist and B. Hansson, General acquisition of human papillomavirus infections of skin occurs in early infancy, *J Clin Microbiol* **41** (2003), 2509–2514.
[73] I. Boxman, R. Berkhout, L. Mulder, M. Wolkers, J. Bouwes Bavinck, B. Vermeer and J. Ter Schegget, Detection of human papillomavirus DNA in plucked hairs from renal transplant recipients and healthy volunteers, *J Invest Dermatol* **108** (1997), 712–715.
[74] I. Boxman, L. Mulder, A. Russell, J. Bouwes Bavinck, A. Green and J. Ter Schegget, Human papillomavirus type 5 is commonly present in immunosuppressed and immunocompetent individuals, *Br J Dermatol* **141** (1999), 246–249.
[75] I. Boxman, A. Russell, L. Mulder, J. Bouwes Bavinck, J. Ter Schegget, A. Green and Collaborators of the Nambour Prevention Study, Case-control study in a subtropical Australian population to assess the relation between non-melanoma skin cancer and Epidermodysplasia verruciformis human papillomavirus DNA in plucked eyebrow hairs, *Int J Cancer* **86** (2000), 118–121.
[76] A. Köhler, T. Forschner, T. Meyer, C. Ulrich, M. Gottschling, E. Stockfleth and I. Nindl, Multifocal distribution of cutaneous human papillomavirus types in hairs from different skin areas, *Br. J. Dermatol* (in press).
[77] L. Tieben, J. Ter Schegget, R. Minnaar, J. Bouwes Bavinck, R. Berkhout, B. Vermeer, M. Jebbink and H. Smits, Detection of cutaneous and genital HPV types in clinical samples by PCR using consensus primers, *J Virol Methods* **42** (1993), 265–279.

[78] V. Shamanin, H. Delius and E.M. de Villiers, Development of a broad spectrum PCR assay for papillomaviruses and its application in screening lung cancer biopsies, *J Gen Virol* **75** (1994), 1149–1156.

[79] R. Berkhout, L. Tieben, H. Smits, J. Bouwes Bavinck, B. Vermeer and J. Ter Schegget, Nested PCR approach for detection and typing of Epidermodysplasia verruciformis-associated human papillomavirus types in cutaneous cancers from renal transplant recipients, *J Clin Microbiol* **33** (1995), 690–695.

[80] C. Harwood, P. Spink, T. Surentheran, I. Leigh, E.-M. de Villiers, J. McGregor, C. Proby and J. Breuer, Degenerate and nested PCR: A highly sensitive and specific method for detection of human papillomavirus infection in cutaneous warts, *J Clin Microbiol* **37** (1999), 3545–3555.

[81] O. Forslund, A. Antonsson, P. Nordin, B. Stenquist and B. Hansson, A broad range of human papillomavirus types detected with a general PCR method suitable for analysis of cutaneous tumours and normal skin, *J Gen Virol* **80** (1999), 2437–2443.

[82] T. Meyer, R. Arndt, E. Christophers and E. Stockfleth, Frequency and spectrum of HPV types detected in cutaneous squamous-cell carcinomas depend on the HPV detection system: A comparison of four PCR assays, *Dermatology* **201** (2000), 204–211.

[83] D. O'Connor, E. Kay, M. Leader, G. Murphy, G. Atkins, and M. Mabruk, Altered *p53* expression in benign and malignant skin lesions from renal transplant recipients and immunocompetent patients with skin cancer: Correlation with human papillomaviruses? *Diagn Mol Pathol* **10** (2001), 190–199.

[84] A. Brink, B. Lloveras, I. Nindl, D. Heideman, D. Kramer, R. Pol, M. Fuente, C. Meijer and P. Snijders, Development of a general-primer-PCR-reverse-line-blotting system for detection of beta and gamma cutaneous human papillomaviruses, *J Clin Microbiol* **43** (2005), 5581–5587.

[85] M. de Koning, W. Quint, L. Struijk, B. Kleter, P. Wanningen, L. van Doorn, S. Weissenborn, M. Feltkamp and J. Ter Schegget, Evaluation of a novel highly sensitive, broad-spectrum PCR-reverse hybridization assay for detection and identification of beta-papillomavirus DNA, *J Clin Microbiol* **44** (2006), 1792–1800.

[86] G. Astori, D. Lavergne, C. Benton, B. Hockmayr, K. Egawa, C. Garbe and E. de Villiers, Human papillomaviruses are commonly found in normal skin of immunocompetent hosts, *J Invest Dermatol* **110** (1998), 752–755.

[87] C. Harwood, T. Surentheran, J. McGregor, P. Spink, I. Leigh, J. Breuer and C. Proby, Human papillomavirus infection and non-melanoma skin cancer in immunosuppressed and immunocompetent individuals, *J Med Virol* **61** (2000), 289–297.

[88] T. Meyer, R. Arndt, E. Christophers, I. Nindl and E. Stockfleth, Importance of human papillomaviruses for the development of skin cancer, *Cancer Detect Prev* **25** (2001), 533–547.

[89] O. Forslund, H. Ly, C. Reid and G. Higgins, A broad spectrum of human papillomavirus types is present in the skin of Australian patients with non-melanoma skin cancers and solar keratosis, *Br J Dermatol* **149** (2003), 64–73.

[90] H. Pfister, P. Fuchs, S. Majewski, S. Jablonska, I. Pniewska and M. Malejczyk, High prevalence of Epidermodysplasia verruciformis-associated human papillomavirus DNA in actinic keratoses of the immunocompetent population, *Arch Dermatol Res* **295** (2003), 273–279.

[91] U. Wieland, A. Ritzkowsky, M. Stoltidis, S. Weissenborn, S. Stark, M. Ploner, S. Majewski, S. Jablonska, H. Pfister and P. Fuchs, Papillomavirus DNA in basal cell carcinomas of immunocompetent patients: an accidental association? *J Invest Dermatol* **115** (2000), 124–128.

[92] D. O'Connor, E. Kay, M. Leader, G. Atkins, G. Murphy and M. Mabruk, *p53* codon 72 polymorphism and human papillomavirus associated skin cancer, *J Clin Pathol* **54** (2001), 539–542.

[93] O. Forslund, A. Antonsson, G. Higgins, H. Ly, H. Delius, A. Hunziker and E.-M. de Villiers, Nucleotide sequence and phylogenetic classification of candidate human papilloma virus type 92, *Virology* **312** (2003), 255–260.

[94] I. Nindl, A. Köhler, T. Meyer, T. Forschner, C. Meijer, P. Snijders, W. Sterry and E. Stockfleth, Detection of human papillomavirus DNA in primary squamous cell carcinoma and metastases, *Br J Dermatol* **154** (2006), 797–799.

[95] S. Weissenborn, I. Nindl, K. Purdie, C. Harwood, C. Proby, J. Breuer, S. Majewski, H. Pfister and U. Wieland, Human papillomavirus-DNA loads in actinic keratoses exceed those in non-melanoma skin cancers, *J Invest Dermatol* **125** (2005), 93–97.

[96] L. Struijk, J. Bouwes Bavinck, P. Wanningen, E. van der Meijden, R. Westendorp, J. Ter Schegget and M. Feltkamp, Presence of human papillomavirus DNA in plucked eyebrow hairs is associated with a history of cutaneous squamous cell carcinoma, *J Invest Dermatol* **121** (2003), 1531–1535.

[97] J. Bouwes Bavinck, S. Stark, A. Petridis, M. Marugg, J. Ter Schegget, R. Westendorp, P. Fuchs, B. Vermeer and H. Pfister, The presence of antibodies against virus-like particles of Epidermodysplasia verruciformis-associated human-papillomavirus type 8 in patients with actinic keratoses, *Br J Dermatol* **142** (2000), 103–109.

[98] C. Masini, P. Fuchs, F. Gabrielli, S. Stark, F. Sera, M. Ploner, C. Melchi, G. Primavera, G. Pirchio, O. Picconi, P. Petasecca, M. Cattaruzza, H. Pfister and D. Abeni, Evidence for the association of human papillomavirus infection and cutaneous squamous cell carcinoma in immunocompetent individuals, *Arch Dermatol* **139** (2003), 890–894.

[99] S. Stark, A. Petridis, S. Ghim, A. Jenson, J. Bouwes Bavinck, G. Gross, E. Stockfleth, P. Fuchs and H. Pfister, Prevalence of antibodies against virus-like particles of Epidermodysplasia verruciformis-associated HPV8 in patients at risk of skin cancer, *J Invest Dermatol* **111** (1998), 696–701.

[100] M. Feltkamp, R. Broer, F. di Summa, L. Struijk, Meijden van der, B. Verlaan, R. Westendorp, J. Ter Schegget, W. Spaan and J. Bouwes Bavinck, Seroreactivity to Epidermodysplasia verruciformis-related human papillomavirus types is associated with nonmelanoma skin cancer, *Cancer Res* **63** (2003), 2695–2700.

[101] M. Karagas, H. Nelson, P. Sehr, T. Waterboer, T. Stukel, A. Andrew, A. Green, J. Bouwes Bavinck, A. Perry, S. Spencer, J. Rees, L. Mott and M. Pawlita, Human papillomavirus infection and incidence of squamous cell and basal cell carcinomas of the skin, *J Natl Cancer Inst* **98** (2006), 389–395.

[102] J. Boyle, R. Mackie, J. Briggs, B. Junor and T. Aitchison, Cancer, warts, and sunshine in renal transplant patients. A case-control study, *Lancet* **1** (1984), 702–705.

[103] J. Bouwes Bavinck, B. Vermeer, F. Van der Woude, J. Vandenbroucke, G. Schreuder, J. Thorogood, G. Persijn and F. Claas, Relation between skin cancer and HLA antigens in renal-transplant recipients, *N Engl J Med* **325** (1991), 843–848.

[104] S. Birkeland, H. Storm, L. Lamm, L. Barlow, I. Blohme, B. Forsberg, B. Eklund, O. Fjeldborg, M. Friedberg and L.

Frodin, Cancer risk after renal transplantation in the Nordic countries, 1964–1986, *Int J Cancer* **60** (1995), 183–189.

[105] M. Hartevelt, J. Bouwes Bavinck, A. Kootte, B. Vermeer and J. Vandenbroucke, Incidence of skin cancer after renal transplantation in The Netherlands, *Transplantation* **49** (1990), 506–509.

[106] J. Bouwes Bavinck, D. Hardie, A. Green, S. Cutmore, A. MacNaught, B. O'Sullivan, V. Siskind, F. Van der Woude and I. Hardie, The risk of skin cancer in renal transplant recipients in Queensland, Australia. A follow-up study, *Transplantation* **61** (1996), 715–721.

[107] K. Blessing, K. McLaren, E. Benton, B. Barr, M. Bunney, I. Smith and G. Beveridge, Histopathology of skin lesions in renal allograft recipients-an assessment of viral features and dysplasia, *Histopathology* **14** (1989), 129–139.

[108] S. Euvrard, Y. Chardonnet, C. Pouteil Noble, J. Kanitakis, M. Chignol, J. Thivolet and J. Touraine, Association of skin malignancies with various and multiple carcinogenic and noncarcinogenic human papillomaviruses in renal transplant recipients, *Cancer* **72** (1993), 2198–2206.

[109] V. Shamanin, M. Glover, C. Rausch, C. Proby, I. Leigh, H. zur Hausen and E.-M. de Villiers, Specific types of human papillomavirus found in benign proliferations and carcinomas of the skin in immunosuppressed patients, *Cancer Res* **54** (1994), 4610–4613.

[110] L. de Jong-Tieben, R. Berkhout, H. Smits, J. Bouwes Bavinck, B. Vermeer, F. Van der Woude and J. Ter Schegget, High frequency of detection of Epidermodysplasia verruciformis-associated human papillomavirus DNA in biopsies from malignant and premalignant skin lesions from renal transplant recipients, *J Invest Dermatol* **105** (1995), 367–371.

[111] E.-M. de Villiers, D. Lavergne, K. McLaren and E. Benton, Prevailing papillomavirus types in non-melanoma carcinomas of the skin in renal allograft recipients, *Int J Cancer* **73** (1997), 356–361.

[112] R. Berkhout, J. Bouwes Bavinck and J. Ter Schegget, Persistence of human papillomavirus DNA in benign and (pre)malignant skin lesions from renal transplant recipients, *J Clin Microbiol* **38** (2000), 2087–2096.

[113] L. de Jong-Tieben, R. Berkhout, J. Ter Schegget, B. Vermeer, J. de Fijter, J. Bruijn, R. Westendorp and J. Bouwes Bavinck, The prevalence of human papillomavirus DNA in benign keratotic skin lesions of renal transplant recipients with and without a history of skin cancer is equally high: A clinical study to assess risk factors for keratotic skin lesions and skin cancer, *Transplantation* **69** (2000), 44–49.

[114] K. Purdie, T. Surentheran, J. Sterling, L. Bell, J. McGregor, C. Proby, C. Harwood and J. Breuer, Human papillomavirus gene expression in cutaneous squamous cell carcinomas from immunosuppressed and immunocompetent individuals, *J Invest Dermatol* **125** (2005), 98–107.

[115] C. Dang, A. Köhler, T. Forschner, P. Sehr, K. Michael, M. Pawlita, E. Stockfleth and I. Nindl, E6/E7 expression of human papillomavirus types in cutaneous squamous cell dysplasia and carcinoma in immunosuppressed organ transplant recipients, *Br J Dermatol* **155** (2006), 129–136.

[116] T. Iftner, S. Bierfelder, Z. Csapo and H. Pfister, Involvement of human papillomavirus type 8 genes E6 and E7 in transformation and replication, *J Virol* **62** (1988), 3655–3661.

[117] T. Kiyono, K. Nagashima and M. Ishibashi, The primary structure of major viral RNA in a rat cell line transfected with type 47 human papillomavirus DNA and the transforming activity of its cDNA and E6 gene, *Virology* **173** (1989), 551–565.

[118] T. Kiyono, A. Hiraiwa and M. Ishibashi, Differences in transforming activity and coded amino acid sequence among E6 genes of several papillomaviruses associated with Epidermodysplasia verruciformis, *Virology* **186** (1992), 628–639.

[119] A. Hiraiwa, T. Kiyono, K. Segawa, K. Utsumi, M. Ohashi and M. Ishibashi, Comparative study on E6 and E7 genes of some cutaneous and genital papillomaviruses of human origin for their ability to transform 3Y1 cells, *Virology* **192** (1993), 102–111.

[120] T. Yamashita, K. Segawa, Y. Fujinaga, T. Nishikawa and K. Fujinaga, Biological and biochemical activity of E7 genes of the cutaneous human papillomavirus type 5 and 8, *Oncogene* **8** (1993), 2433–2441.

[121] A. Schmitt, J. Harry, B. Rapp, F. Wettstein and T. Iftner, Comparison of the properties of the E6 and E7 genes of low- and high-risk cutaneous papillomaviruses reveals strongly transforming and high *Rb*-binding activity for the E7 protein of the low-risk human papillomavirus type 1, *J Virol* **68** (1994), 7051–7059.

[122] S. Caldeira, I. Zehbe, R. Accardi, I. Malanchi, W. Dong, M. Giarre, E.-M. de Villiers, R. Filotico, P. Boukamp and M. Tommasino, The E6 and E7 proteins of the cutaneous human papillomavirus type 38 display transforming properties, *J Virol* **77** (2003), 2195–2206.

[123] K. Purdie, J. Pennington, C. Proby, S. Khalaf, E.-M. de Villiers, I. Leigh and A. Storey, The promoter of a novel human papillomavirus (HPV77) associated with skin cancer displays UV responsiveness, which is mediated through a consensus *p53* binding sequence, *EMBO J* **18** (1999), 5359–5369.

[124] E. de Villiers, A. Ruhland and P. Sekaric, Human papillomaviruses in non-melanoma skin cancer, *Semin Cancer Biol* **9** (1999), 413–422.

[125] A. Ruhland and E.-M. de Villiers, Opposite regulation of the HPV 20-URR and HPV 27-URR promoters by ultraviolet irradiation and cytokines, *Int J Cancer* **91** (2001), 828–834.

[126] S. Jackson and A. Storey, E6 proteins from diverse cutaneous HPV types inhibit apoptosis in response to UV damage, *Oncogene* **19** (2000), 592–598.

[127] S. Jackson, C. Harwood, M. Thomas, L. Banks and A. Storey, Role of *Bak* in UV-induced apoptosis in skin cancer and abrogation by HPV E6 proteins, *Genes Dev* **14** (2000), 3065–3073.

[128] T. Iftner, M. Elbel, B. Schopp, T. Hiller, J. Loizou, K. Caldecott and F. Stubenrauch, Interference of papillomavirus E6 protein with single-strand break repair by interaction with XRCC1, *EMBO J* **21** (2002), 4741–4748.

[129] S. Giampieri and A. Storey, Repair of UV-induced thymine dimers is compromised in cells expressing the E6 protein from human papillomaviruses types 5 and 18, *Br J Cancer* **90** (2004), 2203–2209.

[130] S. Giampieri, R. Garcia-Escudero, J. Green and A. Storey, Human papillomavirus type 77 E6 protein selectively inhibits *p53*-dependent transcription of proapoptotic genes following UV-B irradiation, *Oncogene* **23** (2004), 5864–5870.

[131] L. Chow and T. Broker, *In vitro* experimental systems for HPV: Epithelial raft cultures for investigations of viral reproduction and pathogenesis and for genetic analyses of viral proteins and regulatory sequences, *Clin Dermatol* **15** (1997), 217–227.

[132] I. Boxman, L. Mulder, F. Noya, V de Waard, S. Gibbs, T. Broker, F. ten Kate, L. Chow and J. Ter Schegget, Trans-

duction of the E6 and E7 genes of Epidermodysplasia-verruciformis-associated human papillomaviruses alters human keratinocyte growth and differentiation in organotypic cultures, *J Invest Dermatol* **117** (2001), 1397–1404.
[133] B. Akgül, R. Garcia-Escudero, L. Ghali, H. Pfister, P. Fuchs, H. Navsaria and A. Storey, The E7 protein of cutaneous human papillomavirus type 8 causes invasion of human keratinocytes into the dermis in organotypic cultures of skin, *Cancer Res* **65** (2005), 2216–2223.
[134] M. Campo, M. Moar, W. Jarrett and H. Laird, A new papillomavirus associated with alimentary cancer in cattle, *Nature* **286** (1980), 180–182.
[135] M. Campo, M. Moar, M. Sartirana, I. Kennedy and W. Jarrett, The presence of bovine papillomavirus type 4 DNA is not required for the progression to, or the maintenance of, the malignant state in cancers of the alimentary canal in cattle, *EMBO J* **4** (1985), 1819–1825.
[136] M. Campo, B. O'Neil, R. Barron and W. Jarrett, Experimental reproduction of the papilloma-carcinoma complex of the alimentary canal in cattle, *Carcinogenesis* **15** (1994), 1597–1601.
[137] M. Jackson, M. Campo and J. Gaukroger, Cooperation between papillomavirus and chemical cofactors in oncogenesis, *Crit Rev Oncog* **4** (1993), 277–291.
[138] H. Pfister, B. Fink and C. Thomas, Extrachromosomal bovine papillomavirus type 1 DNA in hamster fibromas and fibrosarcomas, *Virology* **115** (1981), 414–418.
[139] N. Otten, C. von Tscharner, S. Lazary, D. Antczak and H. Gerber, DNA of bovine papillomavirus type 1 and 2 in equine sarcoids: PCR detection and direct sequencing, *Arch Virol* **132** (1993), 121–131.
[140] G. Chambers, V. Ellsmore, P. O'Brien, S. Reid, S. Love, M. Campo and L. Nasir, Association of bovine papillomavirus with the equine sarcoid, *J Gen Virol* **84** (2003), 1055–1062.
[141] L. Bogaert, A. Martens, C. De Baere and F. Gasthuys, Detection of bovine papillomavirus DNA on the normal skin and in the habitual surroundings of horses with and without equine sarcoids, *Res Vet Sci* **79** (2005), 253–258.
[142] H. Bernard, I. Calleja-Macias and S. Dunn, Genome variation of human papillomavirus types: phylogenetic and medical implications, *Int J Cancer* **118** (2006), 1071–1076.
[143] F. Wettstein, M. Barbosa and M. Nasseri, Identification of the major cottontail rabbit papillomavirus late RNA cap site and mapping and quantitation of an E2 and minor E6 coding mRNA in papillomas and carcinomas, *Virology* **159** (1987), 321–328.
[144] S. Watts, R. Ostrow, W. Phelps, J. Prince and A. Faras, Free cottontail rabbit papillomavirus DNA persists in warts and carcinomas of infected rabbits and in cells in culture transformed with virus or viral DNA, *Virology* **125** (1983), 127–138.
[145] J. Brandsma, Z. Yang, S. Barthold and E. Johnson, Use of a rapid, efficient inoculation method to induce papillomas by cottontail rabbit papillomavirus DNA shows that the E7 gene is required, *Proc Natl Acad Sci USA* **88** (1991), 4816–4820.
[146] S. Jeckel, E. Huber, F. Stubenrauch and T. Iftner, A transactivator function of cottontail rabbit papillomavirus E2 is essential for tumor induction in rabbits, *J Virol* **76** (2002), 11209–11215.
[147] E. Amtmann, M. Volm and K. Wayss, Tumour induction in the rodent *Mastomys natalensis* by activation of endogenous papilloma virus genomes, *Nature* **308** (1984), 291–292.
[148] H. Müller and L. Gissmann, *Mastomys natalensis* papilloma virus (MnPV), the causative agent of epithelial proliferations: characterization of the virus particle, *J Gen Virol* **41** (1978), 315–323.
[149] R. Rudolph, H. Müller, M. Reinacher and W. Thiel, Morphology of experimentally induced so-called keratoacanthomas and squamous cell carcinomas in 2 inbred-lines of *Mastomys natalensis*, *J Comp Pathol* **91** (1981), 123–134.
[150] C. Tan, R. Tachezy, M. Van Ranst, S. Chan, H. Bernard and R. Burk, The *Mastomys natalensis* papillomavirus: Nucleotide sequence, genome organization, and phylogenetic relationship of a rodent papillomavirus involved in tumorigenesis of cutaneous epithelia, *Virology* **198** (1994), 534–541.
[151] E. Amtmann, M. Volm and K. Wayss, The *Mastomys natalensis* papillomavirus, in: *The Papoviridae,* N. Salzmann and P. Howley, eds, Plenum Publishing Corporation, 1987, pp. 187–198.
[152] J. Nafz, A. Köhler, M. Ohnesorge, I. Nindl, E. Stockfleth and F. Rösl, Presence and distribution of *Mastomys natalensis* papillomavirus in its natural host, submitted (2007).
[153] J. Tinsley, C. Fisher and P. Searle, Abnormalities of epidermal differentiation associated with expression of the human papillomavirus type 1 early region in transgenic mice, *J Gen Virol* **73** (1992), 1251–1260.
[154] I. Schaper, G. Marcuzzi, S. Weissenborn, H. Kasper, V. Dries, N. Smyth, P. Fuchs and H. Pfister, Development of skin tumors in mice transgenic for early genes of human papillomavirus type 8, *Cancer Res* **65** (2005), 1394–1400.
[155] W. Dong, U. Kloz, R. Accardi, S. Caldeira, W. Tong, Z. Wang, L. Jansen, M. Durst, B. Sylla, L. Gissmann and M. Tommasino, Skin hyperproliferation and susceptibility to chemical carcinogenesis in transgenic mice expressing E6 and E7 of human papillomavirus type 38, *J Virol* **79** (2005), 14899–14908.

Disease Markers 23 (2007) 261–272
IOS Press

HPV infection in men

Joel M. Palefsky*
Department of Medicine, University of California, San Francisco, CA 94143, USA

Abstract. While much is known about the natural history of cervical human papillomavirus (HPV) infection and its consequences, including cervical intraepithelial neoplasia and cervical cancer, relatively little is known about the natural history of anogenital HPV infection and diseases in men. In part this reflects difficulties in penile sampling and visual assessment of penile lesions. Anal HPV infection and disease also remain poorly understood. Although HPV is transmitted sexually and infects the genitals of both sexes, the cervix remains biologically more vulnerable to malignant transformation than does the penis or anus in men. An understanding of male HPV infection is therefore important in terms of reducing transmission of HPV to women and improving women's health. However, it is also important due to the burden of disease in men, who may develop both penile and anal cancer, particularly among HIV-positive men who have sex with men. Improved sampling techniques of the male genitalia and cohort studies in progress should provide important information on the natural history of anogenital HPV infection and disease in men, including risk factors for HPV acquisition and transmission. The impact of HPV vaccination in women on male anogenital HPV infection will also need to be assessed.

Keywords: Penile HPV infection, anal HPV infection, penile intraepithelial neoplasia, anal intraepithelial neoplasia, penile cancer, anal cancer, condyloma, HIV

1. Introduction

The most common cause of HPV-associated mortality is cancer of the cervix, and most of the attention of clinicians and researchers has appropriately been directed toward this disease and its precursors. However, HPV infection of men is of great importance as well given that sexual transmission is the primary mode of spread to women. An understanding of anogenital HPV infection in men is therefore critical to reducing the risk of HPV transmission to women. Moreover, similar to women, men suffer the consequences of anogenital HPV infection in the form of anogenital condyloma, intraepithelial neoplasia and cancer. Recognition and treatment of anogenital HPV-associated lesions in men is critical to reducing the burden of disease in men and treatment of penile lesions has the potential, albeit as yet unproven, to reduce the risk of HPV transmission to women.

The recent success of HPV vaccination to prevent initial HPV infection in women begs the question as to whether men should be vaccinated. Consistent with the above, the benefits could include reduced HPV transmission to women and increase in "herd immunity", as well as reduced penile and anal cancer incidence. Studies have not yet been published documenting efficacy of the vaccine in men, but these are in progress. Even in the absence of vaccinating men, however, a high penetrance of the vaccine in women would likely affect the prevalence and incidence of male anogenital disease in the future, and this will need to be the subject of further study.

2. HPV infection and disease of the penis

2.1. *Epidemiology of penile HPV infection*

Understanding the epidemiology of penile HPV infection and HPV-associated diseases has been challenging for a number of reasons. Unlike sampling a moist

*Address for correspondence: Joel Palefsky, M.D., 505 Parnassus Ave Room M1203, Box 0126, Department of Medicine, University of California, San Francisco, San Francisco, CA 94143, USA. Tel.: +1 415 476 1574; Fax: +1 415 476 0986; E-mail: joel.palefsky@ucsf.edu.

ISSN 0278-0240/07/$17.00

surface such as the cervix, reliable sampling of the dry, keratinized surface of the penis to obtain adequate numbers of cells has been difficult and poorly reproducible. Recently however, several investigators have been using better methods to collect cells, including the use of sandpaper or emery paper to loosen cells, resulting in better yields. This has improved our understanding of the prevalence and risk factors for penile HPV infection.

In one study of penile swabs obtained from 436 men attending a sexually transmitted disease clinic, the prevalence of HPV was 28.2%. Oncogenic HPV types were found in 12.0% of participants, nononcogenic types were found in 14.8% of participants, multiple types were found in 6.1% of participants, and unknown types were found in 5.9% of participants [1]. In a study of male partners of women positive for HPV using the non-amplification-based Hybrid Capture™ II (HCII) method, HC II analysis of penile brushings showed that 24% were positive in the glans, 44% in the prepuce internal surface, 30% in the distal urethra, 24% in the prepuce external surface, 12% in the scrotum and 8% in the anus [2].

In a study of 779 Mexican men requesting a vasectomy, exfoliated cells were obtained from the scrotum, the shaft of the penis and the top of the penis including the coronal sulcus, the glans and the opening of the meatus. Using PCR, the prevalence of any type of HPV was somewhat lower than in the 8.7% and the most commonly found HPV types were HPV59, 51, 6, 16 and 58. HPV positivity was highest among men below age 25 (13.6%), and lowest among men aged 40 years or older (6.0%). Lifetime number of sexual partners was associated with HPV positivity. Condom use with both regular and sex-worker partners, and circumcision were inversely associated with HPV positivity [3]. Likewise, circumcision in another study was associated with reduced risk for detection of both oncogenic and non-oncogenic HPV types [4].

Even less is known about penile HPV infection in HIV-positive men. The risk of penile cancer is elevated in HIV-positive men compared with the general population [5] but little is known about the natural history of penile disease in this population. A high prevalence of high-risk HPV types was present in the anus, penis and mouth (78, 36 and 30%, respectively) and was detected in a cohort of HIV-infected men without evidence of pathology in these areas [6].

2.2. *Diagnosis of HPV-associated lesions of the penis*

In addition to the problems associated with penile sampling, methods to diagnose penile lesions have been problematic. There is no standardized method to do so, but it is commonly accepted that magnification with application of acetic acid, similar to its use in the cervix, will result in improved diagnostic sensitivity, albeit at the expense of specificity [7,8]. Penile HPV infections may be latent, or may lead to subclinical or clinical disease. Latent infection is defined as the presence of HPV DNA within the tissue in the absence of any changes seen on visualization under magnification or histologic changes. A lesion, clinical or subclinical, is defined as the clinically visible and histologic modifications occurring due to HPV infection. Subclinical lesions are defined as those lesions visible only after application of acetic acid. Clinical lesions are defined as those visible to the naked eye without acetic acid.

The clinical examination should be carried out carefully on the entire anogenital region, including the penis, scrotum and perianal region with the help of a strong light and a magnifying lens (at least 4-fold). Subclinical lesions may be visualized after application of 5% acetic acid. While a colposcope may provide light and magnification, most acetowhite reactions will be detected by a hand-held magnifying lens.

The biological basis of acetowhitening is unknown. In lesions of external genitalia, areas with surface nuclear activity (parakeratosis) and/or increased cellular density will react. Acetic acid may be applied with a cotton ball mounted on a sponge-holding forceps, a scopette or by self-application of a gauze soaked in acetic acid. Acetic acid should be applied generously and the clinician must wait two to three minutes before beginning the examination. While recognized as a valuable aid to the diagnosis of penile disease, routine use of these techniques to examine at-risk men has not been advocated by professional organizations. In part, this reflects the absence of standardized training in this technique, limited specificity of acetowhitening and its unknown negative and positive predictive value in populations at different level of risk. Paradoxically, the areas of the penis that turn acetowhite the fastest are most often those with non-specific conditions such as inflammation and abrasion, and there is concern for over-treatment of non-HPV-related lesions.

Accurate identification may lead to better diagnosis of lesions and improved treatment, but the effect of treatment of penile disease has not been proven to reduce mortality among either men or women. Treatment of high-grade penile intraepithelial neoplasia may well reduce the incidence of penile cancer but this has not yet been demonstrated. Although condom use in male partners of women with CIN has been shown to increase regression of CIN [9], there are no data showing that treatment of HPV-associated disease reduces the risk of disease or infection in their female partners. For these reasons, routine screening of men with magnification and acetic acid has never become standard of practice.

With these caveats in mind, examination of men with these techniques may be useful under certain circumstances. These include identification of small, clinically inapparent or subclinical lesions in men who present to the clinician with genital warts. Men who present with symptoms such as itching or pain, or signs such as erythema must also be examined to rule out cancer or high-grade penile intraepithelial neoplasia.

Once identified, a penile biopsy may be needed to exclude the existence of penile cancer or penile intraepithelial neoplasia, or to confirm the diagnosis of HPV-associated lesions. Anesthesia, typically in the form of subcutaneous lidocaine is applied. A punch biopsy such as a Kevorkian, a 4 mm disposable Keyes punch, forceps and scissors, or a knife may be used. To use the Keyes punch, the clinician maintains the pressure and rotation until subcutaneous tissue is reached. The depth of the biopsy also depends on epidermal thickness. When the dermis is entered, there is a sensation of decreased resistance. The dermal tissue is cut with a small scalpel or scissors and the elliptical defect can be cauterized with Monsell's solution (ferric subsulfate) or sutured. Forceps can also be used to lift anesthetized skin or mucosa, and sharp scissors used to snip the biopsy.

2.3. Histopathology of penile HPV-associated lesions

Condyloma acuminata, commonly known as "warts", are exophytic, white grayish protuberances on keratinized skin, with a lobulated or irregular surface. Papillae may be prominent with finger-like projections that exhibit punctate and/or loop-like patterns visible with magnification unless the lesion is heavily keratinized. Some warts will be highly keratinized, thus appearing white. Their number varies from one to 50 or more lesions, and the sizes vary from 0.2 to 1.0 cm, but they may become confluent involving large areas of genitalia. In uncircumcised men warts are most prevalent on the inner aspect of the prepuce and at the frenulum and coronal sulcus. In circumcised men the shaft is often involved. Warts may be present on the meatal lips of the urinary meatus or the distal area of the urethra up to 10–28% of men.

Condylomata acuminata must be distinguished from other papillomatous lesions in this area. On the penis, a variant of normal known as pearly penile papules may simulate warts [10]. These are hypertrphic papillae that form rows of discrete acuminate structures distributed circumferentially around the coronal sulcus. Reactive hyperplasia may also be associated with papillary structures in circumcised men. In these structures, the surface is the same as that of the surrounding skin and no vascular structures are detected. Condylomata lata of secondary syphilis should be distinguished from condylomata acuminata. Some warts may be pigmented, and in such cases may be difficult to distinguish from pigmented papules of high-grade penile intraepithelial neoplasia.

HPV types 6 and 11 are detected in 70–95% of condylomata acuminata, independent of the location, extent and duration of lesions. Oncogenic HPVs are not usually detected in typical warts in immunocompetent individuals.

HPV-associated lesions may also take the form of non-pigmented papules. These lesions have the color of normal skin or are occasionally brown and have a round or dome-shaped, slightly hyperkeratotic or smooth surface [11,12]. HPV-associated papules can be easily distinguished from the umbilicated pink-gray papules of molluscum contagiosum. Sebaceous glands of the prepuce should not be mistaken for HPV-associated papules. These are grey-yellow in color and magnification permits the identification of their structure [12].

Examination of the penis with acetic acid and magnification may also reveal subclinical macules consisting of smooth, flat, well demarcated acetowhite areas of normal epithelium with obvious capillary loops. They are usually found on mucosal surfaces such as the prepuce and glans and occasionally on the keratinized skin of the external genitalia. The differential diagnosis includes balanitis in which the acetowhitening is more diffuse, avascular and irregular; and yeast infection, in which multiple isolated acetowhite areas are often detected. In yeast infection capillaries are evident diffusely and are not restricted to the acetowhite areas. Other causes of acetowhitening includes traumatic microabrasions. While colposcopic examination often permits the clinician to distinguish subclinical HPV-associated lesions from infection or inflammation, it may not always be possible to do so, and local anti-inflammatory treatment may be given to men prior to further work-up.

The term "Bowenoid papulosis" is used to describe papular or maculopapular lesions that show histolog-

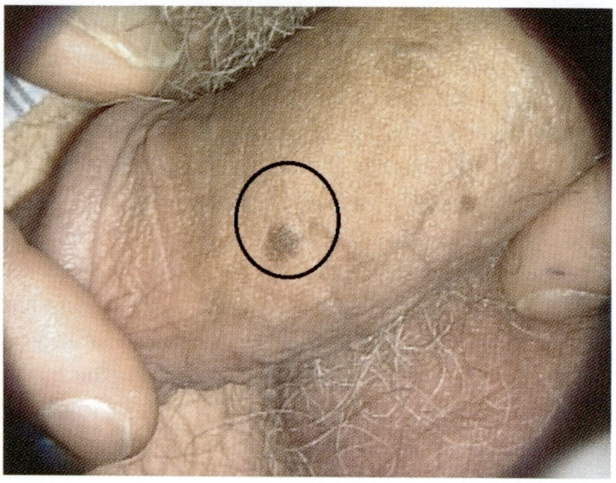

Fig. 1. Lesion with biopsy-confirmed penile intraepithelial neoplasia II-III. The lesion, shown in the black circle is flat and hyperpigmented.

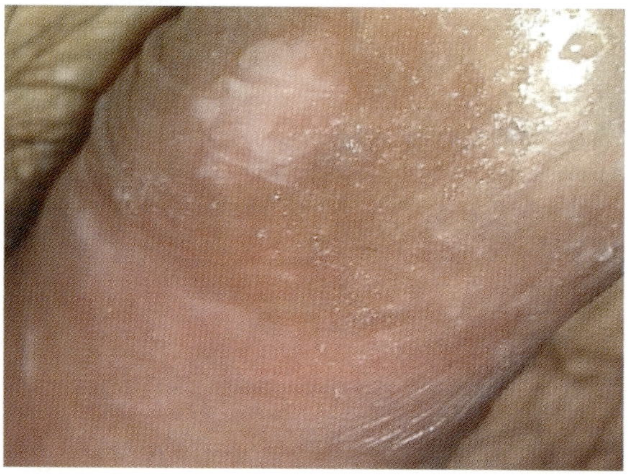

Fig. 2. Lesion with biopsy-confirmed penile intraepithelial neoplasia II. This lesion is from a different patient from that of Fig. 1, and shows a flat, well circumscribed, acetowhite lesion after application of 5% acetic acid.

ical features of high-grade intraepithelial neoplasia or carcinoma in situ [13,14]. These papules are usually hyperpigmented and are often flat despite the term "papulosis". They may be red or slightly brown with a smooth, glistening surface (Figs 1 and 2). They range in number from single lesions to about 30 and may coalesce to form plaques and they may exhibit strong acetowhitening. The differential diagnosis of Bowenoid papules includes pigmented warts, lentigo, naevi and melanoma, seborrheic warts, angiokeratomas, lichen planus and localized psoriatic lesions.

The histology of penile intraepithelial neoplasia in young adults shows features typical of other sites in the male and female genital tracts, including epithelial proliferation, hyperkeratosis and parakeratosis [15]. The cell nuclei are hyperchromatic, clumped and show loss of organization, maturation and cohesion. Mitotic figures are generally numerous and abnormal forms are often present. Potentially oncogenic HPV types are usually associated with these lesions and the most frequently identified type is HPV16 [14–16].

The prevalence of penile intraepithelial neoplasia is much lower in studies from the United States than in Europe. This may be linked to higher rates of circumcision, since circumcised male partners of women with CIN have a lower rate of penile intraepithelial neoplasia than uncircumcised men [17]. Circumcised men also have a lower prevalence of subclinical disease since many of these are often localized to the prepuce.

The natural history of high-grade penile intraepithelial neoplasia in young adults is not well known since natural history studies have not been done. It is likely however that conversion to invasive penile cancer is a rare event. In older patients, high-grade penile intraepithelial neoplasia mostly consists of Bowen's disease and Erythroplasia of Queyrat. These are believed to be precursor lesions of basaloid and warty carcinomas of the penis [18]. Consistent with the high prevalence of HPV in these lesions, their associated cancers have a high prevalence of HPV (Table 1). Precursors of predominantly HPV-negative keratinizing and verrucous penile carcinomas are not established.

Clinically, high-grade penile intraepithelial neoplasia in patients older than 50 years may be slightly elevated, plaque-like (Bowen's disease) or totally flat (Erythroplasia of Queyrat). Erythroplastic lesions appear as bright, velvet-red areas while the leucoplastic form appears as a white plaque, with a smooth or verrucous surface. Localized at first, these lesions may extend to large areas of external genitalia, including the perineum and perianal areas. These lesions may persist for long time and the risk of progression to cancer, although not precisely known, is higher than in penile intraepithelial neoplasia of young adults. The differential diagnosis includes lichen sclerosus, lichen simplex and psoriasis. Erosive or ulcerated areas and atypical vessels within the lesions are suggestive of invasion. Penile intraepithelial neoplasia in older patients is associated with the same HPV types found in intraepithelial neoplasia in younger patients [11].

Penile cancer is an uncommon cancer, but its incidence varies widely in different countries [19]. It is a rare cancer in North America, where circumcision is more common than in other regions of the world. Similar to vulvar cancer there may be two separate pathways to development of penile cancer. As described

Table 1
Prevalence of HPV DNA using PCR in selected penile cancer case series (⩾5 cases)

Reference	Study area	Detection method	Number of cases	Overall HPV positivity (%)
Rubin 2001 [69]	USA and South America	PCR SPF 10 primers, LIPA genotyping	106 Keratinizing SCC 5 Warty SCC 15 basaloid SCC	34.9% 100% 80%
Levi 1998 [70]	South America	PCR GH20/PCO4 primers MY09/MY11 PCR primers with probing for	64 50	28% 56%
Carter 2001 [71]	USA	PCR L1 consensus primers and type specific primers for 6/18	33	81.8%
Cupp, 1995 [72]	USA	MY09/MY 11 L1 primers and E6 primers for 16/18	42 squamous cell cancers 13 carcinoma in situ	54.8% 92.3%
Picconi, 2000 [73]	Argentina	GP5/GP6 primers, typing by SCCP analysis	34	52.9%
Bezerra, 2001 [74]	Brazil	L1 primer PCR	11 warty carcinoma 60 SCC	45.5% 26.7%
Gregoire, 1995 [75]	USA and Paraguay	PCR with specific priming for HPV16 (E6), 18 (E6), 6/11 (E1), also E1 priming for wide range including 16, 18, 31, 33, 35, 52	45 SCC 12 basaloid 10 papillary 9 warty 6 verrucous 8 Mixed SCC, other 19 Mixed SCC, warty or basaloid	11.1% 75.0% 0% 22.2% 0% 0% 47.4%

above, basaloid and warty penile cancers are frequently HPV-associated (about 80–100%), in contrast to a smaller proportion of keratinizing and verrucous penile carcinomas (Table 1). Overall, about 50% of penile cancers contain HPV DNA. HPV16 is the most common HPV type detected in penile cancer. HPV31 or 33 were described only rarely. Giant condylomata acuminata, also known as Buschke-Lowenstein tumors, may precede the development of verrucous carcinomas in some cases and may contain HPV6 or 11.

2.4. Treatment of HPV-associated penile disease

The definitive diagnosis of HPV-related penile disease requires a biopsy, but this is usually unnecessary. Typical warts, papillomas and non-pigmented papules do not need to be biopsied. For subclinical lesions, in case of doubt, local anti-inflammatory treatment should be given in an effort to induce regression of non-specific acetowhite areas. Lesions with features suggesting intraepithelial neoplasia should be biopsied to confirm the diagnosis and to exclude the existence of invasive cancer. This is particularly true in patients older than 40, since the risk of progression to invasion of intraepithelial neoplasia is higher in this group.

There is general consensus about the need for treatment of clinically detectable warts and penile intraepithelial neoplasia. There is less consensus on the need for treatment of subclinical lesions. In choosing the treatment modality, factors to consider are differences in size, location, number and histology of the lesions [20]. Other factors to consider include whether the lesions are newly diagnosed or recurrent, and the patient's compliance and pain threshold. Small warts may be treated topically. Patient-applied therapies such as podophyllotoxin or imiquimod cream are useful first approaches. They have the advantage of allowing patients to treat themselves, but have the disadvantages of requiring several weeks or more for therapeutic responses. Patients must also be able to visualize the lesions to know where to apply the creams. Topical treatment with 80% trichloracetic acid (TCA) or liquid nitrogen are acceptable options but must be applied by the treating clinician. This may be preferable for lesions that are too small or inaccessible for self-treatment by the patient, and have the advantage of inducing a therapeutic response quickly. Use of TCA is preferable on non-keratinized mucosal lesions, since liquid nitrogen is painful at those locations. Liquid nitrogen is preferred by some clinicians for cutaneous and hyperkeratinized mucosal lesions. Both treatments often require multiple applications by clinicians, typically 1–2 weeks apart. Second-line therapies that can be used include interferon, 5 fluorouracil, electrocautery and laser surgery. Lesions persisting after local treatment should be considered for surgical or laser ablation.

Treatment of penile intraepithelial neoplasia should be performed after biopsies have excluded invasive penile cancer. The choice of ablative therapy will depend on the size and location of the lesions. A physician may remove it with laser vaporisation or electrosurgery. These lesions can also be treated with TCA and liquid nitrogen. Treatment with podophyllotoxin or imiquimod isn't currently recommended as these drugs have only been approved for treatment of genital warts.

As with all cancers, penile cancer is treated by stage, type, the patient's age and overall condition. For Stage I (localized cancer) the cure rate is high and may involve wide local excision. If the tumor begins in the glans and involves other tissues, treatment may involve partial penectomy and lymph node removal, external radiation therapy and microsurgery. In Stage II, cancer cells have spread to the glans and shaft of the penis, and surgery involving partial, total, or radical penectomy is usually the first approach, or radiation therapy followed by penectomy. Stage III involves cancer that has spread beyond the penis. In addition to penectomy, lymph node removal on both sides of the groin, radiation therapy and chemotherapy may be required. A variety of different chemotherapy drugs have been used in penile cancer in combination with radiation therapy. For stage IV, the cancer has metastasized to other parts of the body. Penectomy, wide local excision, and microsurgery may be used as well as chemotherapy and radiation therapy.

2.5. Relationship between penile HPV infection and HPV-associated disease in women

Since the penis is the presumed source of most HPV infection that is transmitted to women, there has been increasing interest in determining concordance of HPV types between sexual partners. Consistent with a relationship between penile and cervical HPV infection, male condom use has been shown to promote regression of human papillomavirus-associated penile lesions in male sexual partners of women with cervical intraepithelial neoplasia [9], and male circumcision is associated with a reduced risk of cervical cancer in their current female partners [21]. Consistent condom use has recently been shown to reduce the risk of transmission by about 70% [22].

In one study of women with CIN, penile lesions were seen in 68% of male partners, and most lesions were flat and subclinical. HPV was detected in 59% of the penile scrapings and contained mainly oncogenic HPV types [23]. However the degree of concordance of HPV types between sexual partners has varied considerably between different studies. In one study of husbands of women with invasive cervical carcinoma or cervical carcinoma in situ, 18% of the husbands of women with invasive cervical carcinoma, and 21% of the husbands of women with cervical carcinoma in situ were positive for penile HPV DNA, and concordance of HPV types was low between husband and wife [24]. In a more recent study, among couples in which both partners were HPV-positive, 57.8% of the men had the same HPV type as their partners [25]. In another study of male partners of women positive for HPV using the HCII method, using HCII on penile brushings, 32% were positive for one or more HPV types in the high-risk HPV group, 14% in the low-risk HPV group and 24% in both groups [2]. Using PCR in a study of university students in South Korea, HPV DNA was detected more frequently in female students (15.2%) than in male students (8.7%). Among those students who reported being sexually active, the prevalence of HPV was 38.8% in females and 10.6% in males [26]. In contrast, in a study of Mexican men attending vasectomy clinics, the prevalence of HPV in Mexican men was similar to that of Mexican women of the same age [3].

3. HPV infection and disease of the anus in men

3.1. Epidemiology of anal HPV infection and HPV-associated anal neoplasia

Anal HPV infection is remarkably common in men who have sex with men (MSM) and HIV-positive men regardless of sexual orientation [27]. HPV infection is most common in HIV-positive MSM [27,28]. Almost all HIV-positive MSM have anal HPV infection, frequently with multiple HPV types. HIV-positive heterosexual men also have a high prevalence of anal HPV infection [29], as do HIV-negative MSM [27].

Anal HPV infection is the most significant risk factor for the development of anal intraepithelial neoplasia (AIN), the precursor lesion to anal cancer. Consistent with their high prevalence of anal HPV infection, the prevalence of AIN in men is highest in HIV-positive MSM [30] followed by HIV-negative MSM [27,31] and HIV-positive heterosexual men [29]. The incidence of high-grade AIN is also high both HIV-positive and HIV-negative MSM [32–35]. Among HIV-positive MSM this has also been observed despite the introduction of highly active antiretroviral therapy (HAART) [36,37]. In HIV-positive men, anal HPV infection and lower

Table 2
Prevalence of HPV DNA using PCR in selected anal cancer case series (⩾5 cases)

Reference	Study area	Detection method	Number of cases	Overall HPV positivity (%)
Carter J 2001 [71]	USA	PCR L1 consensus primers	64	93.8%
Frisch, 1999 [76]	Denmark and Sweden	GP5+/GP6+	331	83.7% for HR group 4% for low-risk group
Daling, 2004 [43]	USA	MY09/MY11 PCR	119 men 81 SCC 6 Cloacogenic /basaloid 8 Adenocarcinoma 187 women 98 SCC 35 Cloacogenic /basaloid 12 Adenocarcinoma	92.6% 100% 25% 91.8% 97.1% 50.0%
Poletti, 1998 [77]	Switzerland	PCR with PU-1M primers for 16/18/31/33/52/58 and PU-31B primers for 6/11	33	39.4%
Frisch, 1997 [46]	Sweden and Denmark	GP5+/GP6+ primers	388	87.6%
Shroyer, 1995 [78]	USA	MY0/MY11 primers	11 basaloid cancer 16 non-basaloid cancers	90.9% 75.0%

CD4+ cell count are the main risk factors associated with prevalent and incident AIN [30]. In a study of AIN in HIV-negative MSM, risk factors included number of receptive anal sex partners and injection drug use, but HPV infection, and a higher number of HPV types detected were the strongest risk factors for AIN [31]. Similar risk factors were found in an earlier study [30].

Despite evidence that immunosuppression as measured by CD4+ level is linked to the development of AIN, the role of immunosuppression in the progression from high-grade AIN to invasive cancer is unclear. Unlike other HIV-related malignancies such as Kaposi's sarcoma and non-Hodgkin's lymphoma, there is no significant increase in anal cancer after an AIDS diagnosis [38]. Other factors such as host genomic mutations, rather than intrinsic immunosuppression, may be more important in progression to invasive cancer [39].

Like cervical cancer, anal cancer is strongly associated with HPV infection [40] (Table 2). While less common than cervical cancer, anal cancer is increasing in incidence in both women and men, from about 10 cases per million to 20 cases per million from 1973 to 2000 [41]. Some of this increase is attributable to a rising incidence among MSM. Before the HIV epidemic, it was estimated that the incidence of anal cancer among MSM was estimated to be as high as 37 per 100,000 person years, comparable to the incidence of invasive cervical cancer in women prior to the introduction of cervical cytology screening [42].

Similar to cervical cancer, HPV infection is one of the most important risk factors for anal cancer and HPV16 is the most common HPV type isolated in anal cancer [43]. Sexual activity was shown in early studies to be a risk factor for anal cancer [43–45]. In a Scandinavian study, independent risk factors for anal cancer in men included higher numbers of sexual partners and a history of other sexually transmitted infections [46]. Cigarette smoking was a risk factor for anal cancer in at least three studies [43,45,47].

Immunocompromise is another key risk factor, particularly HIV-associated immunocompromise. Data from matching cancer and AIDS registries show that the relative risk of invasive anal cancer was 37 in HIV-positive MSM compared with the general population [5], and the incidence of anal cancer among HIV-positive MSM is estimated to be double that of HIV-negative MSM. Consistent with the data on AIN and HAART, recent data also show that the incidence of anal cancer is continuing to increase in HIV-positive MSM since the introduction of HAART [48–50]. Other immunocompromised patients such as transplant recipients are also at increased risk of anal cancer [51–54].

3.2. Diagnosis of anal HPV-associated anal neoplasia

Given the similarity between anal and cervical cancer, and because cervical Pap testing has been successful in cervical cancer screening, Palefsky and others have proposed an anal cancer screening program that incorporates many of the principles of cervical cancer screening [55]. Anal cancer screening is recommended for populations at high risk of anal cancer. These include all HIV-positive women and men, MSM, women with a history of vulvar or cervical cancer and organ transplant recipients. Anal cytology testing every year to two years has been projected to be a cost-effective intervention to prevent anal cancer in HIV-positive [56] and HIV-negative MSM [57].

Abnormal anal cytology should be followed with measures to diagnose anal disease histologically and to exclude anal cancer. All patients at risk for anal cancer should also have a digital rectal examination to detect palpable lesions consistent with cancer. Lesions are typically visualized using high-resolution anoscopy (HRA). HRA is similar to cervical colposcopy and uses identical equipment (a powerful light source and binocular lenses). Using HRA, lesions that have contributed to abnormal cytologic findings can be visualized and biopsied. 3% acetic acid can be used to assist in the visualization of abnormal tissue, similar to the changes induced by acetic acid in the cervix and on the penis. HPV-infected lesions turn white relative to surrounding normal tissue. Other signs of AIN include abnormal vasculature with features such as punctation, mosaicism and atypical vessels [58] (Fig. 3). The application of Lugol's (iodine) solution can also increase specificity. Abnormal tissue remains unstained or appears light yellow, unlike adjacent normal tissue which stains dark brown or mahogany due to the presence of glycogen in the cells.

The sensitivity of anal cytology to detect biopsy proven AIN is 50 to 80% [59], similar to the sensitivity of cervical Pap tests to detect biopsy-proven CIN. Anal cytology is more sensitive in HIV-positive men compared with HIV-negative men in detecting AIN, most likely reflecting the presence of more extensive HIV-associated disease in the HIV-positive population.

3.3. *Histopathology of anal intraepithelial neoplasia*

Similar to the classification system used for cervical cytology, anal cytology is classified as normal, atypical squamous cells of undetermined significance (ASC-US), atypical squamous cells- cannot rule out high-grade disease (ASC-H), low-grade squamous intraepithelial lesions (LSIL), high-grade squamous intraepithelial lesions (HSIL) and invasive carcinoma. The histologic correlate of CIN is AIN, which is a precursor to anal cancer [60–62]. The grading system reflects the degree of histologic abnormality observed. AIN I is not likely to progress to anal cancer whereas AIN II and AIN III are believed to be the true anal cancer precursors. Like CIN 1, AIN 1 shows signs of replicative HPV infection, including koilocytosis and few signs of cellular atypia. AIN II and AIN III, like their cervical counterparts, show progressively increasing proliferation and replacement of the normal epithelium by cells with a basal morphology and large nuclear-cytoplasmic ratios, and mitoses in the more superficial cell layers.

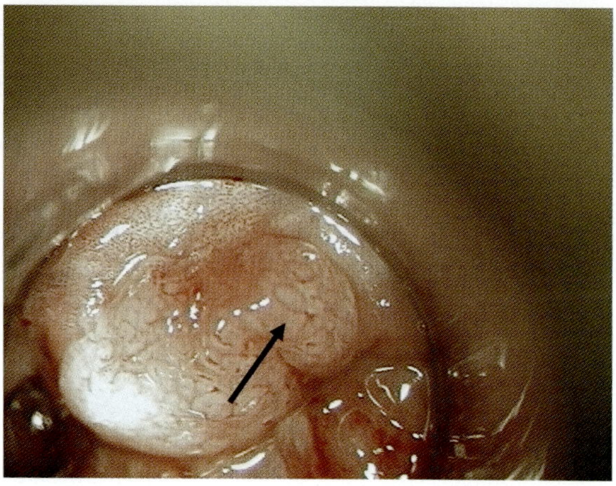

Fig. 3. Lesion with biopsy-confirmed anal intraepithelial neoplasia III. Flat, plaque-like lesion in the anal canal is shown with a black arrow and demonstrates atypical blood vessels.

3.4. *Treatment of HPV-associated anal neoplasia*

3.4.1. *AIN and condyloma*

Because of anatomical challenges such as hemorrhoids and crypts, it can be more difficult to treat AIN compared with CIN. Recent guidelines were published for the treatment of AIN in the setting of HIV infection [55,63]. As in cervical disease, histology, lesion size, lesion location and HIV-status are the main determinants that may influence treatment modalities and treatment goals. While AIN I likely does not progress directly to cancer, treatment may of AIN 1 reduce the risk of enlargement which may preclude the use of topical agents, decrease the risk of progression to AIN II or AIN III, and may provide symptomatic or psychological relief. AIN II and AIN III should be treated whenever possible to prevent cancer. Some experts have a lower threshold to treat HIV-positive men with minimal AIN I in HIV-positive men since there is a faster rate of progression to AIN II or AIN III compared with HIV-negative men [35].

Smaller lesions are generally easier to treat than larger lesions. Topical therapy can be used for relatively flat intra-anal (85% trichloroacetic acid, liquid nitrogen) or perianal lesions (imiquimod, podophyllotoxin,

85% trichloroacetic acid, liquid nitrogen) smaller than 1 cm^2 at the base. Large circumferential intra-anal lesions, particularly in HIV-positive men, have a high recurrence rate if removed rate [64]. Because treatment of extensive intra-anal lesions may require multiple staged procedures and may be associated with a high morbidity (post-operative pain), and high recurrence rate these individuals may be followed closely without treatment. Large, circumferential intra-anal lesions may be removed surgically if patients are symptomatic or if the goal is to rule out anal cancer. Lesions in the middle-sized category (too big for topical therapy, but not large enough to require surgery) are increasingly being treated with infrared coagulation (Redfield Corporation, Rochelle Park, New Jersey) which has been licensed for treatment of condylomata acuminata and tattoo removal [65]. After local anesthesia with 1% lidocaine with epinephrine, the infrared coagulator is used to destroy the lesion by generating intense heat at the tip of the probe. Coagulative necrosis occurs without a smoke plume. This procedure is well tolerated with fewer complications compared with surgery, with only mild to moderate post-procedure discomfort occurring for a few days. Other therapies for AIN may have promise, including photodynbamic therapy [66] and intra-anal imiquimod [67], but these require further study.

Perianal condyloma may be amenable to local patient-applied therapy such as imiquimod or podophyllotoxin, which are not recommended for intra-anal use. Liquid nitrogen, electrocautery, TCA and IRC may be used in the office by the clinician. Condyloma that are too large for office-based therapy usually require removal in the surgical suite. Perianal high-grade disease may be treated with TCA, IRC or surgery.

3.4.2. Anal cancer

Treatment of anal cancer depends on the stage of the cancer and the patient's age and general health. Stage 0, also classified as anal carcinoma in situ, can be removed locally, similar to the treatment described above for AIN II-III. Stage I cancer, which is smaller than two centimeters in diameter, but has not spread to the muscle tissue, can sometimes be treated by local resection, but the usual therapy is a combination of chemotherapy with radiation therapy. If cancer recurs, abdominoperineal resection may remove the remaining cancer. In Stage II cancer, which is larger than two centimeters in diameter, but has not spread to nearby organs or lymph nodes, the treatment options are the same as for Stage I. For stage III-A cancer, which has spread to the lymph nodes around the rectum or to nearby organs such as the bladder, radiation plus chemotherapy is still an option, but because the cancer has spread to the lymph nodes, surgery may be needed to remove parts of the rectum or colon as well as to perform a lymph node dissection. For Stage III-B cancer, in which the cancer has spread to both lymph nodes and nearby organs, radiation and chemotherapy, followed by surgery is the best combination. The recovery rate from Stage IV metastatic anal cancer is low and most treatments are palliative (designed to relieve symptoms rather than cure the cancer).

The standard of care for the treatment of all but Stage IV invasive anal cancer is thus combined modality therapy (CMT) with both RT and chemotherapy (5-FU and mitomycin used together), with or without surgery as described above. More recently, cis-platinum has been increasingly used in place of mitomycin [68]. CMT avoids the morbidity of abdominoperineal resection (APR) which involves removal of the anorectum and necessitates a permanent colostomy. CMT has also been successfully employed in HIV-positive men [68], including those with low CD4+ level but who have a well-controlled HIV viral load on HAART.

4. Conclusions

The consequences of anogenital HPV infection in men must be measured both in terms of their ability to spread HPV infection to their sexual partners, as well as the lesions, including cancers, that affect men directly. Although they share much in common with cervical HPV infection and disease, the natural history of penile and anal HPV infection, intraepithelial neoplasia and cancer is not well understood. Factors that lead to transmission of HPV infection between sexual partners requires further study, as will the effect of prophylactic HPV vaccination of women on male disease. Conversely, prophylactic HPV vaccination of men needs to be studied for its effect on reducing the burden of male disease and protecting the health of women by reducing their exposure to HPV and improving their "herd immunity". As a result of the success of the HPV vaccine in women, more attention than ever is currently being given to the "male factor", and it is expected that these studies will yield important information that will be valuable to the treatment and control of HPV-associated neoplasia in both women and men.

Acknowledgements

The author gratefully acknowledges Ms. Victoria Kuohung and Dr. Michael Berry for the photos in Figs 1 to 3.

References

[1] S.B. Baldwin, D.R. Wallace and M.R. Papenfuss, Human papillomavirus infection in men attending a sexually transmitted disease clinic, *J Infect Dis* **187** (2003), 1064–1070.

[2] S.M. Nicolau, C.G. Camargo and J.N. Stavale, Human papillomavirus DNA detection in male sexual partners of women with genital human papillomavirus infection, *Urology* **65** (2005), 251–255.

[3] S. Vaccarella, E. Lazcano-Ponce and J.A. Castro-Garduno, Prevalence and determinants of human papillomavirus infection in men attending vasectomy clinics in Mexico, *Int J Cancer* **119** (2006), 1934–1939.

[4] S.B. Baldwin, D.R. Wallace, M.R. Papenfuss, M. Abrahamsen, L.C. Vaught and A.R. Giuliano, Condom use and other factors affecting penile human papillomavirus detection in men attending a sexually transmitted disease clinic, *Sex Transm Dis* **31** (2004), 601–607.

[5] M. Frisch, R.J. Biggar and J.J. Goedert, Human papillomavirus-associated cancers in patients with human immunodeficiency virus infection and acquired immunodeficiency syndrome, *J Natl Cancer Inst* **92** (2000), 1500–1510.

[6] G. Sirera, S. Videla and M. Pinol, High prevalence of human papillomavirus infection in the anus, penis and mouth in HIV-positive men, *AIDS* **20** (2006), 1201–1204.

[7] R. Barrasso, J. De Brux, O. Croissant and G. Orth, High prevalence of papillomavirus-associated penile intraepithelial neoplasia in sexual partners of women with cervical intraepithelial neoplasia, *N Engl J Med* **317** (1987), 916–923.

[8] J.M. Palefsky and R. Barrasso, HPV infection and disease in men, *Obstet Gynecol Clin North Am* **23** (1996), 895–916.

[9] M.C. Bleeker, C.J. Hogewoning and F.J. Voorhorst, Condom use promotes regression of human papillomavirus-associated penile lesions in male sexual partners of women with cervical intraepithelial neoplasia, *Int J Cancer* **107** (2003), 804–810.

[10] A.B. Ackerman and R. Kronberg, Pearly penile papules. Acral angiofibromas, *Arch Dermatol* **108** (1973), 673–675.

[11] R. Barrasso and S. Jablonska, Clinical, colposcopic and histologic spectrum of male human papillomavirus-associated genital lesions, *Clin Pract Gynecol* **2** (1989), 73–101.

[12] J. Palefsky and R. Barasso, HPV infection and disease in men, *Obstet Gyn Clin North Am* **23** (1996), 895–916.

[13] T.R. Wade, A.W. Kopf and A.B. Ackerman, Bowenoid papulosis of the penis, *Cancer* **42** (1978), 1890–1903.

[14] S. Obalek, S. Jablonska and G. Orth, HPV-associated intraepithelial neoplasia of external genitalia, *Clin Dermatol* **3** (1985), 104–113.

[15] S. Obalek, S. Jablonska, S. Beaudenon, L. Walczak and G. Orth, Bowenoid papulosis of the male and female genitalia: risk of cervical neoplasia, *J Am Acad Dermatol* **14** (1986), 433–444.

[16] H. Ikenberg, L. Gissmann, G. Gross, E.I. Grussendorf-Conen and H. zur Hausen, Human papillomavirus type-16-related DNA in genital Bowen's disease and in Bowenoid papulosis, *Int J Cancer* **32** (1983), 563–565.

[17] R.U. Levine, C.P. Crum, E. Herman, D. Silvers, A. Ferenczy and R.M. Richart, Cervical papillomavirus infection and intraepithelial neoplasia: a study of male sexual partners, *Obstet Gynecol* **64** (1984), 16–20.

[18] G. Gross and H. Pfister, Role of human papillomavirus in penile cancer, penile intraepithelial squamous cell neoplasias and in genital warts, *Med Microbiol Immunol (Berlin)* **193** (2004), 35–44.

[19] D.M. Parkin, S.L. Whelan, J. Ferlay and H. Storm, Cancer Incidence in Five Continents, *IARC CancerBase* **Lyon No. 7** (2005), I–VIII.

[20] Centers for Disease Control and Prevention. Sexually transmitted diseases treatment guidelines 2002, *MMWR* **51** (2002), RR-6.

[21] X. Castellsague, F.X. Bosch and N. Munoz, Male circumcision, penile human papillomavirus infection, and cervical cancer in female partners, *N Engl J Med* **346** (2002), 1105–1112.

[22] R.L. Winer, J.P. Hughes and Q. Feng, Condom use and the risk of genital human papillomavirus infection in young women, *N Engl J Med* **354** (2006), 2645–2654.

[23] M.C. Bleeker, C.J. Hogewoning and A.J. Van Den Brule, Penile lesions and human papillomavirus in male sexual partners of women with cervical intraepithelial neoplasia, *J Am Acad Dermatol* **47** (2002), 351–357.

[24] S. Franceschi, X. Castellsague and L. Dal Maso, Prevalence and determinants of human papillomavirus genital infection in men, *Br J Cancer* **86** (2002), 705–711.

[25] M.C. Bleeker, C.J. Hogewoning and J. Berkhof, Concordance of specific human papillomavirus types in sex partners is more prevalent than would be expected by chance and is associated with increased viral loads, *Clin Infect Dis* **41** (2005), 612–620.

[26] H.R. Shin, S. Franceschi and S. Vaccarella, Prevalence and determinants of genital infection with papillomavirus, in female and male university students in Busan, South Korea, *J Infect Dis* **190** (2004), 468–476.

[27] J.M. Palefsky, E.A. Holly, M.L. Ralston, M. Da Costa and R.M. Greenblatt, Prevalence and risk factors for anal human papillomavirus infection in human immunodeficiency virus (HIV)-positive and high-risk HIV-negative women, *J Infect Dis* **183** (2001), 383–391.

[28] N. Kiviat, A. Rompalo and R. Bowden, Anal human papillomavirus infection among human immunodeficiency virus-seropositive and -seronegative men, *J Infect Dis* **162** (1990), 358–361.

[29] C. Piketty, T.M. Darragh and M. Da Costa, High prevalence of anal human papillomavirus infection and anal cancer precursors among HIV-infected persons in the absence of anal intercourse, *Ann Intern Med* **138** (2003), 453–459.

[30] J.M. Palefsky, E.A. Holly and M.L. Ralston, Anal squamous intraepithelial lesions in HIV-positive and HIV-negative homosexual and bisexual men: prevalence and risk factors, *J Acquir Immune Defic Syndr Hum Retrovirol* **17** (1998), 320–326.

[31] P.V. Chin-Hong, E. Vittinghoff and R.D. Cranston, Age-related prevalence of anal cancer precursors in homosexual men: the EXPLORE study, *J Natl Cancer Inst* **97** (2005), 896–905.

[32] C.W. Critchlow, C.M. Surawicz, K.K. Holmes et al., Prospective study of high grade anal squamous intraepithelial neoplasia in a cohort of homosexual men: influence of HIV infection, immunosuppression and human papillomavirus infection, *AIDS* **9** (1995), 1255–1262.

[33] C. Piketty, T.M. Darragh and I. Heard, High prevalence of anal squamous intraepithelial lesions in HIV-positive men despite

the use of highly active antiretroviral therapy, *Sex Transm Dis* **31** (2004), 96–99.

[34] J.M. Palefsky, E.A. Holly, M.L. Ralston, N. Jay, J.M. Berry and T.M. Darragh, High incidence of anal high-grade squamous intraepithelial lesions among HIV-positive and HIV-negative homosexual/bisexual men, *AIDS* **12** (1998), 495–503.

[35] J.M. Palefsky, E.A. Holly and C.J. Hogeboom, Virologic, immunologic, and clinical parameters in the incidence and progression of anal squamous intraepithelial lesions in HIV-positive and HIV-negative homosexual men, *J Acquir Immune Defic Syndr Hum Retrovirol* **17** (1998), 314–319.

[36] J.M. Palefsky, E.A. Holly and M.L. Ralston, Effect of highly active antiretroviral therapy on the natural history of anal squamous intraepithelial lesions and anal human papillomavirus infection, *J Acquir Immune Defic Syndr* **28** (2001), 422–428.

[37] J.M. Palefsky, E.A. Holly and J.T. E, Anal intraepithelial neoplasia in the HAART era among HIV-positive men who have sex with men, *AIDS* **19** (2005), 1407–1414.

[38] M. Frisch, R.J. Biggar, E.A. Engels and J.J. Goedert, Association of cancer with AIDS-related immunosuppression in adults, *JAMA* **285** (2001), 1736–1745.

[39] S.E. Gagne, R. Jensen and A. Polvi, High-resolution analysis of genomic alterations and human papillomavirus integration in anal intraepithelial neoplasia, *J Acquir Immune Defic Syndr* **40** (2005), 182–189.

[40] D.M. Parkin, The global health burden of infection-associated cancers in the year 2002, *Int J Cancer* (2006).

[41] L.G. Johnson, M.M. Madeleine, L.M. Newcomer, S.M. Schwartz and J.R. Daling, Anal cancer incidence and survival: the surveillance, epidemiology, and end results experience, 1973–2000, *Cancer* **101** (2004), 281–288.

[42] J.R. Qualters, N.C. Lee, R.A. Smith and R.E. Aubert, Breast and cervical cancer surveillance, United States, 1973–1987, *MMWR* **41** (1992), 1–15.

[43] J.R. Daling, M.M. Madeleine and L.G. Johnson, Human papillomavirus, smoking, and sexual practices in the etiology of anal cancer, *Cancer* **101** (2004), 270–280.

[44] J.R. Daling, N.S. Weiss and T.G. Hislop, Sexual practices, sexually transmitted diseases, and the incidence of anal cancer, *N Engl J Med* **317** (1987), 973–977.

[45] E.A. Holly, A.S. Whittemore, D.A. Aston, D.K. Ahn, B.J. Nickoloff and J.J. Kristiansen, Anal cancer incidence: genital warts, anal fissure or fistula, hemorrhoids, and smoking, *J Natl Cancer Inst* **81** (1989), 1726–1731.

[46] M. Frisch, B. Glimelius and A.J. van den Brule, Sexually transmitted infection as a cause of anal cancer, *N Engl J Med* **337** (1997), 1350–1358.

[47] J.R. Daling, K.J. Sherman and T.G. Hislop, Cigarette smoking and the risk of anogenital cancer, *Am J Epidemiol* **135** (1992), 180–189.

[48] M. Bower, T. Powles and T. Newsom-Davis, HIV-Associated Anal Cancer: Has Highly Active Antiretroviral Therapy Reduced the Incidence or Improved the Outcome? *J Acquir Immune Defic Syndr* **37** (2004), 1563–1565.

[49] E.Y. Chiao, S.E. Krown, E.A. Stier and D. Schrag, A population-based analysis of temporal trends in the incidence of squamous anal canal cancer in relation to the HIV epidemic, *J Acquir Immune Defic Syndr* **40** (2005), 451–455.

[50] M. Bower, C. Palmieri and T. Dhillon, AIDS-related malignancies: changing epidemiology and the impact of highly active antiretroviral therapy, *Curr Opin Infect Dis* **19** (2006), 14–19.

[51] I. Penn, Cancer in the immunosuppressed organ recipient, *Transplant Proc* **23** (1991), 1771–1772.

[52] I. Penn, The changing pattern of posttransplant malignancies, *Transplant Proc* **23** (1991), 1101–1103.

[53] J. Adami, H. Gabel and B. Lindelof, Cancer risk following organ transplantation: a nationwide cohort study in Sweden, *Br J Cancer* **89** (2003), 1221–1227.

[54] H.S. Patel, A.R. Silver and J.M. Northover, Anal cancer in renal transplant patients, *Int J Colorectal Dis* (2005), 1–5.

[55] P.V. Chin-Hong and J.M. Palefsky, Natural history and clinical management of anal human papillomavirus disease in men and women infected with human immunodeficiency virus, *Clin Infect Dis* **35** (2002), 1127–1134.

[56] S.J. Goldie, K.M. Kuntz, M.C. Weinstein, K.A. Freedberg, M.L. Welton and J.M. Palefsky, The clinical effectiveness and cost-effectiveness of screening for anal squamous intraepithelial lesions in homosexual and bisexual HIV-positive men, *JAMA* **281** (1999), 1822–1829.

[57] S.J. Goldie, K.M. Kuntz, M.C. Weinstein, K.A. Freedberg and J.M. Palefsky, Cost-effectiveness of screening for anal squamous intraepithelial lesions and anal cancer in human immunodeficiency virus-negative homosexual and bisexual men, *Am J Med* **108** (2000), 634–641.

[58] N. Jay, E.A. Holly, M. Berry, C.J. Hogeboom, T.M. Darragh and J.M. Palefsky, Colposcopic correlates of anal squamous intraepithelial lesions, *Dis Col Rectum* **40** (1997), 919–928.

[59] J.M. Palefsky, E.A. Holly, C.J. Hogeboom, N. Jay, M. Berry and T.M. Darragh, Anal cytology as a screening tool for anal squamous intraepithelial lesions, *J Acq Immun Defic Syndr* **14** (1997), 415–422.

[60] C. Fenger and V.T. Nielsen, Precancerous changes in the anal canal epithelium in resection specimens, *Acta Pathol Microbiol Immunol Scand [a]* **94** (1986), 63–69.

[61] T.E. Marfing, M.E. Abel and D.M. Gallagher, Perianal Bowen's disease and associated malignancies. Results of a survey, *Dis Colon Rectum* **30** (1987), 782–785.

[62] A.B. Jaeger, A. Gramkow, H. Hjalgrim, M. Melbye and M. Frisch, Bowen disease and risk of subsequent malignant neoplasms: a population-based cohort study of 1147 patients, *Arch Dermatol* **135** (1999), 790–793.

[63] C.A. Benson, J.E. Kaplan, H. Masur, A. Pau and K.K. Holmes, Treating opportunistic infections among HIV-exposed and infected children: recommendations from CDC, the National Institutes of Health, and the Infectious Diseases Society of America, *MMWR Recomm Rep* **53** (2004), 1–112.

[64] G.J. Chang, J.M. Berry, N. Jay, J.M. Palefsky and M.L. Welton, Surgical treatment of high-grade anal squamous intraepithelial lesions: a prospective study, *Dis Colon Rectum* **45** (2002), 453–458.

[65] S.E. Goldstone, A.Z. Kawalek and J.W. Huyett, Infrared coagulator: a useful tool for treating anal squamous intraepithelial lesions, *Dis Colon Rectum* **48** (2005), 1042–1054.

[66] J.H. Scholefield, Treatment of grade III anal intraepithelial neoplasia with photodynamic therapy: report of a case, *Dis Colon Rectum* **46**(11) (2003), 1555–1559.

[67] A. Kreuter, B. Hochdorfer and M. Stucker, Treatment of anal intraepithelial neoplasia in patients with acquired HIV with imiquimod 5% cream, *J Am Acad Dermatol* **50** (2004), 980–981.

[68] J.M. Berry, J.M. Palefsky and M.L. Welton, Anal cancer and its precursors in HIV-positive patients: perspectives and management, *Surg Oncol Clin N Am* **13** (2004), 355–373.

[69] M.A. Rubin, B. Kleter and M. Zhou, Detection and typing of human papillomavirus DNA in penile carcinoma: evidence for multiple independent pathways of penile carcinogenesis, *Am J Pathol* **159** (2001), 1211–1218.

[70] J.E. Levi, P. Rahal, A.S. Sarkis and L. Villa, Human papillomavirus DNA and p53 status in penile carcinomas, *Int J Cancer* **76** (1998), 779–783.

[71] J.J. Carter, M.M. Madeleine and K. Shera, Human papillomavirus 16 and 18 L1 serology compared across anogenital cancer sites, *Cancer Res* **61** (2001), 1934–1940.

[72] M.R. Cupp, R.S. Malek, J.R. Goellner, T.F. Smith and M.J. Espy, The detection of human papillomavirus deoxyribonucleic acid in intraepithelial, in situ, verrucous and invasive carcinoma of the penis, *J Urol* **154** (1995), 1024–1029.

[73] M.A. Picconi, A.M. Eijan and A.L. Distefano, Human papillomavirus (HPV) DNA in penile carcinomas in Argentina: analysis of primary tumors and lymph nodes, *J Med Virol* **61** (2000), 65–69.

[74] A.L. Bezerra, A. Lopes, G. Landman, G.N. Alencar, H. Torloni and L.L. Villa, Clinicopathologic features and human papillomavirus dna prevalence of warty and squamous cell carcinoma of the penis, *Am J Surg Pathol* **25** (2001), 673–678.

[75] L. Gregoire, A.L. Cubilla, V.E. Reuter, G.P. Haas and W.D. Lancaster, Preferential association of human papillomavirus with high-grade histologic variants of penile-invasive squamous cell carcinoma, *J Natl Cancer Inst* **87** (1995), 1705–1709.

[76] M. Frisch, C. Fenger and A.J. van den Brule, Variants of squamous cell carcinoma of the anal canal and perianal skin and their relation to human papillomaviruses, *Cancer Res* **59** (1999), 753–757.

[77] P.A. Poletti, A. Halfon and M.C. Marti, Papillomavirus and anal carcinoma, *Int J Colorectal Dis* **13** (1998), 108–111.

[78] K.R. Shroyer, C.G. Brookes, N.E. Markham and A.L. Shroyer, Detection of human papillomavirus in anorectal squamous cell carcinoma. Correlation with basaloid pattern of differentiation, *Am J Clin Pathol* **104** (1995), 299–305.

Disease Markers 23 (2007) 273–281
IOS Press

HPV detection methods

Antoinette A.T.P. Brink, Peter J.F. Snijders and Chris J.L.M. Meijer*
VU University medical center, Department of Pathology, Section Molecular Pathology, De Boelelaan 1117, 1081 HV Amsterdam, The Netherlands

Abstract. Given the causal relation between a persistent high-risk human papillomavirus (hrHPV) infection and the development of high-grade cervical intraepithelial neoplasia (CIN) and cervical cancer, hrHPV testing has been advocated in addition to cytology for the detection of clinically relevant cervical lesions. HrHPV testing is thought to improve cervical screening algorithms, the management of women with cytologically equivocal smears, and the management of women treated for high grade CIN. In this chapter we discuss different methods for HPV detection and genotyping and their respective applications.

Keywords: Human papillomavirus, polymerase chain reaction, reverse hybridization, hybrid capture, real-time PCR, cervical carcinoma, NASBA, DNA probes, epidemiology

1. Introduction

Cervical cancer is preceded by premalignant lesions termed cervical intraepithelial neoplasia (CIN). Cervical cancer screening largely relies on cytological detection of these premalignant lesions, which can be treated relatively easily and with minor side effects. Given the causal relation between a persistent high-risk human papillomavirus (hrHPV) infection and the development of high-grade CIN and cervical cancer, hrHPV testing has been advocated in addition to cytology for the detection of clinically relevant cervical lesions. HrHPV testing is thought to improve cervical screening algorithms [1], the management of women with cytologically equivocal smears [2,3], and the management of women treated for high grade CIN [4]. In this chapter we elaborate on the different methods for HPV detection and their respective applications.

1.1. HPV phylogeny

HPVs are associated with various benign and malignant epithelial proliferative diseases. Over 100 genotypes of HPV are recognized. An HPV isolate is described as a novel type if the nucleotide sequence of its E6, E7 and L1 genes differs more than 10% from that of any other HPV type. Based on tropism, a distinction can be made between *cutaneous* HPV types that infect the epidermis, and *mucosal* HPV types that infect the epithelia of the anogenital or the aerodigestive tract.

In vitro studies showed that a group of phylogenetically related *mucosal* HPV types have oncogenic potential: their E6 and E7 proteins interfere with cell cycle regulation by mediating degradation of p53 and pRb proteins, respectively [5,6]. Exactly these HPV types are an important causal factor in carcinogenesis of the uterine cervix and are therefore designated *"high-risk"* (hr) [7]. Epidemiological studies have shown that these hrHPVs include types 16, 18, 31, 33, 35, 39, 45, 51, 52, 56, 58, 59, 68, 73 and 82, and probably also types 26, 53 and 66 [8]. In the phylogenetic tree of HPV types, hrHPVs cluster in the groups designated A5, A6, A7, A9 and A11 [9]. Non-oncogenic or *low-risk* genital HPVs (lrHPVs) are phylogenetically distant from the hrHPVs. They include HPV 6, 11, 40, 42, 43, 44, 54, 61, 70, 72, 81, and CP6108. Their E6 and E7 proteins are less competent in interfering with p53 [10] and pRb [11] functions than the E6 and E7 proteins of hrHPVs. LrHPVs can cause benign proliferations such as condylomata acuminata (genital warts). For a number of mucosal HPV types, the risk has not been

*Corresponding author: Prof. Dr. C.J.L.M. Meijer, Dept. Pathology, VU University medical center, PO Box 7057, 1007MB Amsterdam, The Netherlands. Tel.: +31 20 4444070; Fax: +31 20 4442964; E-mail: cjlm.meijer@vumc.nl.

ISSN 0278-0240/07/$17.00

determined yet [8]. However, some of them could be considered as potentially oncogenic due to their phylogenetic relationship with known hrHPV types. For example HPV type 67, which initially was isolated from a vaginal intraepithelial neoplasia (VIN) [12], clusters in the A9 group that contains only hrHPVs such as HPV16 [9].

1.2. The need for HPV genotyping

Many HPV tests rely on cocktails of probes representing 13 or 14 of the most common hrHPV types. It has been suggested that the added value of less frequent hrHPV types to such probe cocktails would be small, probably irrelevant for screening programs, and resulting in a substantial decrease in screening specificity [13,14]. However, the increasing need to distinguish individual hrHPV types is illustrated by several current developments in the field of HPV research. Firstly, there is growing evidence that certain hrHPV types confer increased risks for high-grade CIN and cervical carcinomas. This is discussed in more detail in the next paragraph. Secondly, 20–30% of HPV infections involve multiple HPV types and in those cases typing is necessary to determine the contribution of the individual HPV types. Thirdly, there is an increasing interest in prophylactic HPV vaccination (reviewed in [15]), which entails studies of geographical distribution of HPV types and their associated diseases as a basis for prophylactic vaccination programs. Once vaccination has started, HPV typing remains necessary to monitor the changes in prevalence of the type(s) represented in the vaccines as a measure for vaccine efficacy.

HPV genotyping may also have some advantages and perhaps some prognostic value in monitoring of women who have been treated for CIN3 or cervical cancer, although the treatment itself does not depend on the typing result. Demonstrating the same hrHPV type in the post-treatment specimen as in the primary CIN3 lesion may indicate a recurrent hrHPV infection due to incomplete removal of the lesion or disability of the respective woman to clear a particular hrHPV type [16,17] and might require more intense follow-up or more aggressive treatment.

Finally, the number of known HPV types is still increasing. Although novel HPV types are often isolated from malignancies, their oncogenic potential can only be deduced from a combination of in vitro and epidemiological studies, the latter of which should include typing.

1.3. HrHPV types and risk of high-grade cervical lesions

We showed that in the Dutch screened population [18], HPV types 16 and 33 are more prevalent in women with a cytological reading of moderate dyskaryosis or worse and underlying CIN2 or worse, than in women with normal cytology. This suggests that infection with these types confers an increased risk for development of high-grade cervical lesions [19].

Moreover, HPV type distribution in women with cervical carcinoma as compared with cytologically normal women showed that HPV18 is mainly a risk factor for the development of adenocarcinoma (AdCa) and its precursor adenocarcinoma in situ (ACIS), whereas HPV16 is associated with both squamous cell carcinoma (SCC) and AdCa [20]. In line with the abovementioned findings, an increased risk posed by HPV16 and HPV18 for cervical (pre)cancers of the squamous and adeno-histotypes was shown in a prospective screening cohort of 20810 women followed for up to 10 years [21]. In addition, an increased risk for cervical precancer posed by HPV16 but not by HPV18 was shown in a prospective trial of women with equivocal or mild cervical abnormalities [22]. A likely explanation for increased prevalence of HPV18 in invasive carcinoma but not in high-grade precursor lesions, is an association of HPV18 with a cytopathological effect high in the endocervical canal that is likely to be missed by cytology.

These findings strongly suggest that in particular women who are HPV16 or HPV18 positive should be monitored very closely, even if their smears are cytologically normal.

2. HPV detection methods

Because HPV cannot be cultured, all HPV tests currently in use rely on the detection of viral nucleic acids. HPV detection methods can be divided in target-amplification methods and signal-amplification methods. In the following section, technical aspects of the different currently available HPV detection methods are described.

2.1. Target amplification techniques

2.1.1. Consensus primer polymerase chain reaction (PCR)

In most of the PCR-based HPV detection systems, a broad spectrum of HPV types is amplified by consensus primers, followed by detection with type-specific probes. The consensus primers may be degenerate as in the MY09/11 [23] and CPI/II [24] systems. Alternatively, they may contain mismatches that are accepted under low-stringency PCR conditions as in the GP5+/6+ system [25], they may contain inosine residues at ambiguous base positions such as in the IU/IWDO [26] and SPF [27] primers, or sets of overlapping primers as is the case in the PGMY [28] and Amplicor [29] systems.

2.1.2. Detection and/or genotyping of consensus PCR products

For group-specific detection of HPVs without high-resolution typing, an enzyme immuno assay (EIA) can be applied conveniently using cocktails of e.g. HR- or LR-HPV probes [30,31].

Typing of PCR products was traditionally done by means of dot blotting or Southern blotting and hybridization with type-specific oligonucleotides. More recently, reverse hybridization techniques were introduced. These methods rely on the hybridization of labelled consensus PCR products to HPV-type specific oligos immobilized on filters. Examples are reverse line blot (RLB) analysis following MY09/11 [23] or GP5+/6+ [25] consensus PCR, or a line probe assay (LiPa) following SPF PCR [27]. Detection of the hybridized PCR product is done by a colorimetric reaction [23,27] or by chemiluminescence [25], the latter allowing repeated usage of the same filter [25]. Instead of filters, glass microarrays of HPV type-specific probes can also be used [32]. Recently, a quantitative and high-throughput method was developed [33] based on Luminex suspension array technology. This method relies on detection of consensus primer PCR (GP5+/6+) products with type-specific oligonucleotide probes coupled to fluorescence-labelled polystyrene beads and allows detection of up to 100 different HPV types simultaneously.

Two non-hybridization typing methods following consensus PCR are sequence analysis of the PCR product [34,35] and restriction fragment length polymorphism (RFLP) analysis [36]. RFLP implies the digestion of consensus PCR products with restriction endonucleases, and comparison of the digestion pattern with those of known HPV types. These techniques are useful if unknown types of HPV are present in the specimens, but they have several drawbacks as compared with hybridization methods. For example, RFLP and sequence analysis are not suitable for the detection of infections with multiple HPV types: these will usually give an uninterpretable mix-up of digestion/sequence patterns. In addition, these two methods are less suitable for high-throughput analyses because they are relatively laborious. Finally, RFLP and sequence analysis are less sensitive than hybridization methods because more PCR product is needed to generate a positive signal.

As opposed to typing after consensus PCR, it is also possible to type during the reaction, in real time. Various real-time PCR techniques are available (see also Section 3.2.2), the best known being molecular beacons, the fluorescent 5' exonuclease assay (e.g. Taqman) and fluorescence energy resonance transfer assays (e.g. LightCycler).

At present the only real-time assay that allows consensus HPV-PCR with simultaneous typing is a molecular beacons assay [37]. However, the multiplicity of this technique is limited because the current generation of real-time thermocyclers do not allow for more than six differentially labelled probes. Hence, for typing of multiple HPV infections, reverse hybridization methods are preferred over real-time assays.

2.1.3. Type-specific PCR

If one is interested in a particular HPV type, type-specific PCR can be applied (described in [25,38] among others). Care should be taken when designing primers, because they may still react with other types if chosen in well-conserved regions. Confirmation of the specificity of type-specific PCRs, as with consensus primer PCRs, can be done by (regular or reverse) filter hybridization or by EIA, but also in real-time [39–41]. A great advantage of real-time PCR assays is the possibility to quantify the HPV in the specimen. Several studies have shown that the amount of hrHPV present in a cervical smear (the "viral load") as measured by real-time PCR is predictive for the presence or development of high-grade cervical lesions [42–45]; reviewed in [46]. However, to obtain reliable quantification data DNA extraction is usually necessary, thus increasing the work load.

2.1.4. mRNA amplification

Several recent studies have shown that hrHPV testing can also be done through detection of the viral mRNA. The most relevant transcripts to look for are those encoding the viral oncoproteins E6 and E7. It is hypothesized that the presence of viral E6/E7 mRNA in a cervical smear has a better positive predictive value for high-grade cervical lesions than the presence of viral DNA, because the E6/E7 mRNA represents an active infection with cell- transforming potential whereas the viral DNA may also be present in clinically irrelevant conditions.

Detection of viral mRNA in cervical smears can be done by reverse-transcriptase (RT-) PCR [47] or by nucleic acid sequence-based amplification (NASBA) [48]. For the latter assay type, a commercially available system was recently developed that detects E6/E7 transcripts from the five most common hrHPV types 16, 18, 31, 33 and 45 [49–53]. In hospital-based populations, hrHPV mRNA detection showed a better specificity for the detection of high-grade cervical lesions than hrHPV DNA detection [51,52]. However, this method still needs to be validated for population-based screening and triage of women with smears showing minor cellular abnormalities.

An alternative method relying on hrHPV transcription is the detection of HPV-human fusion transcripts that arise from hrHPV genomes integrated into the host cell genome. This method was designated "amplification of papillomavirus oncogene transcripts" (APOT) [54].

Although this method is rather laborious and therefore not suitable for large-scale hrHPV testing, it can give information that is not obtained using other mRNA amplification techniques. On the one hand, it reveals viral integration, an event that is specific for a real precancerous lesion as opposed to a productive viral infection [55]. On the other hand, it allows the identification of patient-specific fusion transcripts. This may be useful in monitoring of women who have been treated for high-grade lesions, because it will help to determine whether a high-grade lesion occurring after treatment is a recurrence or even a metastasis of the original lesion [56].

2.2. Signal-amplification techniques

2.2.1. Liquid-phase signal amplification techniques

The best known technique in this category is the commercially available, FDA-approved and clinically validated Hybrid Capture 2 (HC2) method [57]. This method uses a mixture of full-length RNA probes representing hrHPV types 16, 18, 31, 33, 35, 39, 45, 51, 52, 56, 58, 59, and 68. Prior to the test, the clinical samples are heat-alkaline-denatured. Hybridization of one or more of the probes to HPV DNA present in the samples is detected by peroxidase-labelled antibodies that recognize the RNA/DNA hybrid, and visualized by chemiluminescence. The analytical sensitivity of this method is 1 pg/ml of cloned HPV16 DNA, which corresponds to approximately 10^5 HPV16 genome copies. This sensitivity is lower than that of most target-amplification methods. Because a mixture of probes is used, HC2 is at present not suitable for high-resolution typing. Some cross reactivity of the HC2 probes with HPV types not represented in the probe mix, including non-oncogenic HPVs, has been described [58].

2.2.2. Morphological signal-amplification techniques

In addition to the abovementioned methods, hrHPV detection can be performed by DNA in situ hybridization (ISH) to cytological slides [59,60] and histological preparations [61]. This can be achieved by fluorescent detection [61] or colored substrate deposition and bright field microscopy. The relatively small size of the HPV genome (7.8 kb) and thus of the probe precludes direct detection of hybrids in case of low viral genome copy numbers and therefore some type of signal amplification is generally necessary. A commercially available HPV ISH system uses an indirect biotin-streptavidin method (Ventana Inform HPV) which at present lacks sufficient sensitivity to detect high-grade cervical lesions [60]. Alternatively, tyramide signal amplification (TSA), also known as catalysed reporter deposition (CARD) can be used, both in fluorescent [61,62] and bright field [62] applications. Also for the CARD method, a commercially available system exists (Dako GenPoint). CARD greatly enhances sensitivity, but in general HPV ISH is too laborious to be used in high-throughput HPV testing.

3. Clinical specimens for HPV detection

The kind of clinical specimens available will determine the choice of the HPV detection method. Most PCR methods mentioned above can be done with any type of clinical material, including formalin-fixed, paraffin-embedded tissue and Pap-stained archival smears. The recent focus on liquid-based cytology (LBC) for cervical cancer screening has initiated numerous studies evaluating the feasibility of different HPV detection methods on cell suspensions destined for LBC, or cell suspensions remaining after LBC preparation. Some of the pros and cons of different types of clinical specimens are discussed below.

3.1. Clinical specimen types suitable for target amplification methods

3.1.1. Specimen types for PCR-based methods

PCR-based HPV DNA detection methods can generally be applied to all kinds of clinical specimens, provided the nucleic acids contained within are not heavily degraded or cross-linked and no putative PCR-inhibiting substances (e.g. organic solvents) are present. Notably, the nucleic acids in formalin-fixed, paraffin-embedded (FFPE) tissue are only amplified in a reliable manner when PCR products are generated that are smaller than 150 bp due to fixative-induced cross links [63]. On the other hand, this type of specimen generally does not contain large amounts of PCR-inhibiting substances, as demonstrated by the fact that a relatively crude extract can be used in the PCR without laborious extraction protocols [64].

As opposed to FFPE material, cervical smears collected in LBC media may show excellent preservation of cell morphology and integrity of nucleic acids. However, to achieve this preservation they usually contain relatively high amounts of organic solvents which will inhibit the PCR and need to be removed by careful extraction. An exception are smears collected in Digene Universal Collection Medium (UCM) [65,66], which can be used directly in the PCR after a simple dilution and freeze-thaw protocol (Hesselink et al., submitted).

Pap-stained archival cervical smears can also be used for PCR purposes, but they also need extraction of nucleic acids to remove remnants of dyes. In addition, the nucleic acids in this type of specimen may also be degraded due to fixation artefacts. For all above-mentioned samples, careful analysis of the nucleic acid quality is recommended to exclude false negative HPV test results due to DNA degradation and/or PCR inhibition. This can be achieved e.g. by a PCR specific for a human single-copy gene [67].

For most reliable PCR results, it is recommended to standardize the amount of input DNA in the PCR. It is self-evident that this can only be done using purified nucleic acids.

3.1.2. Specimen types for mRNA amplification methods

Until recently, hrHPV mRNA testing on cervical smears was hampered by the lack of suitable collection media. The poor RNA quality of samples collected in solutions such as PBS precluded transcription analysis. However, use of LBC is increasing and this is accompanied by the introduction of preservation media that not only safeguard cellular morphology but also the integrity of DNA and mRNA. For example, recent studies have shown that cervical smears collected in PreservCyt LBC medium are of sufficient quality for HPV RT-PCR [68] and NASBA analysis [69].

Alternatively, cervical smears could be collected in a dedicated RNA-preservation buffer [51], but in general these contain chaotropic salts such as guanidinium isothiocyanate and thus destroy cellular morphology.

When hrHPV mRNA is to be detected in cervical biopsy specimens, these should preferably be snap-frozen to guarantee mRNA integrity. However, several groups claim successful mRNA extraction from FFPE material (reviewed in [70]). Provided the use of proper quality controls, this is of course a very interesting source of material, especially for retrospective studies or in situations where snap-freezing is not an option.

3.2. Clinical specimen types suitable for signal-amplification methods

The Digene HC2 method is FDA-approved for use on cervical smears and cervical biopsies collected in Digene's Sample Transport Medium (STM). In addition, the FDA-approval of HC2 includes use on cervical smears collected in Cytyc's ThinPrep medium. However, because this medium preserves cell integrity as opposed to STM, ThinPrep smears require an additional pre-treatment to obtain full cell lysis and release of nucleic acids [71]. With some modifications of the standard protocol, HC2 can also be used on the residual material of cervical smears collected in SurePath fluid (i.e. the suspension that remains after the LBC slides have been prepared) [72–74].

An intermediate between the commercially available LBC media that preserve cell morphology but require pre-treatment steps prior to HC2, and Digene's STM that does not require pre-treatment but destroys cell morphology, is Digene Universal Collection Medium (UCM). This medium can be used for sample transport [66], does not require additional steps prior to HC2 analysis, and because it preserves cell morphology it also allows LBC [65].

4. Considerations regarding test sensitivity and specificity

4.1. Considerations for primary screening and triage

In general, the analytical sensitivities of HPV tests depend on the test system (target amplification versus signal amplification). The sensitivity of the HC2 method is approximately 5,000 copies of the HPV genome per reaction well according to the manufacturer. PCR-based techniques have a much higher analytical sensitivity than HC2, with a slight variation between the methods (reviewed in [46]). For most PCR assays, less than 100 to 1000 HPV genome equivalents in a reaction tube are sufficient to generate a positive PCR signal and to enable typing.

Despite these high analytical sensitivities, currently available hrHPV tests miss a subset of high-grade CIN lesions [75,76]. This may be due to several factors. For PCR-based methods, modification or loss of primer binding sites due to viral integration or naturally occurring sequence variants may be a problem. For HC2 where whole-genome probes are used this is generally not an issue, but then the lower analytical sensitivity of HC2 might preclude detection of lesions with low viral loads. The ideal hrHPV test used in primary screening should combine the high analytical sensitivity of PCR assays with the possibility to detect all configurations and variations of the hrHPV genome, including integrated genomes. Because the intact E6/E7 region of the hrHPV genome is necessary for cellular transformation [77] and is invariably retained upon integration [78], a PCR system detecting this region would be the method of choice [79]. It is self-evident that amplification primers should then be chosen in such a way that they cover all known HPV genomic variations.

On the other hand, a very sensitive hrHPV test consequently has a low clinical specificity, and as a primary screening tool it would result in a substantial increase in referrals for colposcopy and repeat smears. In the Dutch screening population, approximately 5.0% of the women is hrHPV DNA-positive by the GP5+/6+ system [18]. Because even women with hrHPV DNA-positive normal cytology have a 210 times greater risk to develop CIN 3 compared to women with hrHPV negative normal cytology [80], all 5.0% hrHPV DNA-positive women would need follow-up. However, only 10% of them will actually develop CIN3 [81]. This calls for additional stratification of women who have a positive hrHPV DNA test, which can be achieved for example by viral load analysis or HPV mRNA analysis (see Sections 2.1.3 and 2.1.4).

4.2. Considerations for situations not involving triage

For several research questions, clinical specificity of the hrHPV test is not an issue as it is in population-based screening and triage. Methods with high analytical sensitivity are especially suitable for studies in which any HPV infection should be detected, irrespective of its clinical relevance. Examples are epidemiological studies, and studies to determine vaccination efficacy. It is self-evident that HPV genotyping is desired in such studies.

5. Conclusions

As seen in the previous paragraphs, the aim of the study and the clinical material available will determine the choice of the HPV detection method. In general, consensus PCR followed by reverse hybridization is very sensitive and gives the most extensive typing information for many kinds of clinical specimens, including those containing multiple infections.

In general, it is to be expected that future amplification systems will become faster and more automated.

References

[1] A.T. Lorincz and R.M. Richart, Human Papillomavirus DNA Testing as an Adjunct to Cytology in Cervical Screening Programs, *Arch Pathol Lab Med* **127** (2003), 959–968.

[2] J. Cuzick, A. Szarewski, H. Cubie et al., Management of women who test positive for high-risk types of human papillomavirus: the HART study, *Lancet* **362** (2003), 1871–1876.

[3] A.G. Bais, M. Rebolj, P.J. Snijders et al., Triage using HPV-testing in persistent borderline and mildly dyskaryotic smears: Proposal for new guidelines, *Int J Cancer* **116** (2005), 122–129.

[4] G.D. Zielinski, A.G. Bais, T.J. Helmerhorst et al., HPV testing and monitoring of women after treatment of CIN 3: review of the literature and meta-analysis, *Obstet Gynecol Surv* **59** (2004), 543–553.

[5] M. Scheffner, B.A. Werness, J.M. Huibregtse, A.J. Levine and P.M. Howley, The E6 oncoprotein encoded by human papillomavirus types 16 and 18 promotes the degradation of p53, *Cell* **63** (1990), 1129–1136.

[6] N. Dyson, P.M. Howley, K. Munger and E. Harlow, The human papilloma virus-16 E7 oncoprotein is able to bind to the retinoblastoma gene product, *Science* **243** (1989), 934–937.

[7] F.X. Bosch, A. Lorincz, N. Munoz, C.J. Meijer and K.V. Shah, The causal relation between human papillomavirus and cervical cancer, *J Clin Pathol* **55** (2002), 244–265.

[8] N. Munoz, F.X. Bosch, S. de Sanjose et al., Epidemiologic classification of human papillomavirus types associated with cervical cancer, *N Engl J Med* **348** (2003), 518–527.

[9] E.M. de Villiers, C. Fauquet, T.R. Broker, H.U. Bernard and H. zur Hausen, Classification of papillomaviruses, *Virology* **324** (2004), 17–27.

[10] B.A. Werness, A.J. Levine and P.M. Howley, Association of human papillomavirus types 16 and 18 E6 proteins with p53, *Science* **248** (1990), 76–79.

[11] J.R. Gage, C. Meyers and F.O. Wettstein, The E7 proteins of the nononcogenic human papillomavirus type 6b (HPV-6b) and of the oncogenic HPV-16 differ in retinoblastoma protein binding and other properties, *J Virol* **64** (1990), 723–730.

[12] Y. Kirii and T. Matsukura, Nucleotide sequence and phylogenetic classification of human papillomavirus type 67, *Virus Genes* **17** (1998), 117–121.

[13] N. Munoz, F.X. Bosch, X. Castellsague et al., Against which human papillomavirus types shall we vaccinate and screen? The international perspective, *Int J Cancer* **111** (2004), 278–285.

[14] M. Schiffman, M.J. Khan, D. Solomon et al., A study of the impact of adding HPV types to cervical cancer screening and triage tests, *J Natl Cancer Inst* **97** (2005), 147–150.

[15] D.A. Galloway, Papillomavirus vaccines in clinical trials, *Lancet Infect Dis* **3** (2003), 469–475.

[16] A.H. Beskow, M. Moberg and U.B. Gyllensten, HLA class II allele control of HPV load in carcinoma in situ of the cervix uteri, *Int J Cancer* **117** (2005), 510–514.

[17] A.H. Beskow and U.B. Gyllensten, Host genetic control of HPV 16 titer in carcinoma in situ of the cervix uteri, *Int J Cancer* **101** (2002), 526–531.

[18] N.W.J. Bulkmans, L. Rozendaal, P.J. Snijders et al., POBASCAM, a population-based randomised controlled trial for implementation of high-risk HPV testing in cervical screening; Design, methods and baseline data of 44,102 women, *Int J Cancer* **110** (2003), 94–101.

[19] N.W. Bulkmans, M.C. Bleeker, J. Berkhof et al., Prevalence of types 16 and 33 is increased in high-risk human papillomavirus positive women with cervical intraepithelial neoplasia grade 2 or worse, *Int J Cancer* **117** (2005), 177–181.

[20] S. Bulk, J. Berkhof, N.W. Bulkmans et al., Preferential risk of HPV16 for squamous cell carcinoma and of HPV18 for adenocarcinoma of the cervix compared to women with normal cytology in The Netherlands, *Br J Cancer* **94** (2006), 171–175.

[21] M.J. Khan, P.E. Castle, A.T. Lorincz et al., The elevated 10-year risk of cervical precancer and cancer in women with human papillomavirus (HPV) type 16 or 18 and the possible utility of type-specific HPV testing in clinical practice, *J Natl Cancer Inst* **97** (2005), 1072–1079.

[22] P.E. Castle, D. Solomon, M. Schiffman and C.M. Wheeler, Human papillomavirus type 16 infections and 2-year absolute risk of cervical precancer in women with equivocal or mild cytologic abnormalities, *J Natl Cancer Inst* **97** (2005), 1066–1071.

[23] P.E. Gravitt, C.L. Peyton, R.J. Apple and C.M. Wheeler, Genotyping of 27 human papillomavirus types by using L1 consensus PCR products by a single-hybridization, reverse line blot detection method, *J Clin Microbiol* **36** (1998), 3020–3027.

[24] L.M. Tieben, J. ter Schegget, R.P. Minnaar et al., Detection of cutaneous and genital HPV types in clinical samples by PCR using consensus primers, *J Virol Methods* **42** (1993), 265–279.

[25] A.J. van den Brule, R. Pol, N. Fransen-Daalmeijer et al., GP5+/6+ PCR followed by reverse line blot analysis enables rapid and high-throughput identification of human papillomavirus genotypes, *J Clin Microbiol* **40** (2002), 779–787.

[26] L. Gregoire, M. Arella, J. Campione-Piccardo and W.D. Lancaster, Amplification of human papillomavirus DNA sequences by using conserved primers, *J Clin Microbiol* **27** (1989), 2660–2665.

[27] B. Kleter, L.J. van Doorn, L. Schrauwen et al., Development and clinical evaluation of a highly sensitive PCR-reverse hybridization line probe assay for detection and identification of anogenital human papillomavirus, *J Clin Microbiol* **37** (1999), 2508–2517.

[28] P.E. Gravitt, C.L. Peyton, T.Q. Alessi et al., Improved amplification of genital human papillomaviruses, *J Clin Microbiol* **38** (2000), 357–361.

[29] J. Monsonego, J.M. Bohbot, G. Pollini et al., Performance of the Roche AMPLICOR human papillomavirus (HPV) test in prediction of cervical intraepithelial neoplasia (CIN) in women with abnormal PAP smear, *Gynecol Oncol* **99** (2005), 160–168.

[30] M.V. Jacobs, P.J. Snijders, A.J. van den Brule et al., A general primer GP5+/GP6(+)-mediated PCR-enzyme immunoassay method for rapid detection of 14 high-risk and 6 low-risk human papillomavirus genotypes in cervical scrapings, *J Clin Microbiol* **35** (1997), 791–795.

[31] B. Kleter, L.J. van Doorn, J. ter Schegget et al., Novel short-fragment PCR assay for highly sensitive broad-spectrum detection of anogenital human papillomaviruses, *Am J Pathol* **153** (1998), 1731–1739.

[32] N.H. Cho, H.J. An, J.K. Jeong et al., Genotyping of 22 human papillomavirus types by DNA chip in Korean women: comparison with cytologic diagnosis, *Am J Obstet Gynecol* **188** (2003), 56–62.

[33] M. Schmitt, I.G. Bravo, P.J. Snijders et al., Bead-based multiplex genotyping of human papillomaviruses, *J Clin Microbiol* **44** (2006), 504–512.

[34] O. Forslund, A. Antonsson, P. Nordin, B. Stenquist and B.G. Hansson, A broad range of human papillomavirus types detected with a general PCR method suitable for analysis of cutaneous tumours and normal skin, *J Gen Virol* **80**(Pt 9) (1999), 2437–2443.

[35] V. Shamanin, M. Glover, C. Rausch et al., Specific types of human papillomavirus found in benign proliferations and carcinomas of the skin in immunosuppressed patients, *Cancer Res* **54** (1994), 4610–4613.

[36] O. Lungu, T.C. Wright Jr. and S. Silverstein, Typing of human papillomaviruses by polymerase chain reaction amplification with L1 consensus primers and RFLP analysis, *Mol Cell Probes* **6** (1992), 145–152.

[37] K. Szuhai, E. Sandhaus, S.M. Kolkman-Uljee et al., A novel strategy for HPV detection and genotyping with SybrGreen and Molecular Beacon PCR, *Am J Pathol* **159** (2001), 1651–1660.

[38] J.M. Walboomers, M.V. Jacobs, M.M. Manos et al., Human papillomavirus is a necessary cause of invasive cervical cancer worldwide, *J Pathol* **189** (1999), 12–19.

[39] A. Josefsson, K. Livak and U. Gyllensten, Detection and quantitation of human papillomavirus by using the fluorescent 5' exonuclease assay, *J Clin Microbiol* **37** (1999), 490–496.

[40] A.T. Hesselink, A.J. van den Brule, Z.M. Groothuismink et al., Comparison of three different PCR methods for quantifying human papillomavirus type 16 DNA in cervical scrape specimens, *J Clin Microbiol* **43** (2005), 4868–4871.

[41] M. Moberg, I. Gustavsson and U. Gyllensten, Real-time PCR-based system for simultaneous quantification of human papillomavirus types associated with high risk of cervical cancer, *J Clin Microbiol* **41** (2003), 3221–3228.

[42] A.M. Josefsson, P.K. Magnusson, N. Ylitalo et al., Viral load of human papilloma virus 16 as a determinant for development of cervical carcinoma in situ: a nested case-control study, *Lancet* **355** (2000), 2189–2193.

[43] N. Ylitalo, P. Sorensen, A.M. Josefsson et al., Consistent high viral load of human papillomavirus 16 and risk of cervical carcinoma in situ: a nested case-control study, *Lancet* **355** (2000), 2194–2198.

[44] M. van Duin, P.J. Snijders, H.F. Schrijnemakers et al., Human papillomavirus 16 load in normal and abnormal cervical scrapes: an indicator of CIN II/III and viral clearance, *Int J Cancer* **98** (2002), 590–595.

[45] P.J. Snijders, C.J. Hogewoning, A.T. Hesselink et al., Determination of viral load thresholds in cervical scrapings to rule out CIN 3 in HPV 16, 18, 31 and 33-positive women with normal cytology, *Int J Cancer* (2006).
[46] P.J. Snijders, A.J. van den Brule and C.J. Meijer, The clinical relevance of human papillomavirus testing: relationship between analytical and clinical sensitivity, *J Pathol* **201** (2003), 1–6.
[47] K. Sotlar, A. Stubner, D. Diemer et al., Detection of high-risk human papillomavirus E6 and E7 oncogene transcripts in cervical scrapes by nested RT-polymerase chain reaction, *J Med Virol* **74** (2004), 107–116.
[48] H.L. Smits, B. van Gemen, R. Schukkink et al., Application of the NASBA nucleic acid amplification method for the detection of human papillomavirus type 16 E6-E7 transcripts, *J Virol Methods* **54** (1995), 75–81.
[49] K.S. Cuschieri, M.J. Whitley and H.A. Cubie, Human papillomavirus type specific DNA and RNA persistence-implications for cervical disease progression and monitoring, *J Med Virol* **73** (2004), 65–70.
[50] I. Kraus, T. Molden, L.E. Erno et al., Human papillomavirus oncogenic expression in the dysplastic portio; an investigation of biopsies from 190 cervical cones, *Br J Cancer* **90** (2004), 1407–1413.
[51] T. Molden, I. Kraus, F. Karlsen et al., Comparison of human papillomavirus messenger RNA and DNA detection: a cross-sectional study of 4,136 women $>$ 30 years of age with a 2-year follow-up of high-grade squamous intraepithelial lesion, *Cancer Epidemiol Biomarkers Prev* **14** (2005), 367–372.
[52] T. Molden, J.F. Nygard, I. Kraus et al., Predicting CIN2+ when detecting HPV mRNA and DNA by PreTect HPV-proofer and consensus PCR: A 2-year follow-up of women with ASCUS or LSIL Pap smear, *Int J Cancer* **114** (2005), 973–976.
[53] T. Molden, I. Kraus, F. Karlsen, H. Skomedal and B. Hagmar, Human papillomavirus E6/E7 mRNA expression in women younger than 30 years of age, *Gynecol Oncol* **100** (2005), 95–100.
[54] R. Klaes, S.M. Woerner, R. Ridder et al., Detection of high-risk cervical intraepithelial neoplasia and cervical cancer by amplification of transcripts derived from integrated papillomavirus oncogenes, *Cancer Res* **59** (1999), 6132–6136.
[55] N. Wentzensen, R. Ridder, R. Klaes et al., Characterization of viral-cellular fusion transcripts in a large series of HPV16 and 18 positive anogenital lesions, *Oncogene* **21** (2002), 419–426.
[56] S. Vinokurova, N. Wentzensen, J. Einenkel et al., Clonal history of papillomavirus-induced dysplasia in the female lower genital tract, *J Natl Cancer Inst* **97** (2005), 1816–1821.
[57] C. Clavel, M. Masure, I. Putaud et al., Hybrid capture II, a new sensitive test for human papillomavirus detection. Comparison with hybrid capture I and PCR results in cervical lesions, *J Clin Pathol* **51** (1998), 737–740.
[58] P.E. Castle, M. Schiffman, R.D. Burk et al., Restricted cross-reactivity of hybrid capture 2 with nononcogenic human papillomavirus types, *Cancer Epidemiol Biomarkers Prev* **11** (2002), 1394–1399.
[59] M.N. Qureshi, R.D. Rudelli, R.R. Tubbs, C.V. Biscotti and L.J. Layfield, Role of HPV DNA testing in predicting cervical intraepithelial lesions: comparison of HC HPV and ISH HPV, *Diagn Cytopathol* **29** (2003), 149–155.
[60] A.T. Hesselink, A.J. van den Brule, A.A. Brink et al., Comparison of hybrid capture 2 with in situ hybridization for the detection of high-risk human papillomavirus in liquid-based cervical samples, *Cancer* **102** (2004), 11–18.
[61] A.H. Hopman, F. Smedts, W. Dignef et al., Transition of high-grade cervical intraepithelial neoplasia to micro-invasive carcinoma is characterized by integration of HPV 16/18 and numerical chromosome abnormalities, *J Pathol* **202** (2004), 23–33.
[62] H.M. Kerstens, P.J. Poddighe and A.G. Hanselaar, A novel in situ hybridization signal amplification method based on the deposition of biotinylated tyramine, *J Histochem Cytochem* **43** (1995), 347–352.
[63] C.C. Impraim, R.K. Saiki, H.A. Erlich and R.L. Teplitz, Analysis of DNA extracted from formalin-fixed, paraffin-embedded tissues by enzymatic amplification and hybridization with sequence-specific oligonucleotides, *Biochem Biophys Res Commun* **142** (1987), 710–716.
[64] R.J. Slebos, L. Boerrigter, S.G. Evers et al., A rapid and simple procedure for the routine detection of ras point mutations in formalin-fixed, paraffin-embedded tissues, *Diagn Mol Pathol* **1** (1992), 136–141.
[65] Mattosinho de Castro Ferraz Mda, S.M. Nicolau, J.N. Stavale et al., Cervical biopsy-based comparison of a new liquid-based thin-layer preparation with conventional Pap smears, *Diagn Cytopathol* **30** (2004), 220–226.
[66] N.S. Taha, J. Focchi, J.C. Ribalta et al., Universal Collection Medium (UCM)® is as suitable as the Standard Transport Medium (STM)® for Hybrid Capture II® (HC-2) assay, *J Clin Virol* **36** (2006), 32–35.
[67] A.M. de Roda Husman, P.J. Snijders, H.V. Stel et al., Processing of long-stored archival cervical smears for human papillomavirus detection by the polymerase chain reaction, *Br J Cancer* **72** (1995), 412–417.
[68] T.A. Tarkowski, M.S. Rajeevan, D.R. Lee and E.R. Unger, Improved detection of viral RNA isolated from liquid-based cytology samples, *Mol Diagn* **6** (2001), 125–130.
[69] A.K. Lie, B. Risberg, B. Borge et al., DNA- versus RNA-based methods for human papillomavirus detection in cervical neoplasia, *Gynecol Oncol* **97** (2005), 908–915.
[70] F. Lewis, N.J. Maughan, V. Smith, K. Hillan and P. Quirke, Unlocking the archive – gene expression in paraffin-embedded tissue, *J Pathol* **195** (2001), 66–71.
[71] Digene Hybrid Capture 2 high-risk HPV DNA test – part 3 (Labelling). http://www.fda.gov/cdrh/pdf/P890064s009c.pdf, 2006.
[72] M.N. Qureshi, D. Bolick, P.J. Ringer, F.L. Spagler and G. Zimmerman, HPV testing in liquid cytology specimens: comparison of analytic sensitivty and specificity for in situ hybridization and chemiluminescent nucleic acid testing, *Acta Cytol* **49** (2005), 120–126.
[73] P. Vassilakos, P. Petignat, M. Boulvain and A. Campana, Primary screening for cervical cancer precursors by the combined use of liquid-based cytology, computer-assisted cytology and HPV DNA testing, *Br J Cancer* **86** (2002), 382–388.
[74] S. Davis-Devine, S.J. Day and G.G. Freund, Test performance comparison of inform HPV and hybrid capture 2 high-risk HPV DNA tests using the SurePath liquid-based Pap test as the collection method, *Am J Clin Pathol* **124** (2005), 24–30.
[75] G.D. Zielinski, L. Rozendaal, F.J. Voorhorst et al., HPV testing can reduce the number of follow-up visits in women treated for cervical intraepithelial neoplasia grade 3, *Gynecol Oncol* **91** (2003), 67–73.
[76] M.A. Nobbenhuis, C.J. Meijer, A.J. van den Brule et al., Addition of high-risk HPV testing improves the current guidelines on follow-up after treatment for cervical intraepithelial neoplasia, *Br J Cancer* **84** (2001), 796–801.

[77] P. Hawley-Nelson, K.H. Vousden, N.L. Hubbert, D.R. Lowy and J.T. Schiller, HPV16 E6 and E7 proteins cooperate to immortalize human foreskin keratinocytes, *EMBO J* **8** (1989), 3905–3910.

[78] K.B. Choo, C.C. Pan and S.H. Han, Integration of human papillomavirus type 16 into cellular DNA of cervical carcinoma: preferential deletion of the E2 gene and invariable retention of the long control region and the E6/E7 open reading frames, *Virology* **161** (1987), 259–261.

[79] A.T. Hesselink, M. Lettink, J. Berkhof, C.J. Meijer and P.J. Snijders, Comparison of a novel consensus high-risk HPV E7 PCR with GP5+/6+ PCR on cervical scrapings. 2006. 6th International Multidisciplinary Congress on Human Papillomavirus Infection and Global Prevention of Cervical Cancer – EUROGIN. Monsonego, J. 23-4-2006.

[80] L. Rozendaal, J. Westerga, J.C. van der Linden et al., PCR based high risk HPV testing is superior to neural network based screening for predicting incident CIN III in women with normal cytology and borderline changes, *J Clin Pathol* **53** (2000), 606–611.

[81] L. Rozendaal, J.M. Walboomers, J.C. van der Linden et al., PCR-based high-risk HPV test in cervical cancer screening gives objective risk assessment of women with cytomorphologically normal cervical smears, *Int J Cancer* **68** (1996), 766–769.

Disease Markers 23 (2007) 283–296
IOS Press

International standard reagents for HPV detection[1]

Sonia R. Pagliusi[a,*] and Suzanne M. Garland[b,c]
[a]*Department of Immunizations, Vaccines and Biologicals, World Health Organization, Av Appia 20, 1211 Geneva 27, Switzerland*
[b]*Department of Microbiology and Infectious Diseases, The Royal Women's Hospital, 132 Grattan Street, Melbourne, Vic., Australia*
[c]*Department of Obstetrics and Gynaecology, University of Melbourne, Vic., Australia*

Abstract. Humam papillomavirus is the commonest genital viral infection in healthy sexually active subjects, and the presence of chronic or persistent HPV types in genital cells may constitute a prognostic marker of underlying, or predict future HPV-associated diseases. A variety of novel tests for detecting the presence of oncogenic HPV types in biological specimens have been reported. These are based on the various stages of infection and viral life cycle. HPV infects squamous epithelium with expression of various gene products intimately linked to epithelial cell differentiation. Hence, there are basically three classes of detectable markers directly derived from HPVs: molecular markers based on detection of nucleic acid sequences, serological markers based on detection of antibodies against viral proteins, and cellular markers based on detection of proteins expressed intracellularly, upon either infection or carcinogenesis. The nature of various assays and the development of international standard reagents for qualitative and quantitative assessment of assay performance are outlined. There is an increasing demand to develop standard tools to assess the quality of HPV detection systems, for regulatory and clinical management purposes. International standard reagents for HPV will help defining the analytical sensitivity and specificity of various detection methods, and will allow assuring that laboratory services used to evaluate disease burden, HPV vaccines, and cancer prevention strategies are accurate and comparable worldwide. The advancement of prophylactic vaccine candidates against HPV infections and related diseases stresses the increasing importance of HPV assays in monitoring the impact of HPV vaccination on disease burden.

Keywords: Papillomavirus, cervical cancer, diagnostic, genital infection, hybridization, PCR, serology, vaccine

1. Introduction

Papillomaviruses are a large family of non-enveloped DNA viruses that within the animal kingdom cause a variety of epithelial lesions, ranging from benign warts to invasive cancers. Of the known human papilomaviruses (HPV) associated cancers [19], cancer of the uterine cervix accounts for 90%, whilst other anothenital cancers (vulvae, vagina, penis, anus) for 5%, with cancers of head and neck corresponding to about 1% [44].

Over the past decades, prevention programmes for cancer of the cervix have been essentially based on the detection and treatment of precursor lesions (high-grade cervical dysplasia) or early cancer by screening women at risk using the cytological method described by Papanicolau, otherwise known as the "Pap smear" [43]. Despite great progress in cancer control through such cervical cytology screening programmes, high coverage and quality control and assurance are crucial in achieving significant reduction in disease burden [13]. However in low resource countries appropriate resources and continuous quality assurance programmes are not always available. In addition, it is recognized that the traditional Pap smear tests can give

[1]The authors only are responsible for the contents of the publication.

*Corresponding author: Dr Sonia R. Pagliusi, Immunization, Vaccines and Biologicals, Family and Community Health, World Health Organization, Avenue Appia 20, 1211 Geneva 27, Switzerland. Tel.: +41 22 791 4265; Fax: +41 22 791 4860; E-mail: pagliusi@who.int.

ISSN 0278-0240/07/$17.00

both false positive as well as false negative results in the screening for precursor lesions and/or cancer. Hence, the scientific community has been actively in search of effective technologies to complement and improve cytology based cervical screening programs.

The causal relationship between HPV infections and cancer of the uterine cervix was first suggested in the 1970's [16], and comprehensively confirmed later, in finding that virtually all cases studied worldwide have at least one of 15 high risk oncogenic types of HPV [63]. Hence, the presence of oncogenic HPV types in cervical epithelium, is recognized as a necessary cause for triggering cancer of the cervix in women. That is, women will not develop cancer of the cervix without a pre-existing infection with the oncogenic HPVs. The corollary however it is not true, as cancer is a rare outcome of this very common viral infection. Indeed the majority of HPV infections are transient, being cleared by immune surveillance usually within one or two years [18]. HPV was also being identified as the aetiological agent of other cancers, namely 70% of anal cancers, 50% of vaginal cancers, and about 25% of head and neck squamous cell carcinomas (HNSCC) contain HPV DNA, mostly type 16 [54].

The natural history of HPV infection is such that the lifetime risk for development of cervical cancer without involvement of any screening programme is in the order of 3% and with annual Pap smears, less than 1%. The success of screening programmes relates in part from the fact that cervical cancer takes several decades to develop from chronic oncogenic HPV infection [1]. Although HPV is the commonest genital viral infection in healthy sexually active subjects, the presence of persistent oncogenic HPV types in tissue samples may constitute a prognostic marker of underlying or predict disease in the future. The corollary however is not true; the presence of HPV DNA alone does not necessarily imply underlying disease.

1.1. Background on the cell biology of HPV

HPV infects squamous epithelium with expression of various gene products intimately linked to epithelial cell differentiation. HPV infection does not cause a systemic infection; it does not kill the keratinocyte and it induces no or a poor, slow, local inflammatory response. Humoral immunity does not appear to be as important as cell-mediated immunity in clearing HPV infection, but rather is important in protecting an individual from becoming infected. Of note, in natural infection, only around 50% of those becoming HPV DNA positive show a systemic neutralizing antibody response. The remainder of individuals clear infection without developing a measurable antibody response [2].

Following infection of basal epithelial cells, the viral genome is maintained as a low-copy number episome in cells of the basal and parabasal layers and is amplified as the infected cell differentiates and migrates towards the epithelial surface. It is only in the most superficial layers of the epithelium, that late genes coding for viral capsid proteins (L1 and L2) are expressed and the amplified genomes then packaged into infectious virions, with release at the epithelial surface during cellular desquamation [32]. It is because of this complex interaction, that HPV cannot be propagated *in vitro* in cell lines, as many other viruses that are cultured for diagnostic purposes. However viral nucleic acid can be detected as episomal genomes by various molecular hybridization assays. It appears from some studies that a productively infected cell expresses early viral proteins E4, E6, E7 during its migration from the basal layer to the epithelial surface [35]. Expression of the major capsid protein L1 appears to follow expression of E4, and is detectable in cells approaching the epithelial surface. During the progression from productive infection to cellular transformation leading to cervical cancer, the viral DNA becomes integrated into the host cell genome (often with large deletions in the L1gene), and loses the ability to produce infectious virions. Productive HPV infection is manifest as changes cytologically /histologically identified as epithelial lesions. If cell mediated immunity fails to induce lesion regression and viral clearance, then persistent infection may result. In low-grade cervical intraepithelial neoplastic (CIN1) lesions all early proteins are expressed, the lesions are genetically stable and regress in around 60% of cases within time, with an appropriate host immune response (median duration of CIN1/LSIL is 6 months), or do remain unchanged for years [42]. In many high-grade cervical intraepithelial neoplastic lesions (CIN 2 and 3) and in cancers however, viral gene expression is dysregulated, with constitutive expression of the early oncogenes E6 and E7 essential for progression to, and maintenance of malignancy. The histological changes from normal epithelium to cervical intraepithelial neoplasias [CIN] grade 1 to 3, following HPV infection, is schematically shown in the cartoon (Fig. 1).

With this knowledge, novel diagnostic tools for detecting the presence of oncogenic HPV DNA or the effects in cervical samples, have been intensively studied. There are basically three classes of detectable markers directly deriving from HPV viruses: Molecular mark-

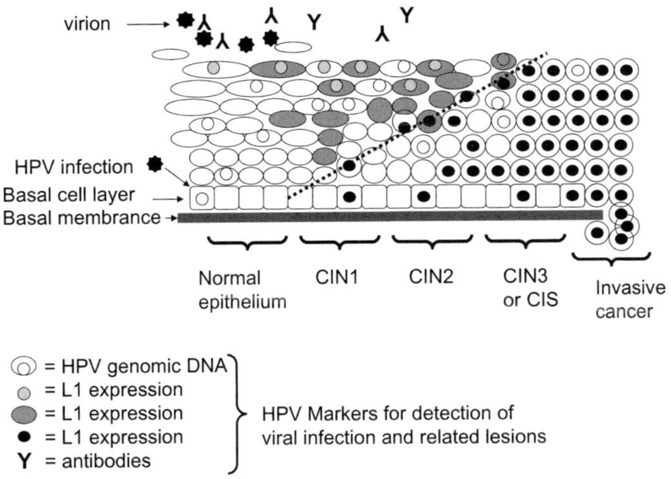

Fig. 1. Schematic representation ofhistological changes followingHPV infection and carcinogenesis. Oncogenic HPV types initiate a productive infection in the basal cells, with detectable expression ofviral DNA, E4,E7, proteins, and L1 expression and virion production and release in the superficial cell layers. E4/L1 expressingcells form low grade lesions. Over time, integrated viral genes express oncoproteins (E6/7) leading to uncontrolled cell growth, to form high grade lesions and invasion.

ers based on detection of viral nucleic acid sequences, serological markers based on immunological responses such as antibodies, and host cellular markers based on proteins expressed upon infection and during oncogenesis. The nature of various assays to detect these three distinct markers of HPV infections and related diseases, their standardization, and potential applications are outlined below.

Because carcinogenesis is triggered by this infectious agent, it has been possible to develop prophylactic vaccine candidates to prevent infection, its related diseases, especially life-threatening cancers [12]. The prophylactic HPV vaccines may have implications not only in the prevention of cancer of the cervix, but also of a substantial fraction of other ano-genital cancers, and potentially head and neck squamous cell carcinomas [45]. The applications of HPV detection methods with respect to vaccines evaluation is discussed below.

Regression of lesions is accompanied by a CD4 T cell dependent delayed type hypersensitivity response. Cell mediated assays are currently used for assessment of HPV induced immune responses upon infections, disease, and vaccination. The methods include mostly proliferation assays, cytokine release assays (ELISPOT or cell culture supernatant), and *in vivo* delayed type hypersensitivity (DTH) assays. Given the many clinical trials assessing therapeutic effects of vaccination with HPV antigens, it would be desirable to have standard reagents for use in assays determining cell-mediated responses. It was suggested to develop and evaluate standard positive control reagents (substrates) for cell-mediated immunity assays [70]. However, we will focus here only on markers specific and directly derived from HPV-expressed molecules. T-cell based assays may not be appropriate for characterization of prophylactic vaccine responses.

1.2. HPV detection methods and standard reagents

Clinical diagnostic is characterized by the application of methods to a clinical activity, allowing clinicians to extract valuable information from biological samples submitted for various assays and to make a definitive diagnosis. For this purpose available tests need to be validated, i.e. determine their capacity to correctly classify an individual within his/her health/disease status.

International standard reagents may assist in the qualitative and quantitative assessment of diagnostic tests, to evaluate the performance and the clinical benefit of various detection methods. Since 1950 the World Health Organization (WHO), as part of its constitutional mandate, develops international standards for a wide range of biological substances used for medical purposes. Over the past years, WHO has worked with the scientific community, national regulatory authorities, other standards-setting bodies, and users, through a series of consultations to review the scientific basis of biological products, and develop reference materials or reagents. The published catalogue of WHO biological reference materials includes todate over 300 materials (a list can be found at www.who.int/biologicals). Recently, efforts were directed towards developing specific standard reagents to detect HPV viral genes, their expressed proteins, or their elicited antibody responses [60].

An international standard reagent is a preparation to which an international unit of activity has been assigned, that is traceable to a defined part of the content of an ampoule. International standards must fulfill several criteria, including demonstrating consistent performance, demonstrating long-term stability under selected storage conditions, and being able to perform in a variety of detection assays. Such standards are intended to make estimations of concentration of molecules or potency, of an appropriate test sample, by direct comparison in suitable biological test systems.

2. HPV DNA detection methods, standards and applications

HPV DNA can be detected in biological material containing infected epithelial cells, mostly derived from scrapes from the ectocervix or other genital tract epithelial sites. In laboratory based measurements of HPV DNA we need to distinguish analytical sensitivity and specificity from clinical sensitivity and specificity. The term *analytical* sensitivity refers to the number of HPV-viral genomes that are identified in a sample by a given test or assay, expressed as a given virus amount of analyte or molecules, whereas analytical specificity refers to the genotypes of HPV that are correctly identified by a test result. In contrast, the *clinical* sensitivity refers to the proportion of women with disease, identified by a positive test result, whereas clinical specificity indicates the proportion of positive results that correlate to underlying disease [59]. Here we will discuss mostly the analytical sensitivity and specificity of methods, rather than their clinical aspects.

2.1. Methods of HPV DNA detection: Hybrid capture and amplification

Currently two types of amplification assays are used in determining HPV DNA. One is a target amplification , polymerase chain reaction (PCR) and the other signal amplification following DNA and RNA hybridization and detection by Hybrid Capture 2 (HC2), (Digene Corporation, Gaithersburg, Maryland, USA) [31].

The HC 2 test is the only FDA approved test so far and is used to show the presence or absence of HPV DNA in exfoliated cells from a woman's cervix, usually obtained by gently scraping the surface of the cervix. This assay is based on the principle that HPV DNA isolated from biological specimens, hybridizes in solution with long synthetic RNA probes complementary to the genomic sequences of specific HPV types. The test is currently provided as two available RNA-probe mixtures containing either five low risk (LR) types (6, 11, 42, 43, 44) or 13 high risk (HR) types (16, 18, 31, 33, 35, 39, 45, 51, 52, 56, 58, 59 and 68). To reduce time and cost, most laboratories only use the HR probe mixture, being the relevant probe mix for clinical management. The HC2 provides a semi-quantitative measure of viral load, as measured by the intensity of emitted light, which is proportional to the amount of target DNA present in the specimen. The relative analytical sensitivity of the assay is equivalent to 1 pg of HPV DNA (5000 copies of HPV genome), although the HR probe cocktail may cross-react with HPVs not in the probe mixture (i.e. types 53, 66, 67, 73). Anything below that level indicates either the absence of HPV or HPV-amounts are below the detection level. A new rapid test under development by Digene detects HPV DNA, and processes 10–20 samples in one batch within two hours. The sensitivity of this test is comparable to the currently available HC 2. A chemiluminescent substrate is used and signal output can be read by a Luminometer readout at a central laboratory, and may be relevant for use in field conditions, health enters or clinical practice.

PCR is a selective amplification assay, increasing exponentially and reproducibly the target HPV sequences present in biological specimens, and theoretically capable of producing one billion copies from a single double stranded DNA molecule, following 30 cycles of amplification. The sensitivity and specificity of PCR-based methods can vary, depending on the primer sets chosen, the size of the PCR product, reaction conditions and performance of the polymerase enzymes used in the reaction, the spectrum of HPV DNA amplified and ability to detect multiple types [20]. Most primer sets used for HPV-PCR are designed to target the L1 gene, but primers targeting the oncogenes E6 and E7 have also been used in clinical studies [28]. The choice of the viral genomic sequences used for PCR has implications for analytical sensitivity, and hence HPV screening strategies in the clinical diagnosis and management of cervical cancer. Generally, the analytical sensitivity of PCR based methods is higher than hybridization assays only. Most accurate PCR methods can detect the equivalent of 1-10 copies of viral genome per reaction, although the results achieved using the same methods can vary depending on factors intrinsic to laboratory individual performance, which may be linked to handling of samples and reagents [47]. Following PCR, distinction of HPV types can be achieved by sequencing or hybridization with type-specific oligonucleotide probes using various detection methods, including dot blot, microtitre plate, reverse line blot strip and microchip formats.

Recently, Roche Diagnostics (Indianapolis, IN, USA) have developed an HPV ELISA based AMPLICOR HPV kit with CE marking ("Conformité Européene") for *in-vitro* diagnostics and is the first commercially available PCR-based test for the detection of HPV. This new test, identifies the same13 high-risk genotypes of HPV as the HC2 test, and will allow diagnostic laboratories to detect HPV DNA by PCR, although not to discriminate genotypes [36]. The "Linear array®" assay, also developed by Roche, allows detection of 37 different HPV genotypes. It detects amplified type specific HPV DNA with oligonucleotides immobilized onto a nylon membrane, an easy to perform detection method. The advantages of this method are speed, with a turn around time of 1 day, plus ease in interpreting individual and/or multiple genotypes, yet without requiring expensive, specialized instrumentation [27].

The development of a quantitative and sensitive hightroughput procedure for the identification of multiple high and low-risk genital HPV genotypes in a single reaction has been recently reported as multiplex papillomavirus genotyping (MPG) [53]. MPG is based on the amplification of HVP DNA by a general primer PCR (GP5+/6+) and the subsequent detection of the products with type-specific oligoucleotide probes coupled to fluorescence-labeled polystyrene beads (luminex suspension array technology). Theoretically, MPG can detect up to 100 different HPV types simultaneously, and appears to be suitable for large scale epidemiological studies and vaccination trials, as well as for routine diagnostic purposes, though it remains to be validated.

A novel HPV oligonucleotide microarray has been developed (Biomedlab, Seoul, Korea), which allows for detection of 22 HPV types using an aldehydederivatized slide glass. PCR products are generated in the presence of fluorescein-tagged nucleotides and hybridized onto the chip and scanned by laser fluorescence, thus able to detect multiple infections with one hybridization step [55]. Ideally, a larger number of HPV type-specific oligonucleotides could be spotted on the Chip, although this method requires the presence of expensive equipment and may not be suitable for many laboratories. Utility of real-time and quantitative PCR in detection of HPV has also been investigated in a number of studies and can provide tools for ready quantitation of various HPV genotypes in specimens [22].

A test for identification of mRNA encoding HPV oncogenes (PreTect HPV-Proofer, Norchip, Norway) intended for diagnostic purposes has been described [30]. E6/E7 mRNA will be present when the virus is actively transcribing and producing oncogene proteins, thus the test is designed to detect RNAs from the E6 and E7 region of the viral genome. Larger scale, population based studies are necessary to evaluate the predictive values of this HPV test.

Finally, a protocol for the amplification of papillomavirus oncogene transcripts (APOT) from cervical specimens has been proposed that allows the distinction of episomal from integrated HPV mRNAs [26]. In most cervical carcinomas, human papillomavirus (HPV) genomes are integrated into host cell chromosomes, such that transcribed mRNAs encompass viral and cellular sequences. In contrast, in early preneoplastic lesions, HPV genomes persist as episomes, and derived transcripts contain exclusively viral sequences. Thus, detection of integrated-derived HPV transcripts in cervical swabs or biopsy specimens by the APOT assay points to advanced dysplasia or invasive cervical cancer. However, because the assay is based on RT-PCR protocols, sequencing steps, and is type specific it has not been adapted readily to use in the routine diagnostic testing.

With a variety of assays for HPV DNA detection, and new and improved methodologies under way, there is increasing demand to standardize the measurement tools to assess the performance of molecular tests and methodologies, for both regulatory and clinical management purposes.

2.2. *Standards for HPV DNA reagents*

The goal of accurate detection of infectious agents is to provide consistent and meaningful results in the research and clinical setting to help target and focus resources in disease prevention and control. An intrinsic part of using such technology should be the use of well-characterized standards. To assess the quality of molecular detection methods, international standard reagents are already widely used for several other viruses including hepatitis A, B, and C and human immunodeficiency virus (HIV) [21,49,51]. Ideally standard reagents should mimic properties of biological samples under measurement and, allow evaluation of the full laboratory sample processing procedures. It would be desirable that HPV DNA standards should contain full HPV genomes to allow identification of any genomic region to be targeted in detection assays, and should be presented in a human genomic background.

Historically, international standards in the form of nucleic acids have been isolated from pools of biological material infected with the virus of interest [71]. As HPV is not a plasma derived virus, there is no such abundant source of biological material to generate HPV DNA standard reagents. Epithelial cells derived from cervical scrapes or small genital biopsy specimens, obtained for diagnosis, provide only low numbers of HPV genomes and often harbor multiple HPV types.

Therefore recombinant plasmids representing double-stranded full genomic, cloned DNA sequences of HPV types were proposed as standards for HPV detection [69]. Such material is renewable and hence readily available. An international collaborative study demonstrated the feasibility of this approach using a variety of HPV DNA detection assays, and the results of this study support the concept that recombinant HPV DNA constructs can be used to develop international standard reagents [47]. The international collaborative study group recommended that the priority for international standard reagents be for HR types HPV 16 and 18 as related to around 70% cancer cases, and then expand to the next most prevalent HR HPV types: HPV types 31, 33, 35, 45, 52, and 58 [6]. For HPV DNA, it is desirable to develop monovalent or individual HPV type standards, allowing unequivocal calibration of individual HPV DNA material and assessment of potential interference when multiple HPV types are present [60].

PCR primers directed at the E6 or E7 regions, encoding oncogenic proteins, have been described as preferable, whereas those targeting the L1 or E1 region may miss advanced disease, because the L1/E1 regions are often lost during integration of viral DNA into host genomic DNA [28]. The plasmid materials proposed by WHO to be developed as international standard reagents contain the full genome sequence of HPV virus types and could be useful in tests targeting both late and early viral genes.

Although such standards are not widely available yet, preliminary studies are being performed to verify material stability and reliability, including titration of the plasmid, as well as stability of the plasmid during a freeze-dry process. In addition, it may be best to designate international standard reagents using arbitrary international units, and the HPV DNA international standard unit remains to be established. Future studies need to determine if HPV DNA candidate standards can also assess the full spectrum of sample processing schemes that would mimic diagnostic sample preparation including DNA extraction, precipitation, or centrifugation procedures.

2.3. Applications of HPV DNA detection assays

The applications of HPV DNA standard reagents will vary depending on the setting in which they are used. Detection assays for HPVDNA with high analytical sensitivity have been crucial in demonstrating the aetiological role of oncogenic HPV presence in cervical cancer [37]. Similary, in prevalence surveys for HPV related cancer cases, as well as among general population, the analytical sensitivity of genotyping assays must be set for accurate discrimination of differences in the distribution of viral types in various geographical areas [5]. Methods with high analytical sensitivity are crucial in order to accurately evaluate that vaccine candidates are preventing the viral infections, and related diseases. In clinical trials of prophylactic or therapeutic vaccines for example, molecular detection methods based on PCR are proven useful in monitoring the efficacy of prophylactic vaccination [14,33,61]. Moreover, it is expected that upon vaccination, a reduction in the prevalence of the types included in vaccine preparations should be measurable in vaccinated cohorts. Sensitive type specific assays are therefore key in the evaluation of vaccination impact on prevalence of vaccine related genotypes, or potential genoptype replacement in post-vaccination periods.

In contrast, the use of HPV testing as a tool for cervical cancer screening programmes, needs to be thoroughly considered in a context of diagnostic algorithms, and may have to take into account the cost-effectiveness and the long-term benefits of such programmes. Detection of oncogenic HPV DNA is considered a predictor of underlying high grade dysplasia of the uterine cervix, at risk for potential invasive disease, but may depend on other factors such as age, viral load [74], other concomitant genital infections [58], high parity and environmental factors [3,7]. Therefore, algorithms of care including HPV testing are being developed and have been endorsed by various expert groups (IARC, ACOG, NHMRC) for use in different combinations and situations adapted locally. These applications include the option of HPV DNA testing with or without Pap, triage of ASCUS/border line lesions, and/or of treatment for cervical dysplasia as reliable predictor for residual disease [8,72]. With the appreciation of the role of HPVs in cervical cancer, the American College of Obstetricians and Gynecologists recently published a new guideline for cytology screening of cervical samples that incorporates the use of HPV detection in women $\geqslant$ 30 years of age as an important adjunct [73].

Most of the published studies to date have been conducted utilizing HC2, with studies based on PCR detection of HPV DNA only just coming to light. In the recently published ALTS study when HPV genotyping was evaluated, authors concluded that ASCUS and LSIL patients who have a positive HPV16 result by genotyping are at significantly greater risk for detection of high-grade abnormalities during a 2-year follow-up period when compared to those who test positive for another oncogenic type of HPV or who are HPV-negative [4]. Furthermore, HPV DNA testing, in particular PCR, can be performed on self-collected samples; these have similar sensitivity to clinician-collected samples [72]. Finally, application of HPV DNA testing may be useful as a rapid intermediate end point for monitoring the efficacy of surgical treatment of CIN usually results in clearance of HPV infection [10].

Despite their high clinical sensitivity for high grade cervical intraepithelial neoplasias, the clinical specificity of HPV DNA tests that have been applied in longitudinal studies is not ideal: It has been hypothesized that some HPV DNA detection methods, with very high analytical sensitivity, will show a higher positivity rate in women that will not be at risk for developing disease and may increase the number of referrals. Hence the clinical management of genital HPV related diseases has suggested that less sensitive HPV assays may be appropriate [59]. Conversely, an HPV test with too low analytical sensitivity will miss individuals positive for the viral DNA, thus at risk. A balance must be found, and viral load threasholds must be defined for HPV tests to be used in screening programs, triage of abnormal cytology, or for post-treatment monitoring. In practical terms, a definitive diagnosis should rely on the combined results of several tests, including histopathology if possible.

3. HPV antibodies detection methods, standards and applications

Multiple serological assays for HPV antibodies have been developed such as enzyme-linked immunoabsorbent assay [ELISA], including sandwich ELISA and radio immuno assays (RIA), competitive ELISA, neutralization and pseudovirion based *in vitro* neutralization methods.

Practically, HPV infections will result in detectable antibodies in only 50–60% of sera from individuals with HPV DNA infection [2]. Up to half of women with cervical cancer have at diagnosis sera antibodies to the HPV oncoproteins E6 and E7, which are rarely found among healthy women; however these are not validated markers of occult cervical cancer [29]. Anti-HPV antibodies are not only detected in serum but also in other body fluids, such as oral and vaginal lavage [38, 39].They may be considered in some circumstances markers of disease, as for instance IgA antibodies to HPV in oral fluid were also reported to correlate with cervical disease [34]. However the diagnostic value of detection of HPV specific antibodies in body fluids other than serum, to determine HPV immune responses, remains to be established.

3.1. Methods of HPV antibody detection: HPV ELISA assays and neutralization assays

Antibody detection methods are mostly directed to antibodies produced against the major capsid protein L1, often released upon productive viral infections. The antibody based methodology has so far shown insufficient sensitivity, complicated by determination of an appropriate cut-off, resulting in low specificity. HPV VLP-based ELISA assays to L1 are type-restricted measures of present or past genital HPV infections. The biological relevance of immune responses should correlate to neutralizing antibodies. These can be assessed in sera of subjects either by some type specific ELISA or biological assay systems able to recognize neutralizing epitopes of HPV.

HPV capsids are composed of two proteins, the major capsid protein L1 and the minor capsid protein L2 [50]. L1 protein when expressed in eurakyotic cells, has the capacity to spontaneously form the three dimensional structure necessary to aggregate as pentameric structures, also called capsomers [40], and finally to self assemble into VLPs that are similar to authentic virions, and can induce high titers of antibodies that neutralize papillomavirus infection *in vitro* [24]. Both capsomers and capsids have been used as antigenic components for vaccination, as well as substrates for immunoassays (Fig. 2).

Most assays depend on the conformation of the antigen used as substrate for antibody detection. Some assays rely on VLPs, and these prove to be necessarily of high purity and quality, and are consequently expensive

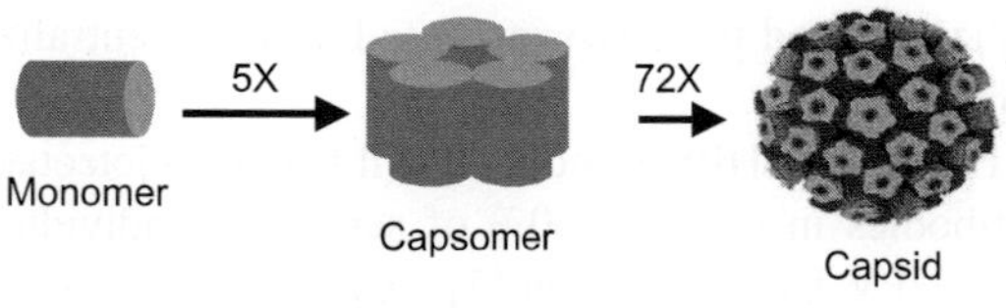

Fig. 2. Schematic representation of monomeric recombinant L1 proteins that self-assembly in pentameric structures as capsomers, and subsequently aggregate to form virus like particles (VLPs), similar to empty viral capsids (courtesy of Dr John Nieland).

to produce. The use of capsomers, which give conformational antigens in the form of pentamers of the viral capsid proteins, is being studied as an alternative. Additionally, assays detecting antibodies to the early proteins E6 and E7 have been also described [29].

Approaches to improve the assay have been the inclusion of Heparin to the ELISA plates, to capture properly folded L1 [64], or the use of an alternative antigen, such as the Glutathione S-transferase (GST)-L1 fusion proteins [54]. These antigens are used in a multiplex bead assay and allow for the detection of antibodies against multiple types [65], though non-specific background remains an issue [66]. Characterization of the assay has been limited and 20% differences have been reported between the VLP and GST assays.

A human papillomavirus (HPV) multiplexed competitive Luminex immunoassay first described by Opalka and colleagues [41], was optimized to increase both the analytical sensitivity and the clinical specificity of the assay [9], to more effectively discriminate the low-titer antibody response of HPV-infected persons from non-infected individuals. The new version is based on conjugation of VLPs to microspheres and the use of specific monoclonal antibody to neutralizing epitopes of viral particles. The assay was automated by use of a TECAN Genesis Workstation, thus improving assay throughput, reproducibility, and operator safety. The assay was validated then using several distinct serum panels from individuals known to be at low and high risk for HPV infection. This high-throughput assay has proven useful for performing epidemiology studies and evaluating the efficacy of prophylactic HPV vaccines.

Previously available HPV neutralization assays were insensitive, cumbersome and/or time-consuming [48]. A surrogate assay relies on hemaglutination inhibition, based on the observation that VLPs crosslink mouse red blood cells that could be reduced or abolished in the presence of an inhibiting L1-specific antibody. The disadvantage of the hemaglutination inhibition assay is that only a subset of neutralizing antibodies prevents agglutination. A similar limitation applies in the case of competitive radioimmunoassay and the multiplex assay, as only a subset of antibodies is able to compete in the assay.

Recently, a simple and high throughput pseudovirus-based *in-vitro* neutralization assay was developed [46]. Neutralization is monitored by measuring the activity of secreted alkaline phosphatase (SEAP), which is expressed from a SEAP gene that is included in the pseudovirus as a reporter gene. The approach is easy to scale up, as pseudovirus stocks are not a limiting step. The SEAP neutralization and VLP-ELISA assays have comparable sensitivity for detecting capsid antibodies generated after natural HPV infections and chemiluminescent detection improves the dynamic range of the assay sensitivity. The SEAP assay appears more specific in detecting type-restricted antibody responses to VLP vaccination, and available data suggest good inter-laboratory reproducibility. The limitations of SEAP neutralization assay are that there may be non-specific inhibition at low sera-dilutions, it requires cell culture, and chemiluminescent reagents are expensive.

3.2. Standards for HPV antibody detection

Following natural infections with HPV, antibodies responses are usually of relatively low titers. In contrast, following vaccination with prophylactic viral like particles (VLPs), circulating neutralizing antibodies appear to be the basis for protection against vaccine related HPV infectious and disease. Hence, type-specific antibody detection will play a key role in determining efficacy, quality, potency and duration of immune responses to HPV vaccination and eventually correlates of protection.

Standard reagents based on antibodies are intended for use in the estimation of potency of an appropriate test sample, by direct comparison in suitable biological test systems, and are usually established in the context of international collaborative studies. In order to develop standards for HPV antibody detection, the World Health Organization has coordinated an international collaborative study among laboratories implicated either in clinical studies or vaccine development [11]. Briefly, the study was aimed to assess the specificity and sensitivity of assays currently in use for measuring antibodies to the major viral capsid protein L1 to HPV, and to determine whether the use a standard reagent and the expression of titers in identical arbitrary units would improve reproducibility of results in various laboratories . Further, we assessed whether the expression of the titers in identical arbitrary units would improve comparability of results between laboratories. Samples studied included sera from individuals naturally infected with HPV 6/11, 16 and 18, a negative serum from a virgin woman, and sera from recipients of HPV vaccine candidates under clinical development, in a total of 12 samples.

The study showed that the range of titers for HPV 16 antibodies in assays expressed by the participating laboratories varied up to 25 fold for one sample. However, when the expression of HPV 16 antibody concentration in each sample was calculated relative to a single arbitrary serum sample assigned the unitage of "1" (one), the comparability of measurements was improved between laboratories, reducing the variability range to 2 to 3 fold. Therefore, the results of the collaborative study suggest that establishment of International Standard reagents for antibodies to HPV would facilitate the comparison of HPV antibody measurements between assays and laboratories worldwide.

Up to half of women with cervical cancer have been reported to show at diagnosis, sera antibodies to the HPV oncoproteins E6 and E7, which are rarely found among healthy women [57]. However, standard reagents for measuring antibody responses to other HPV proteins such as L2, E6 or E7, have not been assessed by an international collaborative study so far. In addition, operating procedures and quality control of the assays have not been fully resolved and standardized [11].

3.3. Applications of HPV antibody standard reagents

HPV standard reagents for serology will be crucial for improving the sensitivity of antibody assays, the consistency of results worldwide, as well as improving inter-laboratory and inter-assays variability, as suggested in comparative studies [11] and thus have a number of applications, as their use would improve assays performance, allow valid comparison of results, among laboratories, and facilitate monitoring of vaccine effectiveness.

There is currently no single "gold standard" for measuring the HPV serological responses, and different assays may be preferable depending on the questions being asked. The presence of anti-HPV antibodies in sera of individuals is mostly a marker for previous infections, not necessarily correlating to present infection or disease, as serological evidence for the association between HPV 16 infection and carcinomas is weak. In addition, HPV seropositivity may result from previous viral infections that have been efficiently cleared or may be present as asymptomatic infections that deserve no clinical management. Consequently, serological assays have not proven their clinical diagnostic value thus far.

Nevertheless, HPV serology has proven valuable in epidemiological studies based on seropositivity for HPV, in understanding the natural history of infections and cancer. Importantly, antibody based immune responses to HPV using various methods has contributed notably to understanding the protection conferred by neutralizing antibodies and allowed important advancements in the area of prophylactic vaccine development, as well as their evaluation by ELISA [15].

In the context of vaccination, serological assays are used to screen volunteers for vaccine trials as to previous exposure to HPV, and evaluating seroconversion in vaccinees. Moreover, the use of international standard reagents in the quality assurance of future recombinant VLP-based HPV vaccines, may be valuable in potency assays used for lot release, if immunogenicity assays are used for this purpose.In post vaccination studies monitoring vaccination performance (immunogenicity) and vaccination coverage, and surveillance of correlates of protection in vaccinated cohorts, are potential areas for using antibody based measurements in the near future.

In conclusion, for assessment of cumulative exposure to genital HPV infection prior to vaccination, the preferred assay to use may be the VLP ELISA, since it is the best validated assay, easier and less expensive to conduct than the pseudovirus assay. However, the availability of high quality VLPs may be a limiting factor. The SEAP assay measures all classes of antibodies relevant to protection, is type-restricted in measuring VLP-induced antibodies, is relatively simple and high throughput, and therefore could be used to monitor vaccine performance in central laboratories or locally after shipment/storage of sera. It might be particularly useful in the attempt to study immune correlates of protection.

4. Detection of HPV derived proteins

The viral proteins E6 and E7, which are selectively expressed in HPV-associated cancers, display potent transforming and tumourigenic activities in tissue culture and transgenic mouse models, respectively. Of particular importance is their ability to promote genetic instability through induction of cellular proliferation, disruption of cell-cycle checkpoints, inhibition of apoptosis and induction of telomerase. For oncogenesis to occur, host immune surveillance, intracellular specific cell signalling cascade regulation, and paracrine regulation of viral gene activity must be breached [17]. Based on this concept, additional biomarkers have been proposed that may be useful in identifying precancerous lesions at risk for malignant progression, instead of regression. Such markers identified recently are, for example, the human cyclin-dependent kinase inhibitor, p16INKa4, the retinoblastoma protein (Rb), the p53 protein, the KI-67 [23], the minichromosome maintainance protein (MCM), and cyclins, which are not usually expressed above the basal layers in normal epithelium [35]. Potential proliferation- and differentiation-related markers of progression are under investigation that may distinguish non-neoplastic lesions from different neoplastic grades, and could predict the risk of progression to cancer. These findings may have significant influence on novel strategies in cervical cancer diagnosis and screening in the near future. Indeed the continous and deregulated expresson of early HPV viral oncoproteins E6 and E7 have been studied at the nucleic acid level to ascertain cervical infections, and their detection at protein level has been proposed as diagnostic marker [25].

4.1. Methods of HPV-derived protein detection

HPV oncoproteins have been mostly detected by immunostaining of cytological or histological preparations, using monoclonal or polyclonal antibodies targeting molecules expressed during the mechanism of cellular transformation and malignancy. Immune responses associated to progressing lesions are preferentially specific early HPV proteins. Biochemical methods detecting oncogenic proteins, such as the early HPV proteins E6 and E7 are in early stages of development as rapid assays for diagnostic purposes.

One E6 detection assay is based on a lateral flow platform, and on the observation that E6 proteins of oncogenic HPVs bind to PDZ proteins [25]. Noteworthy, it has been reported that E6 and E7 proteins of high risk types, such as 16 and 18, can bind specifically to human cellular proteins containing a PDZ domain-protein *in vitro*, also known as repeat sequences in the Drosophila discs large protein, the post synaptic density protein PSD.95/SAP 90, and the epithelial tight junction protein ZO-1, hence PDZ. The binding is strong for E6 proteins from oncogenic types as opposed to non-oncogenic types. Thus, it was hypothesized that the interactions between E6 or E7 and PDZ domain proteins could be used as an assay to detect oncogenic E6 expressing cervical lesions, at risk to progression to cancer.

Overexpression of p16INK4a, induced by the viral oncoprotein E7, distinguishes dysplastic lesions from benign changes, and is also being studied and validated as a method to detect advanced lesions [62]. Similarly, PCR primers directed at the E6 or E7 regions, were suggested to be preferable, whereas those targeting the L1 or E1 region can be unreliable and may miss more advanced disease, because the LI/E1 regions are lost during integration of viral DNA into host genomic DNA.

4.2. Standard reagents for HPV oncogenic proteins and applications

Standard reagents for use in assays directly detecting cellular oncogenic proteins, virus derived or cell derived, would require the development of specific protein or corresponding antibody standard reagents. The need for such development will depend on the validation and of such tests in clinical settings, and remains to be defined.

5. Conclusion

Technology advancements based on detection of viral nucleic acid (sequences), antibodies and cellular biomarkers of disease progression have contributed to changing the landscape of cancer causing infections. Consequently, there is a need to develop quality assurance system for novel HPV products used in a variety of settings for cancer prevention programmes, for disease surveillance, for product improvements, or clinical diagnosis. International standard reagents for HPV would be able to contribute to assure that laboratory services used in evaluation of HPV diseases and preventive interventions are accurate worldwide.

International standard reagents provide a helpful tool for quality assurance of *in vitro* HPV amplification, detection, genotyping, diagnosis. On one hand, this strategy allows laboratories to measure their results in relation to other groups and improve their performance in HPV detection. High analytical specificity and sensitivity of methods are crucial for both epidemiological surveys and vaccine evaluation, as well as for future monitoring of vaccines performance upon deployment in populations. On the other hand, the usefulness of HPV detection in a diagnostic context should be based on its clinical sensitivity and specificity in identifying early disease. The availability of international standards may also allow to compare the various assays, assuring that they have the required sensitivity, so that a negative result assures the safety of a product worldwide.

Once international standard reagents are established, national and local/ or working standards can be derived and calibrated against international units for routine use in the laboratory. It may also be necessary to establish reference panels to aid in the evaluation of diagnostic tests and laboratory proficiency. Indeed, a reference panel of 10 individual genotypes of HIV-1 has been previously established, to help assess the specificity of nucleic acid amplification technology-based assays for HIV-1.[2]

National health authorities need to be prepared to review clinical data, decide on products registration, and control for quality, safety and efficacy of HPV diagnostics, vaccines and therapeutics, for the users within various countries. The national control laboratories need to be prepared to manage the issues related to evaluation of HPV diseases and diagnostic tools, as well as novel HPV vaccines that may arise in the near future. In any event, following approval of any product for general use, quality assurance of HPV antibody measurement kits is important, and national control laboratories should have access to validated reagents to test for quality and eventually for vaccine potency tests, if needed.

Provision of international standard reagents for global use would facilitate the assessment of product and improve the confidence of regulatory authorities on data provided for review. In the mean time, international standard reagents will be useful in determining analytical sensitivity of various methods, in assessing the laboratory performance and in calibrating diagnostic test kits. It is recognized that some international standards may be used for qualitative rather than quantitative purposes.

References

[1] J.G. Baseman and L.A. Koutsky, The epidemiology of human papillomavirus infections, *J Clin Virol* **1** (2005), 16–24.

[2] J.J. Carter, M.M. Madeleine, K. Shera, S.M. Schwartz, K.L., Cushing-Haugen, G.C. Wipf, P. Porter, J.R. Daling, J.K. McDougall and D.A. Galloway, Human papillomavirus, 16and 18 L1 serology compared across anogenital cancer sites, *Cancer Res* **61** (2001), 1934–1940.

[3] X. Castellsague and N. Munoz, Cofactors in human papillomavirus carcinogenesis-role of parity, oral contraceptives, and tobacco smoking, *J Natl Cancer Inst Monogr* **31** (2003), 20–28.

[4] P.E. Castle, D. Solomon, M. Schiffman and C.M. Wheeler for the ALTS Group, Human papillomavirus type 16 infections and 2-year absolute risk of cervical precancer in women with equivocal or mild cytologic abnormalities, *J Nat Can Inst* **97** (2005), 1066–1071.

[5] G.M. Clifford, S. Gallus, R. Herrero, N. Munoz, P.J. Snijders, S. Vaccarella, P.T. Anh, C. Ferreccio, N.T. Hieu, E. Matos, M. Molano, R. Rajkumar, G. Ronco, S. de Sanjose, H.R. Shin, S. Sukvirach, J.O. Thomas, S. Tunsakul, C.J. Meijer and S. Franceschi, IARC HPV Prevalence Surveys Study Group, Worldwide distribution of human papillomavirus types in cytologically normal women in the International Agency for Research on Cancer HPV prevalence surveys: a pooled analysis, *Lancet* **366** (2005), 991–998.

[6] G.M. Clifford, J.S. Smith, M. Plummer, N. Munoz and S. Franceschi, Human papillomavirus types in invasive cervical cancer worldwide: a meta-analysis, *Br J Cancer* **88** (2003), 63–73.

[7] R. Closas Garcia, X. Castellsague, X. Bosch and C.A. Gonzalez, The role of diet and nutrition in cervical carcinogenesis: a review of recent evidence, *Int J Cancer* **117** (2005), 629–637.

[8] J. Cuzick, A. Szarewski, H. Cubie, G. Hulman, H. Kitchener, D. Luesley, E. McGoogan, U. Menon, G. Terry, R. Edwards, C. Brooks, M. Desai, C. Gie, L. Ho, I. Jacobs, C. Pickles and P. Sasieni, Management of women who test positive for high-risk types of human papillomavirus: the HART study, *Lancet* **362** (2003), 1871–1876.

[9] D. Dias, J. Van Doren, S. Schlottmann, S. Kelly, D. Puchalski, W. Ruiz, P. Boerckel, J. Kessler, J.M. Antonello, T. Green, M. Brown, J. Smith, N. Chirmule, E. Barr, K.U. Jansen and M.T. Esser, Optimization and validation of a multiplexed luminex assay to quantify antibodies to neutralizing epitopes on human papillomaviruses 6, 11, 16, and 18, *Clin Diagn Lab Immunol* **8** (2005), 959–969.

[10] K. Elfgren, M. Jacobs, J.M. Walboomers, C.J. Meijer and J. Dillner, Rate of human papillomavirus clearance after treatment of cervical intraepithelial neoplasia, *Obstet Gynecol* **100** (2002), 965–971.

[11] M. Ferguson, A. Heath, S. Johnes, S. Pagliusi and J. Dillner, Results of the first WHO international collaborative study on the standardization of the detection of antibodies to human papillomaviruses, *Int J Cancer* **118** (2005), 1508–1514.

[12] D. Galloway, Papillomavirus vaccines in clinical trials, *Lancet Infect Dis* **8** (2003), 469–475.

[13] L. Gustafsson, J. Pontén, M. Zack and H.-O. Adami, International incidence rates of invasive cervical cancer after introduction of cytological screening, *Cancer Causes Cont* **8** (1997), 755–763.

[14] D.M. Harper, E.L. Franco, C. Wheeler, D.G. Ferris, D. Jenkins, A. Schuind, T. Zahaf, B. Innis, P. Naud, N.S. deCarvalho, C.M. Roteli-Martins, J. Teixeira, M.M. Blattetr, A.P. Korn, W. Quint and G. Dubin, GlaxoSmithKline HPV Vaccine Study Group, Efficacy of a bivalent L1 virus like particle vaccine in prevention of infection with human papillomavirus types 16

[2] WHO Expert Committee on Biological Standardization, Fifty-third Report 2004, http://www.who.int/biologicals/926-Inside%20page.pdf, page 19.

and 18 in young women: a randomized controlled trial, *Lancet* **364** (2004), 1757–1765.

[15] C.D. Harro, Y.Y.Pang, R.B. Roden, A. Hildesheim, Z. Wang, M.J. ReyNOlds, T.C. Mast, R. Robinson, B.R. Murphy, R.A. Karron, J. Dillner, J.T. Schiller and D. Lowy, Safety and immunogenicity trial in adult volunteers of a human papillomavirus 16 L1 virus-like particle vaccine, *J Natl Cancr Inst* **93** (2001), 284–292.

[16] H. zur Hausen, Condylomata acuminata and human genital cancer, *Cancer Res* **36** (1976), 794.

[17] H. zur Hausen, Papillomavirus and cancer: from basic studies to clinical application, *Nat Rev Cancer* **5** (2002), 342–350.

[18] G.Y. Ho, R. Bierman, L. Beardsley, C.J. Chang and R.D. Burk, Natural history of cervicovaginal papillomavirus infection in young women, *N Engl J Med* **338** (1998), 423–428.

[19] IARC Monographs on the Evaluation of Carcinogenic Risks to Humans, 2005, http://monographs.iarc.fr/ENG/Meetings/90-hpv.pdf.

[20] T. Iftner and L.L. Villa, Chapter 12: Human papillomavirus technologies, *J Natl Cancer Inst Monogr* **31** (2003), 80–88.

[21] C. Jennings, S.A. Fiscus, S.M. Crowe, A.D. Danilovic, R.J. Morack, S. Scianna, A. Cachafeiro, D.J. Brambilla, J. Schupbach, W. Stevens, R. Respess, O.E. Varnier, G.E. Corrigan, J.S. Gronowitz, M.A. Ussery and J.W. Bremer, Comparison of Two Human Immunodeficiency Virus (HIV) RNA Surrogate Assays to the Standard HIV RNA Assay, *J Clin Microbiol* **43** (2005), 5950–5956.

[22] A. Josefsson, K. Livak and U. Gyllensten, Detection and quantitation of human papillomavirus by using the fluorescent 5'exonuclease assay, *J Clin Microbiol* **37** (1999), 490–496.

[23] J.T. Keating, A. Cviko, S. Riethdorf, L. Riethdorf, B.J. Quade, D. Sun, S. Duensing, E.E. Sheets, K. Munger and C.P. Crum, Ki-67, cyclin E, and p16INK4 are complimentary surrogate biomarkers for human papilloma virus-related cervical neoplasia, *Am J Surg Pathol* **25** (2001), 884–891.

[24] R. Kirnbauer, Papillomavirus-like particles for serology and vaccine development, *Intervirology* **39** (1996), 54–61.

[25] T. Kiyono, A. Hiraiwa, M. Fujita, Y. Hayashi, T. Akiyama and M. Ishibashi, Binding of high-risk human papillomavirus E6 oncoproteins to the human homologue of the Drosophila discs large tumor suppressor protein, *Proc Natl Acad Sci* **94** (1997), 11612–11616.

[26] R. Klaes, T. Friedrich, D. Spitkovsky, R. Ridder, W. Rudy, U. Petry, G. Dallenbach-Hellweg, D. Schmidt and M. von Knebel Doeberitz, Overexpression of p16(INK4A) as a specific marker for dysplastic and neoplastic epithelial cells of the cervix uteri, *Cancer Res* **59** (1999), 6132–6136.

[27] J.R. Kornegay, M, Roger, P.O. Davies, A.P. Shepard, N.A. Guerrero, B. Lloveras, D. Evans and F. Coutlee, International proficiency study of a consensus L1 PCR assay for the detection and typing of human papillomavirus DNA: evaluation of accuracy and intralaboratory and interlaboratory agreement, *J Clin Microbiol* **41** (2003), 1080–1086.

[28] L.A. Koutsky, K.A. Ault, C.M. Wheeler, D.R. Brown, E. Barr, F.B. Alvarez, L.M. Chiacchierini and K.U. Jansen, Proof of Principle Study Investigators, A controlled trial of a human papillomavirus type 16 vaccine, *N Engl J Med* **347** (2002), 1645–1651.

[29] M. Lehtinen, M. Pawlita, K. Zumbach, K. Lie, M. Hakama, E. Jellum, P. Koskela, T. Luostarinen, J. Paavonen, E. Pukkala, E. Sigstad, S. Thoresen and J. Dillner, Evaluation of antibody response to human papillomavirus early proteins in women in whom cervical cancer developed 1 to 20 years later, *Am J Obstet Gynecol* **188** (2003), 49–55.

[30] A.K. Lie, B. Risberg, B. Borge, B. Sandstad, J. Delabie, R. Rimala, M. Onsrud and S.Thoresen, DNA- versus RNA-based methods for human papillomavirus detection in cervical neoplasia, *Gynecol Onco* **97** (2005), 908–915.

[31] A. Lorincz and J. Anthony, Advances in HPV detection by Hybrid Capture, *Papillomavirus Report* **12** (2001), 145–154.

[32] D.R. Lowy and P.M. Howley, Papillomaviruses, in: *Fields Virology*, D.M. Knipe, P.M. Howley, D.E. Griffin, R.A. Lamb, M.A. Martin, B. Roizman, S.E. Strauss and Pippincott, Chap. 66, 4th edition, eds, Williams & Wilkins, 2001.

[33] C. Mao, L.A. Koutsky, K.A. Ault,C.M. Wheeler, D.R. Brown, D.J. Wiley, F.B. Alvarez, O.M. Bautista, K.U. Jansen and E. Barr, Efficacy of human papillomavirus-16 vaccine to prevent cervical intraepithelial neoplasia: a randomized controlled trial, *Obstet Gynecol* **107** (2006), 18–27.

[34] D.J. Marais, J.M. Best, R.C. Rose, P. Keating, R. Soeters, L. Denny, C.M. Dehaeck, J, Nevin, P. Kay, J.A. Passmore and A.L. Williamson, Oral antibodies to human papillomavirus type 16 in women with cervical neoplasia, *J Med Virol* **65** (2001), 149–154.

[35] K. Middleton, W. Peh, S. Southern, H. Griffin, K. Sotlar, T. Nakahara, A. El-Sherif, L. Morris, R. Seth, M. Hibma, D. Jenkins, P. Lambert, N. Coleman and J. Doorbar, Organization of human papillomavirus productive cycle during neoplastic progression provides a basis for selection of diagnostic markers, *J Virol* **77** (2003), 10186–10201.

[36] J. Monsonego, J.M. Bohbot, G. Pollini, C. Krawec, C. Vincent, I. Merignargues, F. Haroun, P. Sednaoui, L. Monfort, R. Dachez and K. Syrjanen, Performance of the Roche AMPLICOR human papillomavirus (HPV) test in prediction of cervical intraepithelial neoplasia (CIN) in women with abnormal PAP smear, *Gynecol Onco* **99** (2005), 160–168.

[37] N. Munoz, F.X. Bosch, S. de Sanjose, R. Herrero, X. Castellsague, K.V. Shah, P.J. Snijders and C.J. Meijer, International Agency for Research on Cancer Multicenter Cervical Cancer Study Group, Epidemiologic classification of human papillomavirus types associated with cervical cancer, *N Engl J Med* **348** (2003), 518–527.

[38] D. Nardelli-Haefliger, D. Wirthner, J.T. Schiller, D.R. Lowy, A. Hildesheim, F. Ponci and P. De Grandi, Specific antibody levels at the cervix during the menstrual cycle of women vaccinated with human papillomavirus 16 virus-like particles, *J Natl Cancer Inst* **95** (2003), 1128–1137.

[39] M.A. Nobbenhuis, T.J. Helmerhorst, A.J. van den Brule, L. Rozendaal, P.D. Bezemer, F.J. Voorhorst and C.J. Meijer, High-risk human papillomavirus clearance in pregnant women: trends for lower clearance during pregnancy with a catch-up postpartum, *Br J Cancer* **87** (2002), 75–80.

[40] P. Ohlschlager, W. Osen, K. Dell, S. Faath, R.L. Garcea, I. Jochmus, M. Muller, M. Pawlita, K. Schafer, P. Sehr, C. Staib, G. Sutter and L. Gissmann, Human papillomavirus type 16 L1 capsomeres induce L1-specific cytotoxic T lymphocytes and tumor regression in C57BL/6 mice, *J Virol* **77** (2003), 4635–4645.

[41] D. Opalka, C.E. Lachman, S.A. MacMullen, K.U. Jansen, J.F. Smith, N. Chirmule and M.T. Esser, Simultaneous quantitation of antibodies to neutralizing epitopes on virus-like particles for human papillomavirus types 6, 11, 16, and 18 by a multiplexed luminex assay, *Clin Diagn Lab Immunol* **10** (2003), 108–115.

[42] A.G. Östör, Natural history of cervical intraepithelial neoplasia: A critical review, *Int J Gynecol Pathol* **12** (1993), 86–92.

[43] G.N. Papanicolaou and H.F. Traut, The diagnostic value of vaginal smears in carcinoma of uterus, *Am J Obstet Gynecol* **42** (1941), 193–205.

[44] D.M. Parkin, The global health burden of infection-associated cancers in the year 2002, *Int J Cancer* **118** (2006), 3030–3044.
[45] D.M. Parkin, F. Bray, J. Ferlay and P. Pisani, Global cancer statistics 2002, *CA Cancer J Clin* **55** (2005), 74–108.
[46] D.V. Pastrana, C.B. Buck, Y.Y. Pang, C.D. Thompson, P.E. Castle, P.C. FitzGerald, S. Kruger Kjaer, D.R. Lowy and J.T. Schiller, Reactivity of human sera in a sensitive, high-throughput pseudovirus-based papillomavirus neutralization assay for HPV16 and HPV18, Virology **321** (2004), 205–216.
[47] W. Quint, S.R. Pagliusi, N. Lelie, E.-M. de Villiers, C.M. Wheeler and the World Health Organization Human Papillomavirus DNA International Collaborative Study Group, Results of the First World Health Organization International Collaborative Study of Detection of Human Papillomavirus DNA, *J Clin Microbiol* **44** (2006), 571–579.
[48] R.B. Roden, N.L. Hubbert, R. Kirnbauer, N.D. Christensen, D.R. Lowy and J.T. Schiller, Assessment of the serological relatedness of genital human papillomaviruses by hemagglutination inhibition, *J Virol* **70** (1996), 3298–3301.
[49] J. Saldanha, A. Heath, N. Lelie, G. Pisani and M.Y. Yu, Collaborative Study Group, A World Health Organization International Standard for hepatitis A virus RNA nucleic acid amplification technology assays, *Vox Sang* **89** (2005), 52–58.
[50] J.T. Schiller, Papillomavirus-like particle vaccines for cervical cancer, *Mol Med Today* **5** (1999), 209–215.
[51] J. Schirm, A.M. van Loon, E. Valentine-Thon, P.E. Klapper, J. Reid and G.M. Cleator, External quality assessment program for qualitative and quantitative detection of hepatitis C virus RNA in diagnostic virology, *J Clin Microbiol* **40** (2002), 2973–2980.
[52] N.F. Schlecht, Prognostic value of human papillomavirus in the survival of head and neck cancer patients: an overview of the evidence, *Oncol Rep* **14** (2005), 1239–1247.
[53] M. Schmitt, I.G. Bravo, P.J. Snijders, L. Gissmann, M. Pawlita and T. Waterboer, Bead-based multiplex genotyping of human papillomaviruses, *J Clin Microbiol* **44** (2006), 504–512.
[54] P. Sehr, M. Muller, R. Hoepfl, A. Widschwendter and M. Pawlita, HPV antibody detection by ELISA with capsid protein L1 fused to glutathione S-transferase, *J Virol Meth* **106** (2002), 61–70.
[55] S.S. Seo, Y.S. Song, J.W. Kim, N.H. Park, S.B. Kang and H.P. Lee, Good correlation of HPV DNA test between self-collected vaginal and clinician-collected cervical samples by the oligonucleotide microarray, *Gynecol Oncol* **102** (2006), 67–73.
[56] H.R. Shin, S. Franceschi, S. Vaccarella, J.W. Roh, Y.H. Ju, J.K. Oh, H.J. Kong, S.H. Rha, S.I. Jung, J.I. Kim, K.Y. Jung, L.J. van Doorn and W. Quint, Prevalence and determinants of genital infection with papillomavirus, in female and male university students in Busan, South Korea, *J Infect Dis* **190** (2004), 468–476.
[57] I. Silins, E. Avall-Lundqvist, A. Tadesse, K.U. Jansen, U. Stendahl, P. Lenner, K. Zumbach, M. Pawlita, J. Dillner and B. Frankendal, Evaluation of antibodies to human papillomavirus as prognostic markers in cervical cancer patients, *Gynecol Oncol* **85** (2002), 333–338.
[58] J.S. Smith, C. Bosetti, N. Munoz, R. Herrero, F.X. Bosch, J. Eluf-Neto, C.J. Meijer, A.J. Van Den Brule, S. Franceschi and R.W. Peeling, IARC multicentric case-control study, Chlamydia trachomatis and invasive cervical cancer: a pooled analysis of the IARC multicentric case-control study, *Int J Cancer* **111** (2004), 431–439.
[59] P.J. Snijders, A.J. van den Brule and C.J. Meijer, The clinical relevance of human papillomavirus testing: relationship between analytical and clinical sensitivity, *J Pathol* **201** (2003), 1–6.
[60] Technical workshop on international collaborative studies on HPV reagents for laboratory diagnostic procedures: a progress report. http://www.who.int/vaccines-documents/DocsPDF04/www786.pdf.
[61] L.L. Villa, R.L. Costa, C.A. Petta, R.P. Andrade, K.A. Ault, A.R. Giuliano, C.M. Wheeler, L.A. Koutsky, C. Malm, M. Lehtinen, F.E. Skjeldestad, S.E. Olsson, M. Steinwall, D.R. Brown, R.J. Kurman, B.M. Ronnett, M.H. Stoler, A. Ferenczy, D.M. Harper, G.M. Tamms, J. Yu, L. Lupinacci, R. Railkar, F.J. Taddeo, K.U. Jansen, M.T. Esser, H.L. Sings, A.J. Saah and E.Barr, Prophylactic quadrivalent human papillomavirus (types 6, 11, 16, and 18) L1 virus-like particle vaccine in young women: a randomised double-blind placebo-controlled multicentre phase II efficacy trial, *Lancet Oncol* **6** (2005), 271–278.
[62] S. Vinokurova, N. Wentzensen and M. von Knebel Doeberitz, Analysis of p16INK4a and integrated HPV genomes as progression markers, *Methods Mol Med* **119** (2005), 73–83.
[63] J.M. Walboomers, M.V. Jacobs, M.M. Manos, F.X. Bosch, J.A. Kummer, K.V. Shah, P.J. Snijders, J. Peto, C.J. Meijer and N. Munoz, Human papillomavirus is a necessary cause of invasive cervical cancer worldwide, *J Pathol* **189** (1999), 12–19.
[64] X. Wang, M. Sapp, N.D. Christensen and J. Dillner, Heparin-based ELISA reduces background reactivity in virus-like particle-based papillomavirus serology, *J Gen Virol* **85** (2005), 65–73.
[65] T. Waterboer, P. Sehr, K.M. Michael, S. Franceschi, J.D. Nieland, T.O. Joos, M.F. Templin and M. Pawlita, Multiplex human papillomavirus serology based on in situ-purified glutathione s-transferase fusion proteins, *Clin Chem* **51** (2005), 1845–1853.
[66] T. Waterboer, P. Sehr and M. Pawlita, Suppression of non-specific binding in serological Luminex assays, *J Immunol Methods* **309** (2005), 200–204.
[67] N. Wentzensen, C. Bergeron, F. Cas, D. Eschenbach, S. Vinokurova and M. von Knebel Doeberitz, Evaluation of a nuclear score for p16INK4a-stained cervical squamous cells in liquid-based cytology samples, *Cancer* **105** (2005), 461–467.
[68] WHO Expert Committee on Biological Standardization, Fifty-third Report, http://www.who.int/biologicals/926-Inside%20page.pdf.
[69] WHO informal workshop: development of international HPV reference reagents, 2001. http://www.who.int/vaccines-documents/DocsPDF02/www699.pdf.
[70] WHO Technical workshop on cellular mediated immunity to human papillomavirus, 2005. http://www.who.int/vaccies-documents/DocsPDF06/824scxreen.pdf.
[71] WHO Technical Report Series http://whqlibdoc.who.int/trs/WHO_TRS_897.pdf.
[72] T.C. Wright, L. Denny, L. Kuhn, A. Pollack and A. Lorincz, HPV DNA testing of self-collected vaginal samples compared with cytologic screening to detect cervical cancer, *JAMA* **283** (2000), 81–86.
[73] T.C. Wright, M. Schiffman, D. Solomon, J. Cox, F. Garcia, S. Goldie, K. Hatch, K. Noller, N. Roach, C. Runowicz and D. Saslow, Interim guidance for the use of human papillomavirus DNA testing as an adjunct to cervical cytology for screening, *Obstet Gynecol* **103** (2004), 304–309.

[74] N. Ylitalo, P. Sorensen, A.M. Josefsson, P.K. Magnusson, P.K. Andersen, J. Ponten, H.O. Adami, U.B. Gyllensten and M. Melbye, Consistent high viral load of human papillomavirus 16 and risk of cervical carcinoma in situ: a nested case-control study, *Lancet* **355** (2000), 2194–2198.

Disease Markers 23 (2007) 297–313
IOS Press

Papillomavirus life cycle organization and biomarker selection

John Doorbar
National Institute for Medical Research, The Ridgeway, Mill Hill, London, NW7 1AA, UK
Tel.: +44 020 8816 2623; Fax: +44 020 8906 0610; E-mail: jdoorba@nimr.mrc.ac.uk

Abstract. Human papillomaviruses (HPVs) are a diverse group of viruses that cause epithelial lesions of varying severity. Of the 100 or so types that have been identified, around 40 can infect the cervix, with a subset of these causing lesions that can progress to high-grade neoplasia and cervical cancer. These high-risk types are prevalent in the general population, and can predispose to the development of cancer in women who cannot resolve their infection. Virus infection usually leads to the establishment of productive flat warts, or to maintenance of the viral genome in an asymptomatic or latent state. Virus synthesis depends on the ordered expression of viral gene products as the infected basal cell migrates towards the epithelial surface. E7 is expressed in the lower epithelial layers, and is followed eventually by the expression of E4 and L1 closer to the epithelial surface. This ordered pattern changes in characteristic ways during neoplastic progression and latency, and can be irreversibly fixed following integration of the viral genome into the host cell chromosome. Our understanding of expression patterns and their significance, is beginning to explain the nature of disease progression, and offers a rational basis for the selection of biomarkers that may be used to predict disease status and prognostic outcome.

1. The diversity of papillomavirus types that infect humans

Human papillomaviruses (HPV) complete their productive cycle in stratified epithelial tissue such as cutaneous skin or mucosal epithelium. They can infect many epithelial sites and cause a wide variety of epithelial lesions, including common warts, verrucas, laryngeal papillomas, and genital condyloma. The different types of epithelial lesion, are in general, caused by different groups or types of HPV, with some types showing a very restricted tissue tropism [6,34]. This is the case with viruses such as HPV1, which causes cutaneous lesions at palmar and plantar surfaces (Fig. 1A).

DNA sequence analysis over the last 25 years has shown that papillomaviruses are a very diverse group with over 100 human members [34]. Most HPV types belong to the Alpha or Beta genus, with the two groups having quite distinct biology and life cycle patterns. The Alpha papillomaviruses are found only in humans and primates, and it is this group that contains the HPV types that are frequently associated with cervical cancer. HPV16 (α9) causes over 50% of all cervical cancers, while HPV18 (α7) is responsible for around 20% of cases (Fig. 1B). These HPV types are classified as high-risk, and are amongst 20 or so such viruses that infect the cervix (Fig. 1B). The Alpha papillomaviruses also contain low-risk members that infect the cervix, but these are not generally associated with cervical cancer. HPV types such as HPV6 and HPV11 (α10) are the best studied of these, and are also responsible for the production of external genital warts that can be a problem in young adults. Although not generally life threatening, such lesions can be difficult to treat effectively in some patients [94]. The Alpha papillomavirus genus also contains cutaneous HPV types such as HPV2 (α4), which is a prominent cause of common warts in children. The different biology of Alpha papillomavirus members (high-risk, low-risk and cutaneous) is clearly reflected at the level of virus evolution, when whole genomic sequences are compared (Fig. 1B).

Beta papillomaviruses are evolutionarily distinct from the Alpha genus (Fig. 1A), and appear to cause widespread in-apparent or asymptomatic infections in the general population, with children becoming infected at an early age. In immunosuppressed patients,

ISSN 0278-0240/07/$17.00

A

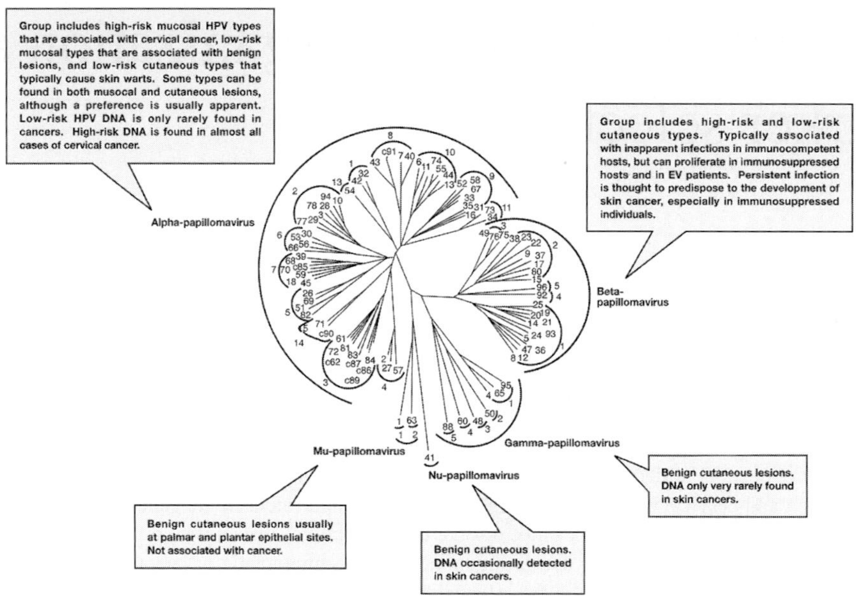

B

Association of Alpha Papillomavirus types with cervical cancer

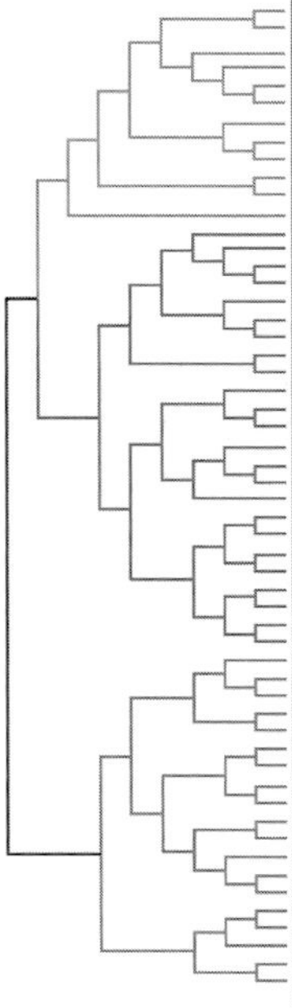

Alpha Type Species		SCC Cervix	Adeno Cervix	Category
HPV6		0.07%		low risk
HPV11		0.07%		low risk
HPV13	10			low risk
HPV74				
HPV44				low risk
HPV55		0.04%		low risk
HPV91				cutaneous (mucosal)
HPV7	8			cutaneous (mucosal)
HPV40				cutaneous (mucosal)
HPV32	1			low risk
HPV42				low risk
HPV54	13			low risk
HPV52		2.25%		high risk
HPV67				
HPV33		2.06%	0.54%	high risk
HPV58	9	1.72%	0.54%	high risk
HPV16		54.38%	41.62%	high risk
HPV31		3.82%	1.08%	high risk
HPV35		1.27%	1.08%	high risk
HPV34	11			high risk
HPV73		0.49%		high risk
HPV59		1.05%	2.16%	high risk
HPV18		11.27%	37.30%	high risk
HPV45		5.21%	5.95%	high risk
HPV70	7			
HPV39		0.82	0.54%	high risk
HPV68		0.37%		high risk
HPV85				
HPV26		0.22%		high risk
HPV69	5			
HPV51		0.75%	0.54%	high risk
HPV82		0.26%		high risk
HPV30				high risk
HPV53	6	0.04%		high risk
HPV56		1.09%		high risk
HPV66		0.19%		high risk
HPV57				cutaneous
HPV2a	4			cutaneous
HPV27				cutaneous
HPV71	15			low risk
HPV90	14			
HPV61				low risk
HPV72				low risk
HPV62				
HPV81		0.04%		low risk
HPV83	3	0.04%		low risk
HPV89				
HPV84				low risk
HPV86				
HPV87				
HPV28				cutaneous
HPV3				cutaneous
HPV10	2			cutaneous
HPV29				cutaneous
HPV77				cutaneous

Fig. 1. The association of papillomaviruses with disease in humans. A. Human Papillomaviruses are contained within five evolutionary groups. HPV types that infect cervical mucosa are contained within the Alpha group. Beta, Gamma, Mu and Nu papillomaviruses typically infect cutaneous sites. The type of lesion associated with each group is shown in the boxes. B. The Alpha papillomaviruses can be subdivided into three categories (high-risk, low-risk and cutaneous), on the basis of DNA sequence analysis. The evolutionary relationships shown on the left are also manifest in their biology. High-risk types come from the Alpha 5, 6, 7, 9 and 11 groups. The frequency with which the different HPV types are found in cervical cancers (squamous cell carcinoma and adenocarcinoma/adenosquamous carcinoma) is shown in the central columns (based on information contained in [79]).

and in individuals suffering from the inherited disease Epidermodysplasia Verruciformis (EV), these viruses can spread unchecked, and have been implicated in the development of non-melanoma skin cancer cancer [55,96]. EV patients carry mutations in their EV-ER1/TMC6 or EVER2/TMC8 genes, which renders them particularly susceptible to these viruses [97,112]. The remaining HPV types come from the Gamma, Mu and Nu genus, and cause visible cutaneous papillomas that do not generally progress to cancer (Fig. 1A). Only two Mu HPV types are known (HPV1 and 63), and the Nu Genus comprises only one member.

2. Similarities in the organization of all papillomavirus genomes

All papillomaviruses consist of a double stranded circular genome of around 8kb containing one coding strand, encapsidated in an icosohedral protein shell made up of a major (L1) and minor (L2) coat protein (Fig. 2A). 360 molecules of L1 and approximately 12 molecules of L2 are needed for the formation of an infectious virion [76]. The L1 and L2 proteins are conserved across widely divergent papillomaviruses, and along with E1 and E2, are key viral gene products that are thought to have been present in the common ancestor of all animal papillomaviruses [113]. Other viral genes, such as E6, E7, E4 and E5, have been acquired or significantly modified during evolution, and are not necessarily present, or may not have the same function in all papillomavirus types [34]. All human papillomaviruses have E6 and E7 open reading frames (ORF), but the Beta papillomaviruses lack an E5 ORF. Avian papillomaviruses lack a clearly recognizable E4 ORF, and do not contain canonical E6 and E7 open reading frames similar to those found in human papillomaviruses [83,113]. The roles of the viral gene products have been most thoroughly worked out for the Alpha HPV types, and more specifically for the high-risk types associated with cervical cancer. While similarities exist amongst HPV types, it is also clear that there are significant differences in the way different papillomaviruses regulate their genes, and in the function of specific viral gene products, and that this reflects the very different biologies of the different viruses.

3. Life cycle organisation and the basis for biomarker selection

Irrespective of their evolutionary origin, all papillomaviruses must complete their life cycle in the epithelial tissue that they infect, and produce infectious particles that are eventually secreted from the epithelial surface. To do this requires the timely and coordinated expression of the different viral gene products as the infected cell moves towards the epithelial surface (Fig. 2B). This highly regulated pattern of gene expression allows the different stages of the virus life cycle to be completed appropriately, and provides a basis for the selection of biomarkers that may be useful in diagnosis. Life cycle events can be divided into a number of phases that are outlined below.

3.1. Primary infection of the epidermis

Papillomavirus infection begins when virus particles gain access to the epithelial basal layer, which in uninfected epidermis contains cells that are mitotically active. Such cells are normally stimulated to divide by growth factors that originate from the underlying stromal tissue, and in uninfected epithelium, it is the continual division of these cells that allows renewal of the epidermis as surface cells exfoliate. It is thought that papillomavirus particles associate with proteoglycans on the cell surface, as well as with secondary receptors that facilitate viral uptake [64,72,91,104]. At most epithelial sites, access to the basal cell layer requires a break in the integrity of the epithelial sheet. Although this may require the presence of microwounds or more obvious damage to the epithelial layer, some papillomaviruses are thought to infect sites where access to the basal layer is naturally facilitated, such as at the base of the hair follicle, or sites where columnar and stratified epithelial cells meet each other (such as at the cervical or anal transformation zone) (Fig. 2B). Successful infection leads to the establishment of the papillomavirus genome as a stable episome that is maintained at low copy number with out integration into the host cell chromosome. Replication of viral DNA in these cells depends on the presence of the cellular replication machinery, with viral DNA replication accompanying cellular DNA replication as the cells progress through S-phase. The only viral proteins that are thought to be necessary in these cells are E1 and E2, which can be expressed from the differentiation-dependent promoter (PL (also referred to as p670 in HPV16)) (Fig. 2B), and which play an important role in viral DNA replication and genome partitioning during cell division. The E2 protein contains a C-terminal DNA binding domain that recognizes a repeated sequence motif in the viral non-coding region [35]. One of these E2-binding motifs is adjacent to the viral origin of replication, and it is

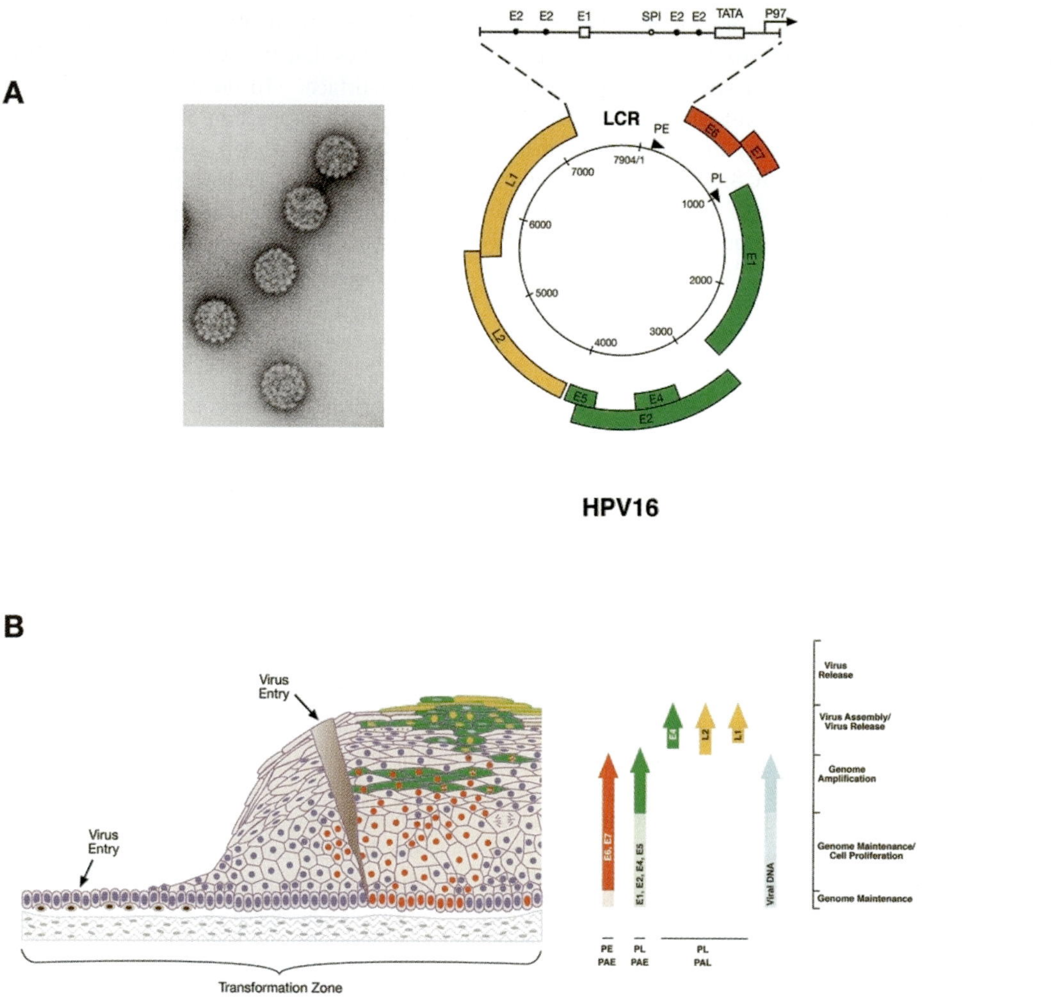

Fig. 2. Life cycle organization amongst human papillomaviruses. A. HPV particles (approx. 55 nm diameter) as visualized by electron microscopy are shown on the left alongside a map of the HPV16 genome (7904 base pairs). The six early open reading frames (E1, E2, E4, E5 (green), and E6 and E7 (red)) are expressed from either the P97 early (PE) or P670 late (PL) promoters during epithelial cell differentiation. The late open reading frames (L1 and L2 (yellow)) are also expressed from P670, following a change in splicing patterns, and a shift in polyadenylation site usage (from PAE (early polyadenylation site) to PAL (late polyadenylation site). All the viral genes are encoded on one DNA strand. The Long Control Region (LCR from 7156 to 84) is enlarged to reveal the E2 binding sites and the P97 promoter. E1 and SP1 binding sites are also shown. B. The part of the transformation zone where the columnar cells of the endocervix meet the stratified squamous cells of the ectocervix is illustrated diagramatically. Virus infection occurs through a microwound, or where access to basal/reserve cells is facilitated (arrows). Cells expressing cell cycle markers are shown with red nuclei. The appearance of such cells above the basal layer is a consequence of E6 and E7 expression. The expression of viral proteins necessary for genome replication occurs in cells expressing E6 and E7 following activation of P670 in the upper epithelial layers (cells shown in green with red nuclei). The L1 and L2 genes (yellow) are expressed in a subset of the cells that contain amplified viral DNA in the upper epithelial layers. Infectious particles are shed from the epithelial surface as the cells are lost through desquamation. The timing and extent of virus gene expression is summarized at the right of the figure using arrows. The consequence of expressing viral gene products in this ordered way is shown at the far right.

thought that E2 recruits E1 to this region by direct binding through its N-terminus. This region of E2 contains binding sites for several viral and cellular proteins such as L2 [57], and in the case of Bovine Papillomavirus type 1, the cellular protein Brd4 [74,122]. The latter interaction is important for the proper segregation of replicated episomes during cell division. Although initially involved in basal cell expansion following infection, the long-term requirement for the viral E6 and E7 proteins is uncertain in cells of the basal layer, as these cells are already able to cycle as a result of their close proximity to the basal lamina. During productive infection, HPV proteins cannot easily be detected in the basal cell layer, although the E7 protein can be seen in cervical neoplasia where expression levels are not properly controlled [44].

3.2. Cell proliferation during productive infection

Papillomavirus entry is though to be followed by a period of cell proliferation, in which the infected cell is driven to divide in order to produce a sheet of basal cells that harbour viral episomes. The HPV E6 and E7 proteins are integral in driving cell proliferation following infection, as well as in stimulating cells to re-enter the cell cycle following their migration towards the epithelial surface (Fig. 2B). The molecular basis of HPV E6/E7 function is now well established, as the deregulation of these gene products is important in the development of cervical neoplasia and eventually cancer. The key function of E7 lies in its ability to associate with the cell cycle regulator pRb (and other members of the pocket protein family), and to disrupt the association between pRb and the E2F family of transcription factors in the absence of growth factor stimulation (Fig. 3). The released E2F can subsequently transactivate cellular genes involved in viral DNA replication such as cyclin A and E, allowing cells above the basal layer to support DNA replication. E7 also associates with histone deacetylases [12], components of the AP1 transcription complex [2], and the cyclin dependent kinase inhibitors p21 and p27 [49], which also regulate cell proliferation. During productive HPV infection, it appears that the level of p21 and p27 is critical in determining whether an infected cell can effectively enter S-phase following migration from the basal layer (Fig. 3). It is thought that high levels of p21 and p27 lead to the formation of inactive complexes with E7 and cyclinE, which stalls the cell in a pre S-phase state and prevents E7-mediated cell proliferation (Fig. 3). The ability of E7 to drive cells into S-phase in differentiating epithelium appears limited to those cells in the lesions which express p21 and p27 at low level, or which express sufficient E7 to overcome the block to cell cycle progression [89]. Immunostaining studies clearly show that cyclinE is detectable in a subset of differentiating epithelial cells during productive infection, and indeed, cyclin E has been proposed as a marker of HPV infection because it is only transiently expressed (and is therefore not readily detectable) during the normal cell cycle. E2F-activated cellular proteins such as cyclinE are regarded as surrogate markers of E7 expression when present above the basal layer in productive lesions. Other E2F activated gene products and/or S-phase proteins such as PCNA, Ki67, p16, MCM and possibly also survivin [11], may serve similar purposes as diagnostic markers, and may be detected above the basal layer during productive papillomavirus infection. The presence of Cyclin E and p16 appears linked to E7 abundance, and may offer additional information (Fig. 3). The function of the HPV E6 protein complements that of E7, and in the high-risk HPV types, the two proteins are expressed together from a single polycistronic mRNA species [107]. A primary role of E6 is its association with p53, which in the case of the high-risk HPV types, mediates p53 ubiquitination and degradation (Fig. 3). This contributes to survivin accumulation [1], and prevents growth arrest or apoptosis in response to E7-mediated cell cycle entry in the upper epithelial layers, which would otherwise occur through activation of the ARF pathway (Fig. 3). E6s general role as an anti-apoptotic protein is further emphasized by the finding that it also associates with Bak [114] and Bax [69]. This role of E6 is important in the development of cervical cancers as it compromises the effectiveness of the cellular DNA damage response, and allows the accumulation of secondary mutations to go unchecked. The E6 protein of the high-risk HPV types also plays a role in mediating cell proliferation independently of E7 through its C-terminal PDZ-ligand domain [115]. E6-PDZ binding can mediate suprabasal cell proliferation [84,85] and may contribute to the development of metastatic tumours by disrupting normal cell-cell contacts. In productive lesions, cells are driven into cycle only in the lower epithelial layers, and extend towards the epithelial surface to varying extents depending on lesion grade and the nature of the infecting HPV type [92]. Genome maintenance and the replication of genomes in the upper epithelial layers appears critically dependent on E6 and E7 expression, as well as the viral proteins involved in origin binding. With the exception of E7 and its surrogate markers however, viral proteins are not readily detectable prior to the onset of genome amplification during normal productive infection [36,44]. The low level expression of viral proteins in the basal layer is thought to reflect, at least in part, the need of the virus to avoid detection by the host's immune system.

3.3. Amplification of viral genomes

The maintenance of viral genomes in the proliferating basal cells, and in cells of the lower epithelium, is a common feature of all papillomaviruses. During productive infection, genome amplification is triggered as the infected cell differentiates and is pushed towards

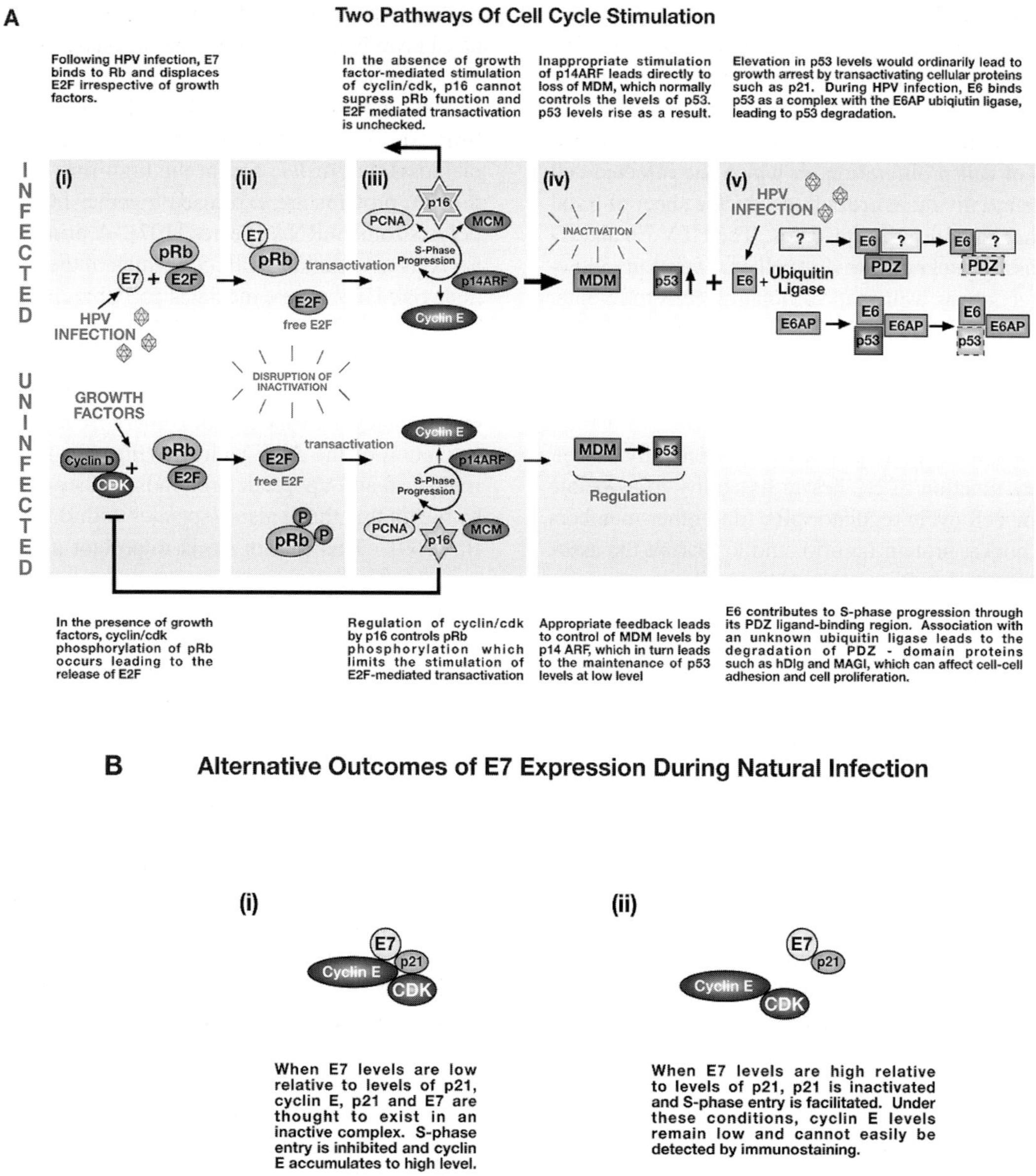

Fig. 3. Molecular basis for the expression of cell cycle markers. A. The regulation of S-phase entry in uninfected cells is shown in the bottom part of the panels, with the effects of HPV infection being shown above. i) In uninfected cells, S-phase entry requires the presence of external growth factors that activate CyclinD/Cdk leading pRb phosphorylation. Following HPV infection, the E7 protein binds to pRb. ii) The consequence of the above is the release of E2F, which can then act as a transcription factor. iii) E2F stimulates the expression of proteins necessary for S-phase entry such as PCNA and MCM. In uninfected cells, p16 regulates the continued expression of these proteins by inhibiting the activation of CyclinD/Cdk. In HPV infected cells, p16 is unable to exert a regulatory effect, as S-phase entry is stimulated by E7 rather than CyclinD/Cdk. iv) The uncontrolled expression of p16 that can sometimes be seen following E7 expression is accompanied by a rise in the levels of p14. This leads to MDM inactivation and to an increase in p53 that is countered by the E6 protein. In uninfected cells, p14 levels are regulated by p16 feedback and p53 levels remain low. v) The E6 protein forms a tripartite complex with E6AP and p53, which leads to the degradation of p53-mediated growth arrest and/or apoptosis. E6 can also stimulate the degradation of PDZ-domain proteins, which affects cell adhesion and signalling. B. The fate of cells expressing E7 can vary during natural infection. i) In the presence of high levels of p21 and lower levels of E7, E7-mediated cell proliferation can be stalled, and CyclinE/Cdk accumulates, probably as an inactive complex. ii) When E7 levels are high, p21-mediated growth arrest is thought to be inhibited as a result of association. In such cells, CyclinE/Cdk exists as a low-level active complex.

the epithelial surface by the division of the cells beneath. The initiation of late events can vary greatly in their timing, and in canine papillomas (caused by COPV), genome amplification begins in a subset of cells in the basal layer [86]. Although the onset of genome amplification in basal cells is not seen with any of the known HPV types, HPV 1 and 63 reproducibly trigger genome amplification in the cell layers immediately above [13,42]. The differences between different HPV types (and indeed evolutionary groups) can be clearly seen when lesions from the same epithelial site are compared. HPV 1, HPV2 and HPV4, which can all cause palmar and plantar warts, come from three different evolutionary groups. HPV2 shows a pattern that is characteristic of the Alpha group, and resembles the HPV types that cause genital warts (e.g. HPV6 and 11) and cervical lesions (HPV16 and 31) in its timing of genome amplification. Lesions from the same site caused by HPV1 and 4 show expression patterns that are clearly distinct [75].

The specific events that trigger the onset of genome amplification are not well understood, but depend in part on changes in the cellular environment as the infected cell migrates towards the epithelial surface. Of key importance is the up-regulation of the differentiation-dependent promoter, which for many HPV types resides within the E7 reading frame (Fig. 2B). Promoter activation, which is not dependent on viral genome amplification [7,106], leads to an increase in the levels of viral proteins necessary for replication, including E1, E2, E4 and E5 (Fig. 2B). Of these, the E4 protein is by far the most abundant, with the protein becoming easily detectable by immunostaining in the upper epithelial layers. In accordance with our understanding of papillomavirus protein function, cells supporting genome amplification stain positive for both E7 and E4, and can be shown to be replication competent using *in vitro* assays (Fig. 4).

Although E1, E2 and E5 expression is thought to accompany the expression of E4 (Fig. 2B), these proteins have proved difficult to detect in HPV-induced lesions. E1 is thought to be a very minor gene product, as codon usage within the E1 ORF is sub-optimal and E1 transcripts are difficult to detect. E2 by contrast, is thought to be expressed more abundantly. The E2 protein has been convincingly localized to cells supporting genome amplification in bovine warts caused by BPV, but its identification in human lesions is currently less conclusive [70,109]. The mRNA species that encode E1, E2 and E4 terminate at the early polyadenylation site and for many of the alpha papillomaviruses, include E5 as their second or third open reading frame. E5 is a transmembrane protein that is localized predominantly in the ER. The E5 protein can associate with the vacuolar proton ATPase and can delay the process of endosomal acidification [37,61,111], which affects the recycling of growth factor receptors on the epithelial surface. The consequence of this is an increase in EGF-mediated receptor signalling, which is thought to contribute (along with E6 and E7) to the maintenance of a replication competent environment during genome amplification [27]. Support for such a role during the virus life cycle comes from the analysis of E5 mutant genomes of HPV16 and 31, which show a lower level of genome amplification than do wild type genomes following propagation in raft culture [43,51]. The detection of E5 by immunostaining is compromised by the fact that the protein is predominantly membrane bound, and that epitope availability is therefore limited. The E5 protein has been detected in lesions induced by BPV where it localises to the basal cell layer and to differentiated epithelial cells supporting genome amplification [17]. In cervical biopsies caused by HPV16, one report has shown the protein to be present in the lower epithelial layers, but not specifically in basal cells [21]. As with E2, there are only a limited number of studies that have investigated E5 distribution *in vivo*, and it is difficult to be certain as to its precise expression pattern.

Although the molecular basis for the role of E1 and E2 in replication is well understood, the role of E4 is not yet fully worked out. Abundant 16E4 can inhibit cell cycle progression by associating with CyclinB/Cdk and CyclinA/Cdk during G2, and this leads to cell cycle arrest at the G2/M boundary by sequestering these proteins in the cytoplasm [31,32]. It has been suggested that the continued expression of E7 in a cell containing abundant E4 (as seen *in vivo*) may lead to the maintenance of an S-phase environment, which allows accumulation of the viral genomes. The correlation between E4 expression and genome amplification is an invariant characteristic of all papillomavirus types that have been analysed [75,92], and in several model systems, the inability to express E4 leads to a reduced ability to support the amplification of viral genomes [82,93, 119]. Although the precise contribution of E4 remains to be established, its association with cyclin dependent kinases [30,31], and with E2 [105], are likely to play important roles. It is intriguing to note, that the increase in E2 that is thought to accompany E4, must eventually down-regulate the viral early promoter that regulates E7 production and entry into S-phase. The steady rise

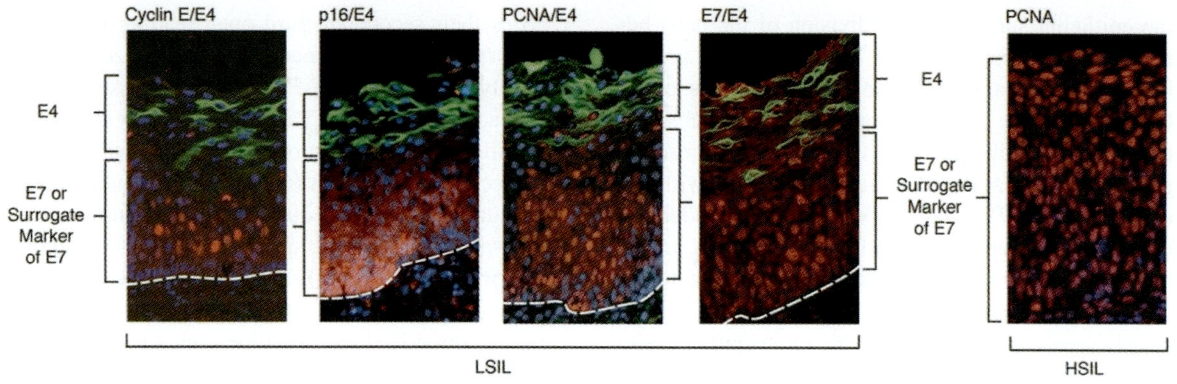

Fig. 4. Expression of E7 surrogates and E4 in cervical neoplasia. The expression of E7, or surrogate markers of E7 (CyclinE, p16, PCNA) are shown in red, and are found in the lower epithelial layers in low-grade lesions caused by HPV16. E4 expression is generally a marker of low-grade disease and is shown in green in the upper epithelial layers. E4 expression is usually lost during progression to high-grade neoplasia and cancer, with surrogate markers of E7 extending to the epithelial surface.

in E2 may act both to initiate genome amplification, and in a timely manner, to turn it off once amplification is complete. Such a scenario is supported by immunostaining data, which shows only a narrow overlap between cells expressing E7 and those expressing E4 (Fig. 4).

3.4. *Virus assembly and release*

The final stage in the virus life cycle involves the packaging of viral genomes into infectious particles that are shed from the epithelial surface. The two virus coat proteins (L1 and L2) are expressed only in cells that have already undergone genome amplification and which contain E4 in their cytoplasm. The E4 protein persists to the epithelial surface and is thought to have an additional role in virus release by associating with cytokeratins [39,98,118] and with the cornified envelope [14,15]. Both L2 and L1 are detectable by immunostaining, with the expression of L2 preceding the expression of L1 [38,47] (Fig. 2B). It appears that the precise timing of capsid synthesis is regulated at the level of RNA processing and protein synthesis [103, 127,130], with a change in splice site usage leading to the production of transcripts that terminate at the late rather than the early polyadenylation site. Important for this is a splicing silencer in the HPV16 L1 gene [129], and the presence of negative regulatory elements that destabilize HPV late transcripts [28,73], and allow the preferential synthesis of early transcripts in proliferating cells. Furthermore, the pattern of codon usage within the late genes is distinct from that of the host cell, and it is thought that this may further contribute to the suppression of L1 expression in the lower epithelial layers [128,130].

In addition to the virion structural proteins, the E2 protein is also thought to be required for the assembly of infectious particles. Both L2 and E2 localize to PML (promyelocytic leukaemia) bodies within the nucleus, with E2 recruiting replicated genomes to this site [16, 33]. Virus assembly occurs when L1 capsomeres enter the nucleus and are recruited to PML structures by L2 [47]. Although papillomavirus particles can assemble in the absence of L2, packaging occurs more efficiently in its presence [108], and viral infectivity is greatly enhanced [100]. In model systems of the virus life cycle, the inability to express L2 leads to a 10-fold reduction in packaging efficiency and a 100 fold reduction in virus infectivity when compared to wild type viral genomes [59]. At a molecular level, the association of L2 with L1 requires hydrophobic sequences near to the C-terminus of the protein that are thought to insert into the central hole of the pentavalent L1 capsomeres [46]. The assembly of caspsids is confined to the nucleus, and is dependent on sequences within the C-terminal region of the L1 protein that are essential for capsomere interactions. These protein-protein interactions are stabilized in the upper epithelial layers by disulphide bonding, which contributes to the stability of the released particles [16,99]. It is thought that the accumulation of virion structural proteins to high level is retarded until the cell reaches the upper epithelial layers in order to limit detection by the host immune response.

4. Abortive infection and neoplastic progression

DNA tumour viruses, such as Polyomaviruses or Adenoviruses, generally cause cancers when their nor-

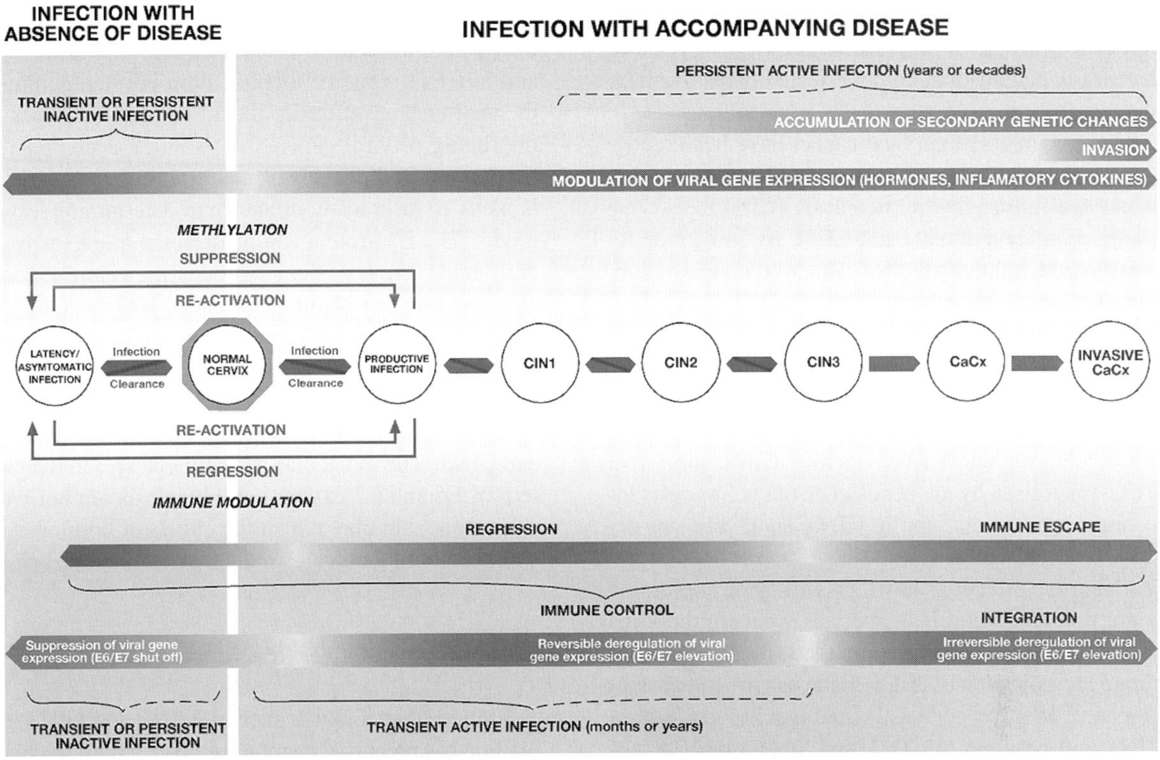

Fig. 5. Different outcomes of human papillomavirus infection. HPV infection at the cervix can have several outcomes. The most straightforward is the establishment of a productive infection that supports the assembly of infectious virions. Such infections can be controlled by the immune system and/or by other factors that regulate viral gene expression. This can lead to viral latency or to viral clearance. The deregulation of viral gene expression can also lead to cervical neoplasia. In the early stages of disease, this is reversible with some CIN2 reverting to CIN1 and below. The long-term deregulation of the viral oncogenes during persistent infection can lead to secondary changes in the cellular genome that contribute to the neoplastic phenotype. Integration of the viral genome into the host cell chromosome, which is thought to be a rare event, can eventually fix E6/E7 expression, predisposing to the accumulation of further genetic abnormalities and the development of cancer.

mal pattern of gene expression is compromised, and in many instances, this is also how papillomavirus-associated cancers can arise. High-risk genotypes such as HPV-16 infect cervical epithelium, with cervical cancer arising within the transformation zone of women who have long-term/persistent infections. The transformation zone is the site where the columnar cells of the endocervix meet the stratified squamous cells of the ectocervix, and this appears to be a particularly unstable site for high-risk HPV types. HPV16 infections can be found at many sites in the anogenital tract, including the vagina, vulva and penis, but despite this widespread distribution, the incidence of cancer at these sites is generally quite low (0.001% of the population). At the cervical transformation zone, the frequency of HPV-associated cancers is around 20 to 40 times higher than this, and in the absence of screening, affects around 30–40 people per 100,000 (depending on the population being studied). Only at the anus, in men who have sex with men, does the incidence of HPV-associated cancer rise to levels that are similar to those found at the cervix, and it is interesting to note that at both these susceptible sites there is a transformation zone [8].

HPV infection of the cervix can have a number of different outcomes, but in most cases it is thought that a period of productive infection is eventually followed by lesion regression and viral clearance (Fig. 5), or by the maintenance of viral genomes as latent episomes in cells of the basal layer. Resolution of infection as a result of a cell-mediated immune response is thought to be the primary mechanism by which infections are cleared, with most women who become infected showing no evidence of the infecting virus type after 18 months [121]. Primary infections are relatively common in young women, and affect between 20–40% depending on the population and geographical location, with the cumulative incidence of exposure over 5 years being as high as 60% [24,29,120]. This high lifetime risk of infection (estimated at approximately 80%) contrasts markedly with the relatively low risk of developing cervical cancer, and it is now well established that cancer progression typically occurs over years or decades in patients that do not effectively resolve their initial infection.

The precursors of cervical cancer have been recognized for many years, and are classified by pathologists as cervical intraepithelial neoplasia (CIN) of varying grade. Flat condylomata and CIN1 are low-grade lesions in which the productive cycle of the virus is supported to some degree, with cells that are being driven through the cell cycle being confined to the lower epithelial layers (Fig. 6). In CIN1, such cycling cells typically occupy the lower third of the epithelium, with mitotic figures being occasionally apparent in these cell layers. High-grade lesions such as CIN2 and CIN3 are characterised by the persistence of cycling cells into higher cell layers, and in CIN3, such cells are detectable at the epithelial surface. Such lesions represent abortive infections in which viral gene expression is not properly controlled, and late events in the virus life cycle are not properly supported (Fig. 6). The accurate identification of lesion grade has prognostic significance, as it has been estimated that around 20% of CIN1 will progress to CIN2, and that around 30% of CIN2 will progress to CIN3 if left untreated. CIN3 are generally considered to be the direct precursors of cervical cancer, and it has been suggested that around 40% of CIN3 lesions will progress to cervical cancer in the absence of intervention [95]. This figure may need to be re-evaluated in light of recent data from vaccination trials, which show that lesions graded as CIN2 or higher can be detected in around 1% of infected women within a few years of infection [54], and it is likely that many of these either regress or revert to lower grade disease rather than progressing to cancer. The aim of cervical screening is to predict the severity of cervical disease from the analysis of cells taken from the epithelial surface, and this approach has been hugely successful in managing cervical cancer in developed countries [95]. The molecular events that cause a productive lesion to progress to neoplasia and eventually to cancer are not precisely understood, but appear to reflect changes in viral gene expression, and in particular, an elevation in the level of E6 and E7 expression [116]. Using molecular markers that can distinguish between key life cycle phases (i.e. cell proliferation, genome amplification and virus synthesis) it appears that these events change in a very ordered way during progression to high-grade neoplasia, with the thickness of the E7-expressing layer increasing markedly with increasing disease severity [75]. This deregulation of early gene expression is accompanied by a concomitant failure to trigger late events until the cells are close to the epithelial surface, and in CIN3, genome amplification is often confined to small pockets at the epithelial surface. Changes in the timing of viral gene expression are accompanied by changes in the levels of the viral proteins, and this is likely to have a key influence in determining lesion grade. The E7 protein can be detected more easily in high-grade neoplasia than in productive lesions [36,44, 45], and this can also be evidenced when staining is carried out with surrogate markers of E7 expression such as $p16^{INK4A}$. Detectable $p16^{INK4A}$ is considered a surrogate marker of elevated E7 expression, and can be detected in some CIN1 lesions as well as in CIN2 and CIN3. The molecular basis for changes in the pattern of E6 and E7 expression in neplasia are not well understood, but may reflect the effects of hormones or cytokines acting on cells in the transformation zone.

5. Development of cervical cancer

High-grade neoplasia such as CIN2 and CIN3 are regarded as precursor lesions that have a high frequency of progressing to cancer. Although it is clear that cervical cancer can sometimes develop rapidly from such lesions, more typically it requires long-term/deregulated expression of the viral oncogenes, which is facilitated by the integration of HPV DNA into the host cell chromosome. Integration is typically a random event, and can occur at any site in the host cell DNA, with different levels of disruption to viral gene expression occurring as a result. Several reports have suggested that integration is favoured at common fragile sites, and in some instances, the expression pattern of cellular genes near to the integration site may contribute to the development of cancer [123]. The most significant consequence of integration however, is the deregulated expression of the viral E6 and E7 genes, which leads to persistent stimulation of S-phase entry, and the loss of the cellular p53 protein as a result of E6 activity. This combination of events predisposes to the accumulation of secondary genetic changes in the host cell genome, and compromises the ability of the cell to effectively repair damaged DNA. Although high-risk papillomaviruses express genes that stimulate cell proliferation and inhibit the p53-mediated DNA damage response, their presence alone is not sufficient to induce cervical cancer. The accumulation of mutations in the host-cell genome is an important and necessary event in the development of cervical cancer, and can occur over

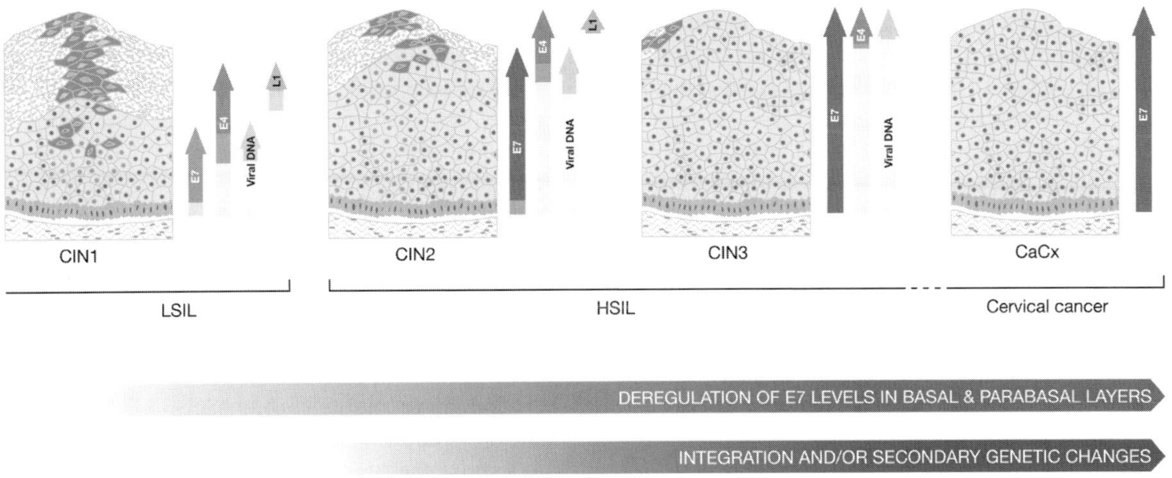

Fig. 6. Changes in expression patterns that accompany cervical cancer progression. Low-grade cervical lesions such as CIN1 (LSIL) are similar to productive infections caused by other HPV types. In such lesions, the three phases in the virus life cycle are distinguishable using antibodies to E7, E4 and L1 (shown diagrammatically on the left). During neoplastic progression (CIN2, CIN3), the levels of E6 and E7 are de-regulated, which facilitates the accumulation of secondary genetic changes that predispose to the development of cervical cancer. Although the order of events is unaltered (E7 then E4 then L1), cells expressing E7 extend closer and closer towards the epithelial surface as the grade of neoplasia increases. In high-grade neoplasia (CIN3), genome amplification is restricted to small pockets of differentiated cells, with the expression of L1 occurring only rarely. The development of cervical cancer typically involves the integration of viral DNA into the host cell genome, which stabilizes E6/E7 expression and facilitates the accumulation of secondary changes in the host cell.

time in women who carry persistent active infections. Such mutations can occur by chance, or can arise as a result of environmental events. Tobacco metabolites, which are present in the cervical secretions of women who smoke, are thought to act as co-factors in the development of cervical cancer [56,58]. Multiparity and the long-term use of oral contraceptives are also associated with increased risk [19,77], as is the presence of additional genital infections such as chlamydia. Given the requirement for secondary genetic changes, it is not difficult to see why cervical cancer develops at the site of infection over the course of years or decades. The average age of women presenting with visible high-grade neoplasia (CIN3) is in the late twenties, whereas the mean age of women with cervical cancer is in the fifties [9].

Integration is an important event in the development of most cervical cancers. The retention of E6 and E7 and the continued expression of these proteins is usually accompanied by the loss of regulatory genes such as E2 and E4, which are thought to antagonize E7-mediated cell proliferation during productive infection [30,31, 48,52,81]. Integration also leads to the loss of negative regulatory elements at the 3' end of HPV early transcripts, which contributes further to the deregulated expression of viral oncogenes [62]. The requirement of these genes for maintenance of the cancer cell phenotype is shown clearly by studies that have aimed to inhibit the expression of these genes in cervical cancer cells. Cell lines such as SiHa and Hela, which have been grown in the laboratory for almost 50 years, undergo apoptosis and cell death following the inhibition of E6 function by various approaches [18,53,63]. This also occurs following the re-introduction of E2, which suppresses the expression of the viral oncogenes by binding to the URR and down-regulating the early promoter [52,88]. Levels of E7 expression can also be affected by exposure to glucocorticoids and progesterone, as well as by methylation, and by changes in chromatin organization [3,65,90].

Although many different HPV types can infect the cervix, they are not all associated with cervical cancer. Most of the high-risk HPV types are contained within a separate evolutionary branch that is clearly distinct from the low-risk cutaneous and mucosal alpha papillomaviruses [102]. Even within the high-risk HPV group, there are however considerable differences in the frequency of cancer association which are not yet fully understood [23,25]. This can be seen from the fact that HPV16 and HPV31, which are closely related at the evolutionary level, are associated with very different levels of cervical cancer (HPV16, 53.5%; HPV31, 2.9%) [79]. Although these differences are not fully understood, the E6 and E7 proteins encoded by the high-risk types are thought to have specific functions that are important in cancer progression. High-risk (but not low-risk) E7 proteins can stimulate the accumulation of centrosomal abnormalities in cell culture and transgenic animals, and it has been suggested that this may increase the chance of genetic errors during each round of cell division [40,41,101]. This function of E7 is not totally dependent on its ability to bind to pRb and other members of the pocket protein family, which is of key importance in driving cell proliferation. High-risk E7 proteins bind pRb more efficiently than the low risk E7 proteins [50,78], and contribute to cancer progression by stimulating their proteosome-mediated degradation [5,10]. Like E7, the E6 proteins also differ in function when low and high-risk viruses are compared. The ability of high-risk E6 proteins to form a tripartite complex involving E6AP and p53 is well documented, and leads to the ubiquitination and degradation of p53 the p53 protein. The low-risk E6 proteins bind p53 with lower affinity, and have no significant ability to bind E6AP and to stimulate the degradation of p53 [60, 110]. The loss of the p53-mediated DNA damage response in cells that are driven into S-phase over years or decades, allows the accumulation of secondary changes in the host cell chromosome that eventually lead to cancer. The high-risk E6 proteins differ from the low-risk proteins in having a PDZ-binding domain at their C-terminus, which allows the binding and degradation of cellular targets containing PDZ motifs, such as hDlg and hScrib, which are involved in the regulation of cell growth and attachment [124]. PDZ binding is a characteristic of high-risk E6 proteins, and it is thought that the loss of cell-cell contacts that is mediated by tight junctions may contribute to the loss of cell polarity seen in HPV-associated cervical cancers [80]. The association with PDZ-domain proteins is distinct from E6's ability to bind and degrade p53, and appears important for cell proliferation in experimental systems [66,85]. High-risk E6 proteins have also been reported to be able to be able to activate the catalytic subunit of telomerase (hTERT (human telomerase reverse transcriptase) [67]. Telomerase activity is usually absent in somatic cells, and leads to the shortening of telomeres as cells divide. E6-mediated hTERT activation stimulates the addition of hexamer repeats to the telomeric ends of chromosomes, which is expected to inhibit cell senescence and extend the lifespan of cells harbouring HPV genomes. Such a function, may predispose to persistent infection.

Most cervical HPV infections do not lead to cervical cancer, with the vast majority causing only transient infections. It has been suggested that HPV16 and 18 may be more persistent than other HPV types [20], with persistence becoming a problem in women over 30 [117]. In experimental models, lesion formation is followed by lesion regression in as little as 5 weeks [22,87], whereas in infected women, most HPVs are thought to be cleared within 18 months with re-infection by the same HPV type being uncommon [121]. The immune system is clearly important in controlling persistence, and patients with immune defects can develop widespread lesions that are refractory to treatment. In model systems and in humans, regressing warts are associated with lymphocyte infiltration and elimination of infected tissue over the course of a few weeks [26,68, 87]. Although papillomavirus persistence is thought to depend in part on the genetic background of the host and the nature of the infecting HPV type, it appears that as a group, the Alpha papillomaviruses have developed characteristics that may enhance the longevity of infection. Amongst these characteristics are the regulation of E-cadherin expression and Langerhans cell density by E6 [71,125], the interference with MHC presentation by E5 [125], and interference with the function of interferon response factor 3 by E7 [4]. The fact that papillomaviruses avoid cell lysis, and express their late proteins only in the upper epithelial layers may further restrict detection by the immune system. The viral early proteins, which are expressed in the lower epithelial layers, are thought to be expressed at levels below those required to effectively trigger a host immune response. The stimulation of a cell-mediated response that can clear infection, appears to depend on the cross-priming of dendritic cells by viral antigens expressed on keratinocytes. It is uncertain whether the virus remains latent in the basal layer following regression, but this is suspected, and may explain the frequent detection of HPV DNA in the absence of disease. It appears that methylation may also play a role in controlling viral gene expression, and that under some circumstances, this may lead to an asymptomatic infection without a preceding productive phase [65] or immune response. Latent infection is thought to require E1 and E2 to allow basal cell replication of viral episomes, but is not thought to depend on the expression of E6 and E7 [126].

6. A consensus view of biomarker expression patterns during infection

Productively infected cells need to express the viral gene products in a defined order for infectious virions to be assembled at the epithelial surface. During productive infection, cell cycle markers such as PCNA and MCM are confined to the lower epithelial layers, with their presence being a direct consequence of E6/E7 activity. A separate and distinct type of biomarker identifies cells that are undergoing genome amplification, with the E4 protein being the most abundant member of this group. Virus assembly follows genome amplification, and is marked eventually by the appearance of capsid proteins (L1 and L2) in the upper epithelial layers. Virion structural proteins represent a third category of biomarker, and identify cells that are completing their productive cycle. Our current theories suggest that infected cells express each of these markers in turn during epithelial differentiation, and that the extent of productive infection can be established by considering the timing and extent of their expression.

During neoplastic progression, it appears that two types of change can occur. Firstly, viral gene expression becomes de-regulated and E6/E7 levels in the basal and parabasal cells increases. Given the known functions of these proteins, this is predicted to be a significant event in stimulating the accumulation of genetic errors in the host cell chromosome. Integration eventually fixes the expression of E6/E7 in the cell, which contributes further to the chance of progression. The second type of change relates to the regulation of late events, which become progressively retarded as the grade of neoplasia increases. This can be seen by immunostaining, as an increase in the thickness of the E7-expressing layers, and a reduction in the extent to which E4 is expressed in the upper layers of the epithelium. Whether these two events are linked remains to be established, as does the precise mechanisms that regulate such activity.

Acknowledgements

JD is a programme leader in the Division of Virology at the MRC National Institute for Medical Research, and is supported by the UK Medical Research Council. The encouragement and advice provided by Sir John Skehel FRS (Director), and Jonathan Stoye (Head of Virology) is gratefully appreciated, as is the commitment of all members of the NIMR Papillomavirus laboratory who have contributed to the ideas presented in this review.

References

[1] D.C. Altieri, Validating survivin as a cancer therapeutic target, *Nat Rev Cancer* **3** (2003), 46–54.

[2] M.J. Antinore, M.J. Birrer, D. Patel, L. Nader and D.J. McCance, The human papillomavirus type 16 E7 gene product interacts with and trans-activates the AP1 family of transcription factors, *EMBO J* **15** (1996), 1950–1960.

[3] J.M. Arbeit, P.M. Howley and D. Hanahan, Chronic estrogen-induced cervical and vaginal squamous carcinogenesis in human papillomavirus type 16 transgenic mice, *Proc Natl Acad Sci USA* **93** (1996), 2930–2935.

[4] P. Barnard, E. Payne and N.A. McMillan, The human papillomavirus E7 protein is able to inhibit the antiviral and anti-growth functions of interferon-alpha, *Virology* **277** (2000), 411–419.

[5] E. Berezutskaya, B. Yu, A. Morozov, P. Raychaudhuri and S. Bagchi, Differential regulation of the pocket domains of the retinoblastoma family proteins by the HPV16 E7 oncoprotein, *Cell Growth Differ* **8** (1997), 1277–1286.

[6] H.U. Bernard, The clinical importance of the nomenclature, evolution and taxonomy of human papillomaviruses, *J Clin Virol* **32**(Suppl 1) (2005), S1–S6.

[7] J.M. Bodily and C. Meyers, Genetic analysis of the human papillomavirus type 31 differentiation-dependent late promoter, *J Virol* **79** (2005), 3309–3321.

[8] F.X. Bosch and S. de Sanjose, Chapter 1: Human papillomavirus and cervical cancer – burden and assessment of causality, *J Natl Cancer Inst Monogr* **31** (2003), 3–13.

[9] F.X. Bosch, Rationale for Human Papillomavirus (HPV) Vaccines, in: *Emerging Issues on HPV Infections. From Science to Practice*, M. Monsonego, ed., 2006, Kager: Basel, pp. 206–216.

[10] S.N. Boyer, D.E. Wazer and V. Band, E7 protein of human papilloma virus-16 induces degradation of retinoblastoma protein through the ubiquitin-proteasome pathway, *Cancer Res* **56** (1996), 4620–4624.

[11] M. Branca, C. Giorgi, D. Santini, L. Di Bonito, M. Ciotti, S. Costa, A. Benedetto, E.A. Casolati, C. Favalli, P. Paba, P. Di Bonito, L. Mariani, S. Syrjanen, D. Bonifacio, L. Accardi, F. Zanconati and K. Syrjanen, Survivin as a marker of cervical intraepithelial neoplasia and high-risk human papillomavirus and a predictor of virus clearance and prognosis in cervical cancer, *Am J Clin Pathol* **124** (2005), 113–121.

[12] A. Brehm, S.J. Nielsen, E.A. Miska, D.J. McCance, J.L. Reid, A.J. Bannister and T. Kouzarides, The E7 oncoprotein associates with Mi2 and histone deacetylase activity to promote cell growth, *Embo J* **18** (1999), 2449–2458.

[13] F. Breitburd, O. Croissant and G. Orth, Expression of Human Papillomavirus type-1 E4 gene products in warts, in: *Cancer Cells 5*. 1987, Cold Spring Harbor Laboratory press: Cold Spring Harbor, New York. 115–122.

[14] D.R. Brown, D. Kitchin, B. Qadadri, N. Neptune, T. Batteiger and A. Ermel, The human papillomavirus type 11 E1–E4 protein is a transglutaminase 3 substrate and induces abnormalities of the cornified cell envelope, *Virology* **345** (2006), 290–298.

[15] J.T. Bryan and D.R. Brown, Association of the human papillomavirus type 11 E1^E4 protein with cornified cell envelopes derived from infected genital epithelium, *Virology* **277** (2000), 262–269.

[16] C.B. Buck, D.V. Pastrana, D.R. Lowy and J.T. Schiller, Efficient intracellular assembly of papillomaviral vectors, *J Virol* **78** (2004), 751–757.

[17] S. Burnett, N. Jareborg and D. DiMaio, Localization of bovine papillomavirus type 1 E5 protein to transformed keratinocytes and permissive differentiated cells in fibropapilloma tissue, *P.N.A.S.* **89** (1992), 5665–5669.

[18] K. Butz, T. Ristriani, A. Hengstermann, C. Denk, M. Scheffner and F. Hoppe-Seyler, siRNA targeting of the viral E6 oncogene efficiently kills human papillomavirus-positive cancer cells, *Oncogene* **22** (2003), 5938–5945.

[19] P.E. Castle, Beyond human papillomavirus: the cervix, exogenous secondary factors, and the development of cervical precancer and cancer, *J Low Genit Tract Dis* **8** (2004), 224–230.

[20] P.E. Castle, D. Solomon, M. Schiffman and C.M. Wheeler, Human papillomavirus type 16 infections and 2-year absolute risk of cervical precancer in women with equivocal or mild cytologic abnormalities, *J Natl Cancer Inst* **97** (2005), 1066–1071.

[21] J.L. Chang, Y.P. Tsao, D.W. Liu, S.J. Huang, W.H. Lee and S.L. Chen, The expression of HPV-16 E5 protein in squamous neoplastic changes in the uterine cervix, *J Biomed Sci* **8** (2001), 206–213.

[22] N.D. Christensen, N.M. Cladel, C.A. Reed and R. Han, Rabbit oral papillomavirus complete genome sequence and immunity following genital infection, *Virology* **269** (2000), 451–461.

[23] G.M. Clifford, J.S. Smith, T. Aguado and S. Franceschi, Comparison of HPV type distribution in high-grade cervical lesions and cervical cancer: a meta-analysis, *Br J Cancer* **89** (2003), 101–105.

[24] G.M. Clifford, J.S. Smith, M. Plummer, N. Munoz and S. Franceschi, Human papillomavirus types in invasive cervical cancer worldwide: a meta-analysis, *Br J Cancer* **88** (2003), 63–73.

[25] G.M. Clifford, R.K. Rana, S. Franceschi, J.S. Smith, G. Gough and J.M. Pimenta, Human papillomavirus genotype distribution in low-grade cervical lesions: comparison by geographic region and with cervical cancer, *Cancer Epidemiol Biomarkers Prev* **14** (2005), 1157–1164.

[26] N. Coleman, H.D.L. Birley, A.M. Renton, N.F. Hanna, B.K. Ryait, M. Byrne et al., Immunological events in regressing genital warts, *Am J Clin Pathol* **102** (1994), 768–774.

[27] K. Crusius, I. Rodriguez and A. Alonso, The human papillomavirus type 16 E5 protein modulates ERK1/2 and p38 MAP kinase activation by an EGFR-independent process in stressed human keratinocytes, *Virus Genes* **20** (2000), 65–69.

[28] S.A. Cumming, M.G. McPhillips, T. Veerapraditsin, S.G. Milligan and S.V. Graham, Activity of the human papillomavirus type 16 late negative regulatory element is partly due to four weak consensus 5' splice sites that bind a U1 snRNP-like complex, *J Virol* **77** (2003), 5167–5177.

[29] K.S. Cuschieri, H.A. Cubie, M.W. Whitley, A.L. Seagar, M.J. Arends, C. Moore, G. Gilkisson and E. McGoogan, Multiple high risk HPV infections are common in cervical neoplasia and young women in a cervical screening population, *J Clin Pathol* **57** (2004), 68–72.

[30] C.E. Davy, D.J. Jackson, Q. Wang, K. Raj, P.J. Masterson, N.F. Fenner, S. Southern, S. Cuthill, J.B. Millar, and J. Doorbar, Identification of a G(2) arrest domain in the E1^E4 protein of human papillomavirus type 16., *J Virol* **76** (2002), 9806–9818.

[31] C.E. Davy, D.J. Jackson, K. Raj, W.L. Peh, S.A. Southern, P. Das, R. Sorathia, P. Laskey, K. Middleton, T. Nakahara, Q. Wang, P.J. Masterson, P.F. Lambert, S. Cuthill, J.B. Millar and J. Doorbar, Human Papillomavirus Type 16 E1^E4-Induced G2 Arrest Is Associated with Cytoplasmic Retention of Active Cdk1/Cyclin B1 Complexes, *J Virol* **79** (2005), 3998–4011.

[32] C.E. Davy, M. Ayub, D.J. Jackson, P. Das, P. McIntosh and J. Doorbar, HPV16 E1^E4 protein is phosphorylated by Cdk2/cyclin A and relocalizes this complex to the cytoplasm, *Virology* (2006).

[33] P.M. Day, R.B.S. Roden, D.R. Lowy and J.T. Schiller, The papillomavirus minor capsid protein, L2, induces localization of the major capsid protein, L1, and the viral transcription/replication protein, E2, to PML oncogenic domains, *J Virol* **72** (1998), 142–150.

[34] E.M. de Villiers, C. Fauquet, T.R. Broker, H.U. Bernard and H. zur Hausen, Classification of papillomaviruses, *Virology* **324** (2004), 17–27.

[35] G. Dell, K.W. Wilkinson, R. Tranter, J. Parish, R. Leo Brady and K. Gaston, Comparison of the structure and DNA-binding properties of the E2 proteins from an oncogenic and a non-oncogenic human papillomavirus, *J Mol Biol* **334** (2003), 979–991.

[36] A.D. Di Lonardo, M.L. Marcante, F. Poggiali, E. Hamsoikova and A. Venuti, Egg yolk antibodies against the E7 oncogenic protein of human papillomavirus type 16, *Arch Virol* **146** (2001), 117–125.

[37] G.L. Disbrow, J.A. Hanover and R. Schlegel, Endoplasmic reticulum-localized human papillomavirus type 16 E5 protein alters endosomal pH but not trans-Golgi pH, *J Virol* **79** (2005), 5839–5846.

[38] J. Doorbar and P.H. Gallimore, Identification of proteins encoded by the L1 and L2 open reading frames of human papillomavirus type 1a, *J Virol* **61** (1987), 2793–2799.

[39] J. Doorbar, S. Ely, J. Sterling, C. McLean and L. Crawford, Specific interaction between HPV-16 E1^E4 and cytokeratins results in collapse of the epithelial cell intermediate filament network, *Nature* **352** (1991), 824–827.

[40] S. Duensing, A. Duensing, E.R. Flores, A. Do, P.F. Lambert and K. Munger, Centrosome abnormalities and genomic instability by episomal expression of human papillomavirus type 16 in raft cultures of human keratinocytes, *J Virol* **75** (2001), 7712–7716.

[41] S. Duensing and K. Munger, Mechanisms of genomic instability in human cancer: insights from studies with human papillomavirus oncoproteins, *Int J Cancer* **109** (2004), 157–162.

[42] K. Egawa, A. Iftner, J. Doorbar, Y. Honda and T. Iftner, Synthesis of Viral DNA and Late Capsid Protein L1 in Parabasal Spinous Cell Layers of Naturally Occurring Benign Warts Infected with Human Papillomavirus Type 1, *Virology* **268** (2000), 281–293.

[43] F. Fehrmann, D.J. Klumpp and L.A. Laimins, Human papillomavirus type 31 E5 protein supports cell cycle progression and activates late viral functions upon epithelial differentiation, *J Virol* **77** (2003), 2819–2831.

[44] M. Fiedler, E. Muller-Holzner, H.P. Viertler, A. Widschwendter, A. Laich, G. Pfister, G.A. Spoden, P. Jansen-Durr and W. Zwerschke, High level HPV-16 E7 oncoprotein expression correlates with reduced pRb-levels in cervical biopsies, *Faseb J* **18** (2004), 1120–1122.

[45] M. Fiedler, S. Ressler, B. Campo-Fernandez, A. Laich, L. Jansen, A. Widschwendter, H.P. Viertler, N. Bacher, D. Morandell, E. Muller-Holzner, M. Durst, P. Jansen-Durr and W. Zwerschke, Expression of the high-risk human papillomavirus type 18 and 45 E7 oncoproteins in cervical carcinoma biopsies, *J Gen Virol* **86** (2005), 3235–3241.

[46] R.L. Finnen, K.D. Erickson, X.S. Chen and R.L. Garcea, Interactions between papillomavirus L1 and L2 capsid proteins, *J Virol* **77** (2003), 4818–4826.

[47] L. Florin, C. Sapp, R.E. Streeck and M. Sapp, Assembly and translocation of papillomavirus capsid proteins, *J Virol* **76** (2002), 10009–10014.

[48] N. Fournier, K. Raj, P. Saudan, S. Utzig, R. Sahli, V. Simanis and P. Beard, Expression of human papillomavirus 16 E2 protein in Schizosaccharomyces pombe delays the initiation of mitosis, *Oncogene* **18** (1999), 4015–4021.

[49] J.O. Funk, S. Waga, J.B. Harry, E. Espling, B. Stillman and D.A. Galloway, Inhibition of CDK activity and PCNA-dependent DNA replication by p21 is blocked by interaction with the HPV16 E7 oncoprotein, *Genes and Development* **11** (1997), 2090–2100.

[50] J.R. Gage, C. Meyers and F.O. Wettstein, The E7 proteins of the nononcogenic human papillomavirus type 6b (HPV-6b) and of the oncogenic HPV-16 differ in retinoblastoma protein binding and other properties, *J Virol* **64** (1990), 723–730.

[51] S.M. Genther, S. Sterling, S. Duensing, K. Munger, C. Sattler and P.F. Lambert, Quantitative role of the human papillomavirus type 16 E5 gene during the productive stage of the viral life cycle, *J Virol* **77** (2003), 2832–2842.

[52] E.C. Goodwin and D. DiMaio, Repression of human papillomavirus oncogenes in HeLa cervical carcinoma cells causes the orderly reactivation of dormant tumor suppressor pathways, *Proc Natl Acad Sci USA* **97** (2000), 12513–12518.

[53] H. Griffin, R. Elston, J. DJ, K. Ansell, M. Coleman, G. Winter and J. Doorbar, Inhibition of papillomavirus protein function in cervical cancer cells by intrabody targeting, *JMB* (2006), in press.

[54] D.M. Harper, E.L. Franco, C.M. Wheeler, A.B. Moscicki, B. Romanowski, C.M. Roteli-Martins, D. Jenkins, A. Schuind, S.A. Costa Clemens and G. Dubin, Sustained efficacy up to 4.5 years of a bivalent L1 virus-like particle vaccine against human papillomavirus types 16 and 18: follow-up from a randomised control trial, *Lancet* **367** (2006), 1247–1255.

[55] C.A. Harwood and C.M. Proby, Human papillomaviruses and non-melanoma skin cancer, *Curr Opin Infect Dis* **15** (2002), 101–114.

[56] H.W. Haverkos, Viruses, chemicals and co-carcinogenesis, *Oncogene* **23** (2004), 6492–6499.

[57] P. Heino, J. Zhou and P.F. Lambert, Interaction of the papillomavirus transcription/replication factor, E2, and the viral capsid protein, L2, *Virology* **276** (2000), 304–314.

[58] D. Hellberg and U. Stendahl, The biological role of smoking, oral contraceptive use and endogenous sexual steroid hormones in invasive squamous epithelial cervical cancer, *Anticancer Res* **25** (2005), 3041–3046.

[59] S.C. Holmgren, N.A. Patterson, M.A. Ozbun and P.F. Lambert, The minor capsid protein L2 contributes to two steps in the human papillomavirus type 31 life cycle, *J Virol* **79** (2005), 3938–3948.

[60] J.M. Huibregtse, M. Scheffner and P.M. Howley, Localization of the E6AP regionsthat direct human papillomavirus E6 binding, association with p53 and ubiquitination of associated proteins, *Mol Cell Biol* **13** (1993), 4918–4927.

[61] E.S. Hwang, T. Nottoli and D. Dimaio, The HPV16 E5 protein: expression, detection, and stable complex formation with transmembrane proteins in COS cells, *Virology* **211** (1995), 227–233.

[62] S. Jeon and P.F. Lambert, Integration of HPV16 DNA into the human genome leads to increased stability of E6/E7 mRNAs: implications for cervical carcinogenesis, *PNAS* **92** (1995), 1654–1658.

[63] M. Jiang and J. Milner, Selective silencing of viral gene expression in HPV-positive human cervical carcinoma cells treated with siRNA, a primer of RNA interference, *Oncogene* **21** (2002), 6041–6048.

[64] J.G. Joyce, J.S. Tung, C.T. Przysiecki, J.C. Cook, E.D. Lehman, J.A. Sands, K.U. Jansen and P.M. Keller, The L1 major capsid protein of human papillomavirus type 11 recombinant virus-like particles interacts with heparin and cell-surface glycosaminoglycans on human keratinocytes., *J Biol Chem* **274** (1999), 5810–5822.

[65] M. Kalantari, I.E. Calleja-Macias, D. Tewari, B. Hagmar, K. Lie, H.A. Barrera-Saldana, D.J. Wiley and H.U. Bernard, Conserved methylation patterns of human papillomavirus type 16 DNA in asymptomatic infection and cervical neoplasia, *J Virol* **78** (2004), 12762–12772.

[66] T. Kiyono, A. Hiraiwa, M. Fujita, Y. Hayashi, T. Akiyama and M. Ishibashi, Binding of high-risk human papillomavirus E6 oncoproteins to the human homologue of the Drosophila discs large tumor suppressor protein, *Proc Natl Acad Sci U S A* **94** (1997), 11612–11616.

[67] A.J. Klingelhutz, S.A. Foster and J.K. McDougall, Telomerase activation by the E6 gene product of human papillomavirus type 16, *Nature* **380** (1996), 79–82.

[68] G. Knowles, B.W. O'Neil and M.S. Campo, Phenotypical characterization of lymphocytes infiltrating regressing papillomas, *J Virol* **70** (1996), 8451–8458.

[69] B. Li and Q.P. Dou, Bax degradation by the ubiquitin/proteasome-dependent pathway: involvement in tumor survival and progression, *Proc Natl Acad Sci U S A* **97** (2000), 3850–3855.

[70] N.J. Maitland, S. Conway, N.S. Wilkinson, J. Ramsdale, J.R. Morris, C.M. Sanders, J.E. Burns, P.L. Stern and M. Wells, Expression patterns of the human papillomavirus type 16 transcription factor E2 in low- and high-grade cervical intraepithelial neoplasia, *J Pathol* **186** (1998), 275–280.

[71] K. Matthews, C.M. Leong, L. Baxter, E. Inglis, K. Yun, B.T. Backstrom, J. Doorbar and M. Hibma, Depletion of Langerhans cells in human papillomavirus type 16-infected skin is associated with E6-mediated down regulation of E-cadherin, *J Virol* **77** (2003), 8378–8385.

[72] N.A. McMillan, E. Payne, I.H. Frazer and M. Evander, Expression of the alpha6 integrin confers papillomavirus binding upon receptor-negative B-cells, *Virology* **261** (1999), 271–279.

[73] M.G. McPhillips, T. Veerapraditsin, S.A. Cumming, D. Karali, S.G. Milligan, W. Boner, I.M. Morgan and S.V. Graham, SF2/ASF binds the human papillomavirus type 16 late RNA control element and is regulated during differentiation of virus-infected epithelial cells, *J Virol* **78** (2004), 10598–10605.

[74] M.G. McPhillips, K. Ozato and A.A. McBride, Interaction of bovine papillomavirus E2 protein with Brd4 stabilizes its association with chromatin, *J Virol* **79** (2005), 8920–8932.

[75] K. Middleton, W. Peh, S.A. Southern, H.M. Griffin, K. Sotlar, T. Nakahara, A. El-Sherif, L. Morris, R. Seth, M. Hibma, D. Jenkins, P.F. Lambert, N. Coleman and J. Doorbar, Organisation of the human papillomavirus productive cycle during neoplastic progression provides a basis for the selection of diagnostic markers, *J Virol* **77** (2003), 10186–10201.

[76] Y. Modis, B.L. Trus and S.C. Harrison, Atomic model of the papillomavirus capsid, *Embo J* **21** (2002), 4754–4762.

[77] J. Moodley, Combined oral contraceptives and cervical cancer, *Curr Opin Obstet Gynecol* **16** (2004), 27–29.

[78] K. Munger, W.C. Phelps, V. Bubb, P.M. Howley and R. Schlegel, The E6 and E7 genes of the human papillomavirus type 16 together are necessary and sufficient for transfor-

mation of primary human keratinocytes, *J Virol* **63** (1989), 4417–4421.
[79] N. Munoz, F.X. Bosch, X. Castellsague, M. Diaz, S. de Sanjose, D. Hammouda, K.V. Shah and C.J. Meijer, Against which human papillomavirus types shall we vaccinate and screen? The international perspective, *Int J Cancer* **111** (2004), 278–285.
[80] S. Nakagawa and J.M. Huibregtse, Human scribble (Vartul) is targeted for ubiquitin-mediated degradation by the high-risk papillomavirus E6 proteins and the E6AP ubiquitin-protein ligase, *Mol Cell Biol* **20** (2000), 8244–8253.
[81] T. Nakahara, A. Nishimura, M. Tanaka, T. Ueno, A. Ishimoto and H. Sakai, Modulation of the cell division cycle by human papillomavirus type 18 E4, *J Virol* **76** (2002), 10914–10920.
[82] T. Nakahara, W.L. Peh, J. Doorbar, D. Lee and P.F. Lambert, Human Papillomavirus Type 16 E1ˆE4 Contributes to Multiple Facets of the Papillomavirus Life Cycle, *J Virol* **79** (2005), 13150–13165.
[83] A. Narechania, M. Terai, Z. Chen, R. DeSalle and R.D. Burk, Lack of the canonical pRB-binding domain in the E7 ORF of artiodactyl papillomaviruses is associated with the development of fibropapillomas, *J Gen Virol* **85** (2004), 1243–1250.
[84] M.L. Nguyen, M.M. Nguyen, D. Lee, A.E. Griep and P.F. Lambert, The PDZ ligand domain of the human papillomavirus type 16 E6 protein is required for E6's induction of epithelial hyperplasia *in vivo*, *J Virol* **77** (2003), 6957–6964.
[85] M.M. Nguyen, M.L. Nguyen, G. Caruana, A. Bernstein, P.F. Lambert and A.E. Griep, Requirement of PDZ-containing proteins for cell cycle regulation and differentiation in the mouse lens epithelium, *Mol Cell Biol* **23** (2003), 8970–8981.
[86] P. Nicholls, J. Doorbar, R.W. Moore, W. Peh, D. Anderson and M. Stanley, Detection of Viral DNA and E4 Protein in Basal Keratinocytes of Experimental Canine Oral Papillomavirus Lesions, *Virology* **283** (2001), 82–98.
[87] P.K. Nicholls, P.F. Moore, D.M. Anderson, R.A. Moore, N.R. Parry, G.W. Gough and M.A. Stanley, Regression of canine oral papillomas is associated with infiltration of CD4+ and CD8+ lymphocytes, *Virology* **283** (2001), 31–39.
[88] A. Nishimura, T. Ono, A. Ishimoto, J.J. Dowhanick, M.A. Frizzell, P.M. Howley and H. Sakai, Mechanisms of human papillomavirus E2-mediated repression of viral oncogene expression and cervical cancer cell growth inhibition, *J Virol* **74** (2000), 3752–3760.
[89] F. Noya, W.-M. Chien, T.R. Broker and L.T. Chow, p21cip1 degradation in differentiated keratinocytes is abrogated by costabilization with cyclin E indced by human papillomavirus E7, *J. Virol* **75** (2001), 6121–6134.
[90] M.M. Pater, G.A. Hughes, D.E. Hyslop, H. Nakshatri and A. Pater, Glucocorticoid-dependent oncogenic transformation by type 16 but not type 11 human papilloma virus DNA, *Nature* **335** (1988), 832–835.
[91] N.A. Patterson, J.L. Smith and M.A. Ozbun, Human papillomavirus type 31b infection of human keratinocytes does not require heparan sulfate, *J Virol* **79** (2005), 6838–6847.
[92] W.L. Peh, K. Middleton, N. Christensen, P. Nicholls, K. Egawa, K. Sotlar, J. Brandsma, A. Percival, J. Lewis, W.J. Liu and J. Doorbar, Life cycle heterogeneity in animal models of human papillomavirus-associated disease, *J Virol* **76** (2002), 10401–10416.
[93] W.L. Peh, J.L. Brandsma, N.D. Christensen, N.M. Cladel, X. Wu and J. Doorbar, The Viral E4 Protein Is Required for the Completion of the Cottontail Rabbit Papillomavirus (CRPV) Productive Cycle *In Vivo*, *J.Virol* **15** (2004), 2142–2151.
[94] G. Persson, K. Andersson and I. Krantz, Symptomatic genital papillomavirus infection in a community. Incidence and clinical picture, *Acta Obstet Gynecol Scand* **75** (1996), 287–290.
[95] J. Peto, C. Gilham, O. Fletcher and F.E. Matthews, The cervical cancer epidemic that screening has prevented in the UK, *Lancet* **364** (2004), 249–256.
[96] H. Pfister, Chapter 8: Human papillomavirus and skin cancer, *J Natl Cancer Inst Monogr* (2003), 52–56.
[97] N. Ramoz, L.A. Rueda, B. Bouadjar, L.S. Montoya, G. Orth and M. Favre, Mutations in two adjacent novel genes are associated with epidermodysplasia verruciformis, *Nat Genet* **32** (2002), 579–581.
[98] S. Roberts, I. Ashmole, S. Rookes and P. Gallimore, Mutational analysis of the human papillomavirus type 16 E1ˆE4 protein shows that the C terminus is dispensable for keratin cytoskeleton association but is involved in inducing disruption of the keratin filaments, *J Virol* **71** (1997), 3554–3562.
[99] R.B. Roden, D.R. Lowy and J.T. Schiller, Papillomavirus is resistant to desiccation, *J Infect Dis* **176** (1997), 1076–1079.
[100] R.B. Roden, P.M. Day, B.K. Bronzo, W.H.t. Yutzy, Y. Yang, D.R. Lowy and J.T. Schiller, Positively charged termini of the L2 minor capsid protein are necessary for papillomavirus infection, *J Virol* **75** (2001), 10493–10497.
[101] A.J. Schaeffer, M. Nguyen, A. Liem, D. Lee, C. Montagna, P.F. Lambert, T. Ried and M.J. Difilippantonio, E6 and E7 oncoproteins induce distinct patterns of chromosomal aneuploidy in skin tumors from transgenic mice, *Cancer Res* **64** (2004), 538–546.
[102] M. Schiffman, R. Herrero, R. Desalle, A. Hildesheim, S. Wacholder, A.C. Rodriguez, M.C. Bratti, M.E. Sherman, J. Morales, D. Guillen, M. Alfaro, M. Hutchinson, T.C. Wright, D. Solomon, Z. Chen, J. Schussler, P.E. Castle and R.D. Burk, The carcinogenicity of human papillomavirus types reflects viral evolution, *Virology* **337** (2005), 76–84.
[103] S. Schwartz, Regulation of human papillomavirus late gene expression, *Ups J Med Sci* **105** (2000), 171–192.
[104] S. Shafti-Keramat, A. Handisurya, E. Kriehuber, G. Meneguzzi, K. Slupetzky and R. Kirnbauer, Different heparan sulfate proteoglycans serve as cellular receptors for human papillomaviruses, *J Virol* **77** (2003), 13125–13135.
[105] R. Sorathia, C. Davy, H. Sterlinko, D. Jackson, Q. Wang, P. McIntosh, W.L. Peh, H. Griffin, C.-M. Chiang, L. Banks and J. Doorbar, The E4 protein of HPV16 interacts with E2 and regulates its nuclear functions. in 21st International Papillomavirus Conference. 2004. Mexico City, Mexico.
[106] K.M. Spink and L.A. Laimins, Induction of the human papillomavirus type 31 late promoter requires differentiation but not DNA amplification, *J Virol* **79** (2005), 4918–4926.
[107] S.N. Stacey, D. Jordan, A.J. Williamson, M. Brown, J.H. Coote and J.R. Arrand, Leaky scanning is the predominant mechanism for translation of human papillomavirus type 16 E7 oncoprotein from E6/E7 bicistronic mRNA, *J Virol* **74** (2000), 7284–7297.
[108] Y. Stauffer, K. Raj, K. Masternak and P. Beard, Infectious human papillomavirus type 18 pseudovirions, *J Mol Biol* **283** (1998), 529–536.
[109] M. Stevenson, L.C. Hudson, J.E. Burns, R.L. Stewart, M. Wells and N.J. Maitland, Inverse relationship between the expression of the human papillomavirus type 16 transcription factor E2 and virus DNA copy number during the progression of cervical intraepithelial neoplasia, *J Gen Virol* **81** (2000), 1825–1832.

[110] A. Storey, M. Thomas, A. Kalita, C. Harwood, D. Gardiol, F. Mantovani, J. Breuer, I.M. Leigh, G. Matlashewski and L. Banks, Role of a p53 polymorphism in the development of human papillomavirus-associated cancer, *Nature* **393** (1998), 229–234.

[111] S.W. Straight, B. Herman and D.J. McCance, The E5 oncoprotein of HPV16 inhibits the acidification of endosomes in human keratinocytes, *J Virol* **69** (1995), 3185–3192.

[112] G. Tate, T. Suzuki, K. Kishimoto and T. Mitsuya, Novel mutations of EVER1/TMC6 gene in a Japanese patient with epidermodysplasia verruciformis, *J Hum Genet* **49** (2004), 223–225.

[113] M. Terai, R. DeSalle and R.D. Burk, Lack of canonical E6 and E7 open reading frames in bird papillomaviruses: Fringilla coelebs papillomavirus and Psittacus erithacus timneh papillomavirus, *J Virol* **76** (2002), 10020–10023.

[114] M. Thomas and L. Banks, Inhibition of Bak-induced apoptosis by HPV-18 E6, *Oncogene* **17** (1998), 2943–2954.

[115] M. Thomas, R. Laura, K. Hepner, E. Guccione, C. Sawyers, L. Lasky and L. Banks, Oncogenic human papillomavirus E6 proteins target the MAGI-2 and MAGI-3 proteins for degradation, *Oncogene* **21** (2002), 5088–5096.

[116] M. von Knebel Doeberitz, New markers for cervical dysplasia to visualise the genomic chaos created by aberrant oncogenic papillomavirus infections, *Eur J Cancer* **38** (2002), 2229–2242.

[117] K.L. Wallin, F. Wiklund, T. Angstrom, F. Bergman, U. Stendahl, G. Wadell, G. Hallmans and J. Dillner, Type-specific persistence of human papillomavirus DNA before the development of invasive cervical cancer, *N Engl J Med* **341** (1999), 1633–1638.

[118] Q. Wang, H. Griffin, S. Southern, D. Jackson, A. Martin, P. McIntosh, C. Davy, P.J. Masterson, P.A. Walker, P. Laskey, M.B. Omary and J. Doorbar, Functional Analysis of the human papillomavirus type 16 E1^E4 protein provides a mechanism for *in vivo* and *in vitro* keratin filament re-organisation, *J Virol* **78** (2004), 821–833.

[119] R. Wilson, F. Fehrmann and L.A. Laimins, Role of the E1–E4 protein in the differentiation-dependent life cycle of human papillomavirus type 31, *J Virol* **79** (2005), 6732–6740.

[120] C.B. Woodman, S. Collins, H. Winter, A. Bailey, J. Ellis, P. Prior, M. Yates, T.P. Rollason and L.S. Young, Natural history of cervical human papillomavirus infection in young women: a longitudinal cohort study, *Lancet* **357** (2001), 1831–1836.

[121] L.F. Xi, G.W. Demers, L.A. Koutsky, N.B. Kiviat, J. Kuypers, D.H. Watts, K.K. Holmes and D.A. Galloway, Analysis of human papillomavirus type 16 variants indicates establishment of persistent infection, *J Infect Dis* **172** (1995), 747–755.

[122] J. You, J.L. Croyle, A. Nishimura, K. Ozato and P.M. Howley, Interaction of the bovine papillomavirus E2 protein with Brd4 tethers the viral DNA to host mitotic chromosomes, *Cell* **117** (2004), 349–360.

[123] T. Yu, M.J. Ferber, T.H. Cheung, T.K. Chung, Y.F. Wong and D.I. Smith, The role of viral integration in the development of cervical cancer, *Cancer Genet Cytogenet* **158** (2005), 27–34.

[124] J. Zeitler, C.P. Hsu, H. Dionne and D. Bilder, Domains controlling cell polarity and proliferation in the Drosophila tumor suppressor Scribble, *J Cell Biol* **167** (2004), 1137–1146.

[125] B. Zhang, P. Li, E. Wang, Z. Brahmi, K.W. Dunn, J.S. Blum and A. Roman, The E5 protein of human papillomavirus type 16 perturbs MHC class II antigen maturation in human foreskin keratinocytes treated with interferon-gamma, *Virology* **310** (2003), 100–108.

[126] P. Zhang, M. Nouri, J.L. Brandsma, T. Iftner and B.M. Steinberg, Induction of E6/E7 expression in cottontail rabbit papillomavirus latency following UV activation, *Virology* **263** (1999), 388–394.

[127] K.N. Zhao, W.J. Liu and I.H. Frazer, Codon usage bias and A+T content variation in human papillomavirus genomes, *Virus Res* **98** (2003), 95–104.

[128] K.N. Zhao, W. Gu, N.X. Fang, N.A. Saunders and I.H. Frazer, Gene codon composition determines differentiation-dependent expression of a viral capsid gene in keratinocytes *in vitro* and *in vivo*, *Mol Cell Biol* **25** (2005), 8643–8655.

[129] X. Zhao, M. Rush and S. Schwartz, Identification of an hnRNP A1-dependent splicing silencer in the human papillomavirus type 16 L1 coding region that prevents premature expression of the late L1 gene, *J Virol* **78** (2004), 10888–10905.

[130] J. Zhou, W.J. Liu, S.W. Peng, X.Y. Sun and I. Frazer, Papillomavirus capsid protein expression level depends on the match between codon usage and tRNA availability, *J Virol* **73** (1999), 4972–4982.

ventive HPV vaccines may have substantial influence on disease prevalence and will increase the demand of screening assays with better predictive values to detect possible vaccination failures and to pick up precursor lesions that are induced by HPV types not covered by current vaccines [35].

2. Current cervical cancer screening approaches

Current cervical cancer screening in industrialized countries is based on the cytology based Pap test. This test has been introduced in the middle of the last century and has not been modified substantially since then.

The major problem of Pap cytology screening is lack of reproducibility of the test results [81]. Many classification systems for cervical cytology have been proposed over the years in different health systems, including the classical Papanicolaou terminology, the Munich classifications that are closely related to the Papanicolaou system (primarily used in Germany), and the histology oriented WHO classification (frequently used in the UK). The most widely used system is the two-tiered Bethesda classification in that abnormal cells are classified as low grade or high grade squamous intraepithelial lesions (LSIL, HSIL) [97].

LSIL mainly represents morphological correlates of active HPV replication (e.g. koilocytes), whereas HSIL is characterized by morphological alterations indicative of transformation, primarily increasing nuclear alterations. A substantial number of atypical specimens can not be attributed to either one of these categories and are referred to as atypical squamous cells of undetermined significance (ASC-US) or atypical squamous cells can not exclude HSIL (ASC-H) that require further evaluation. Due to the many influencing parameters such as different cytology classifications and different guidelines for the management of abnormal cytology, data about the efficacy of Pap based screening are not easily comparable between different health care systems. Accordingly, the sensitivity of Pap testing for the detection of CIN2 or higher varied between 34% and 94% as summarized recently by Wright [126]. In contrast, the specificity of Pap testing is consistently high in the majority of the studies.

In order to compensate the low sensitivity of Pap cytology, the test is frequently repeated.

The main problem of Pap cytology is the large proportion of inconclusive or mildly abnormal test results that may mask a low number of high grade precancerous cases. In the ALTS trial, a two year cumulative diagnosis of CIN3 was found in 8–9% of the ASC-US cases and in about 15% of the LSIL cases.

In order to avoid missing these cases, a lot of effort is necessary to work up borderline test results. Several large studies analyzing the management of ASC-US and LSIL have been performed and were reviewed in a recent meta-analysis [3]. Based on these studies, three management strategies are currently performed: Repeat cytology, direct colposcopy and HPV triage of ASC-US. Currently, HPV testing has not been recommended for LSIL, since the vast majority of these lesions are HPV positive. However, recent studies suggest that a risk stratification by HPV single typing might improve HPV based triage both for ASCUS and LSIL [22].

In the British HART study, primary HPV screening was evaluated and found to be a promising alternative to primary screening using cytology [25]. HPV positive cases could be followed up with cytology, however, depending of the population and age of screening, a large number of HPV-infected women that do not have disease or cervical lesions would still require further more detailed work up under these circumstances. So far, other promising biomarkers have not been assessed in sufficiently large primary screening studies.

In the vast majority of developing countries no organized cervical cancer screening programs exist. Opportunistic screening is rarely offered, because there is limited access to infrastructure that allows performing appropriate cytology. In these countries, the detection of cervical cancer and precancer is mainly based on direct visual inspection. One advantage of the visual screening approach is the direct possibility of treating suspect lesions in the same session [26]. However, it is difficult to detect small ectocervical and endocervical lesions under visual inspection; depending on the screening intervals, lesions might be overseen and develop to invasive cancer. On the other side, many changes observed in VIA are rather unspecific and might lead to substantial overtreatment of women without need for it. This in turn triggers an increased risk of premature birth, delivery complications due to stenosis of the uterine canal after invasive procedures in the cervical region, and increased susceptibility towards transmission of other STDs, especially HIV [37].

3. Potential improvement of cervical cancer screening programs by the use of biomarkers

There are several fields of application for cancer biomarkers, including early detection of cancers, improved reproducibility of the histopathological diagnoses, surveillance of persons at risk and post therapy monitoring. In cervical cancer screening, biomarkers are needed that allow to identify persons at risk to develop cancer at a time point that still allows for a successful curative intervention before invasive cancer develops. Biomarker test performance is characterized by measures of sensitivity, specificity, positive predictive value (PPV), and negative predictive value (NPV). Naturally, it is desirable to have assays with both high sensitivity and specificity. A lack of sensitivity will result in missing cases that require treatment. A lack of specificity results in the identification of false positive cases that have to be worked up despite being disease free. PPV and NPV are both related to the test performance and the disease prevalence. The lower disease prevalence is, the lower will be the PPV of an assay with given sensitivity and specificity. The PPV indicates the proportion of individuals tested positive that really have the disease. The NPV gives an indication how safe an assay is, i.e. how sure one can be that a negative result indicates that disease is not present. It is estimated that the introduction of prophylactic HPV vaccines will reduce the incidence of cervical cancers and precursors and therefore will reduce the PPV of abnormal smears from currently 50–70% down to 10–20% in regions with high vaccination coverage [35].

Currently, besides primary Pap screening, only HPV testing has been assessed as a primary screening marker in larger population based studies [25,86].

While cytology results can be very clear with direct clinical implications (a negative or a high grade result) even without control biopsy [6] there are diagnostic categories that have no direct clinical implication, but need to be followed up with more complex clinical algorithms . Unlike cytology, a positive HPV test would always require a follow up before a clinical diagnosis can be established. Different work-up strategies have been suggested, including cytology triage, repeat HPV testing or type-specific HPV detection [25,86] (Wright unpublished results).

The workup of the primary test result (i.e. the triage) can be the second field of application for novel biomarkers. Currently, HPV testing is recommended as one option to triage ASC-US cytology [125]. A biomarker used in triage should be specifically associated with disease progression. Recently, some novel biomarkers such as HPV mRNA and p16^{INK4a} have been evaluated in initial studies and have shown promising results but are still lacking validation in larger trials and head to head comparison with HPV testing and other markers [24].

In addition to primary and triage screening markers, biomarkers could be used for a risk assessment of detected lesions, to stratify intermediate lesions, to predict progression and to monitor recurrences after treatment. A very interesting field for biomarkers could be the assessment of CIN1 and CIN2 lesions. While CIN1 is usually managed conservatively, CIN2 is frequently treated despite a rather low progression rate. There are ongoing discussions whether to generally treat CIN2 [99,124]. An important field of application for a biomarker could be the discrimination between CIN1+2 with a high risk of progression from those lesions with a high chance to spontaneously regress. Treatment would then be restricted to the high risk CIN1+2 group as indicated by the biomarker.

4. Identification of novel biomarkers for cervical cancer screening

In the past 20 years, substantial efforts have been undertaken to identify novel biomarkers for more efficient and cost effective cervical cancer screening programs. Most of the work has been done on the role of HPV testing. This aspect is extensively reviewed by Meijer and colleagues in this issue. Apart from that, numerous other markers have been evaluated in cervical cancer precursor lesions. Due to the accessibility of the uterine cervix, most approaches have concentrated on identifying markers directly in tissue samples taken from the uterine cervix.

5. Biomarkers derived from the analysis of molecular key events of cervical carcinogenesis

Some promising biomarkers have recently been delineated by studying the major molecular events involved in cervical carcinogenesis. To facilitate the understanding of the basic molecular concepts that lead to the identification of these markers we briefly summarize the most important steps in cervical transformation in the context of biomarker discovery.

The initial event in cervical transformation is an infection with high risk human papilloma viruses (HR-HPV). The majority of HR-HPV infections regress spontaneously, only a small proportion persists and induces cervical intraepithelial neoplasias (CIN). The risk of progression to invasive cancer rises with the lesions' grade [80], Fig. 1.

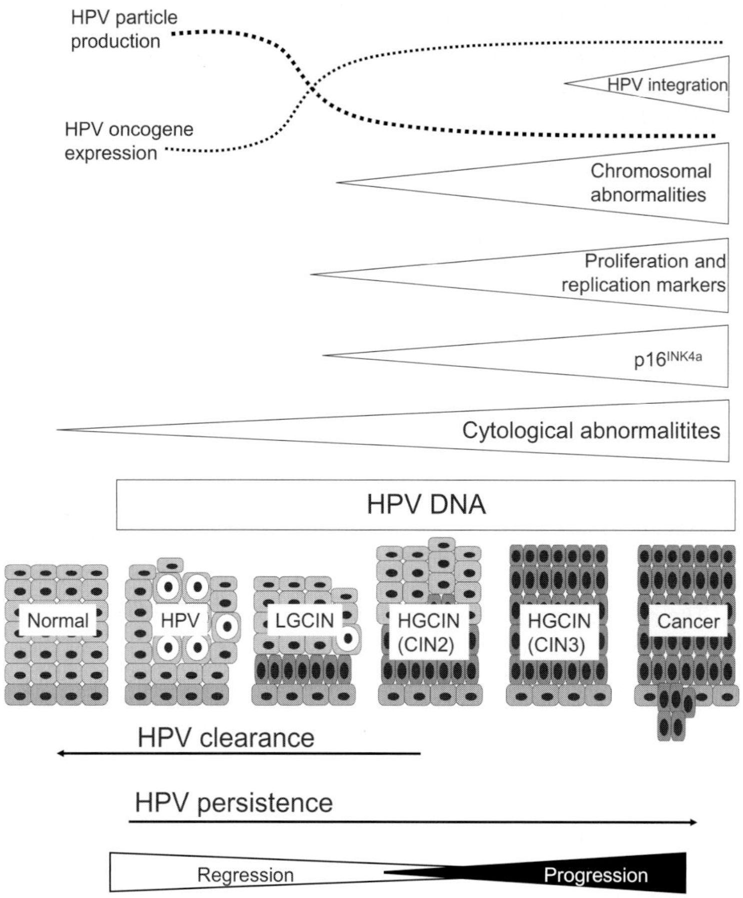

Fig. 1. Progression model of cervical carcinogenesis. During progression from HPV infection to high grade intraepithelial lesions, HPV oncogene expression is substantially increased, while HPV particle production goes down. Deregulated expression of HPV oncogenes induces chromosomal abnormalities, expression of proliferation markers and expression of p16^{INK4a}. HPV integration is a rather late event following the chromosomal instability.

The molecular interactions between HPV proteins and host cell proteins and genome homeostasis have been studied intensely over the past 20 years. The early viral genes encode proteins that are involved in the viral life cycle and the late genes encode the viral envelope proteins L1 and L2. Two early genes, E6 and E7 were found to be the most important factors in cellular transformation induced by high risk HPV. The E6 and E7 gene products target a plethora of cellular functions, with the most important interactions being the inactivation of pRB by E7 and the degradation of p53 by E6. Loss of pRB function leads to E2F mediated cell cycle activation that usually would be counteracted by the activation of apoptotic programs in the host cells. However, induction of apoptosis is counteracted by E6 mediated p53 degradation (Fig. 2). The detailed interactions of E6 and E7 with the regulation of apoptosis and cell cycle of the host cell are summarized in [64, 70,133].

During their normal replication oncogenic papillomaviruses avoid pathogenic effects on their host cells in order to multiply themselves largely unnoticed by the infected host. To achieve this, part of the replication strategy relies on the fact that during the normal viral life cycle, E6 and E7 are selectively expressed in the upper epithelial layers to activate the viral replication machinery [29,102]. By the restriction of viral replication to terminally differentiated cells that have no proliferation capacity, the virus avoids harmful consequences for its host. The expression of E6 and E7 in replication competent basal cells seems to be tightly suppressed by certain cellular factors that have not been identified yet [132]. The major hallmark of progression from HPV infected tissue to dysplastic lesions is the altered expression pattern of the HPV oncogenes. In high

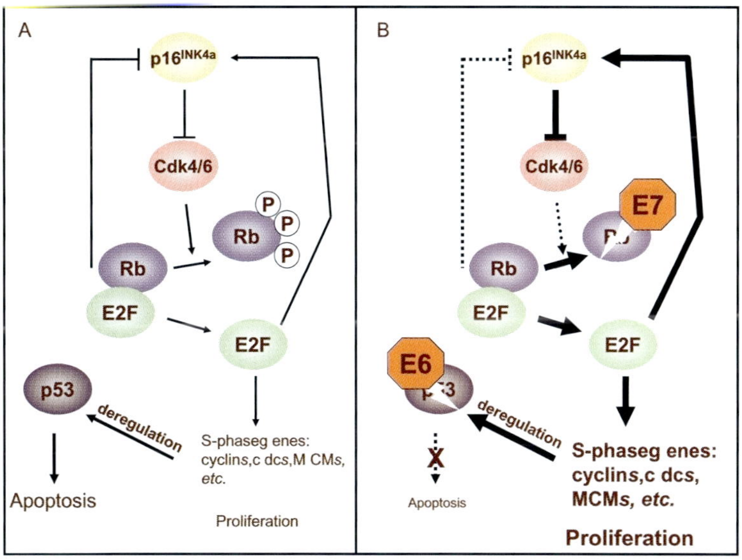

Fig. 2. Schematic diagram of the cellular proteins involved in G1-S phase transition and the interference of HPV oncogenes, adapted from Khleif [54]. A: Strict regulation of E2F in normal cells. Phosphorylation of Rb by Cdk4/6 releases E2F from its binding to Rb and leads to the expression of S-phase genes. Cdk4/6 activity is blocked by p16^{INK4a} that is activated by E2F and blocked by Rb/E2F complexes. Deregulated S-phase activation in normal cells would lead to apoptosis. B: Interference of HPV oncoproteins with G1-S-Phase regulation. E7 leads to disruption of E2F-Rb binding. p16^{INK4a} is strongly overexpressed due to the loss of Rb/E2F repression and the strong activation by free E2F. However, S-phase genes are continuously activated since the p16^{INK4a} mediated repression of Cdk4/6 has no downstream effect on Rb. Apoptosis is abrogated by E6 mediated degradation of p53.

grade CIN lesions, E6 and E7 are strongly expressed in basal epithelial cells and the viral oncogenes interfere substantially with cell cycle control of these replication competent host cells [108]. In the cells uncontrolled proliferation, deregulated cell cycle control, and hence chromosomal instability occurs that results in multiple numeric and structural chromosomal aberrations [27, 28].

In the course of repair processes in chromosomally instable cells, HPV genomes may become integrated into the host cell chromosomes [116,117]. While only a small part of the CIN lesions displays integrated viral genomes, a high percentage of cervical cancers harbors integrated HPV DNA [46,58], suggesting that viral integration is not the cause but rather a consequence of increasing chromosomal instability of HPV transformed cells. During the viral integration process, E2 is usually disrupted and the E6 and E7 genes are conserved. As a result, E6 and E7 expression may be further enhanced [50,51]. Oncogene expression is driven by the viral promoter and can be modulated by surrounding cellular components like cellular promoters, enhancers and repressors or by epigenetic modifications [107]. Recently, it was demonstrated that the E2 binding sites in HPV are differentially methylated indicating that functional inactivation of E2 might be either related to integration or to methylation of the E2 binding site [7]. The most important cellular and viral changes in the course from HPV infection to invasive cancer are schematically summarized in Fig. 1.

5.1. Surrogate biomarkers of deregulated HPV oncogene expression

5.1.1. p16^{INK4a}

The overexpression of the cyclin dependent kinase inhibitor p16^{INK4a} is a direct consequence of deregulated HPV oncogene expression [54]. Usually, binding of pRB to E2F blocks E2F driven cell cycle activation. In replicating cells, E2F is regulated by phosphorylation of RB. Rb phosphorylation is normally mediated by cyclin dependent kinases (CDK4, CDK6) that are controlled by several kinase inhibitors (INKs). Aberrant expression of E7 in basal cells disrupts binding of pRB to E2F that is counteracted by massive expression of p16^{INK4a}, an important CDK inhibitor (Fig. 2). Since E7-dependent E2F release is not mediated by phosphorylation of pRb, the counter-regulatory p16^{INK4a} expression has no effect on the activated cell cycle [89].

Under physiological conditions p16^{INK4a} is expressed when cells undergo a genomic stress situation such as substantial shortening of telomeres in ageing

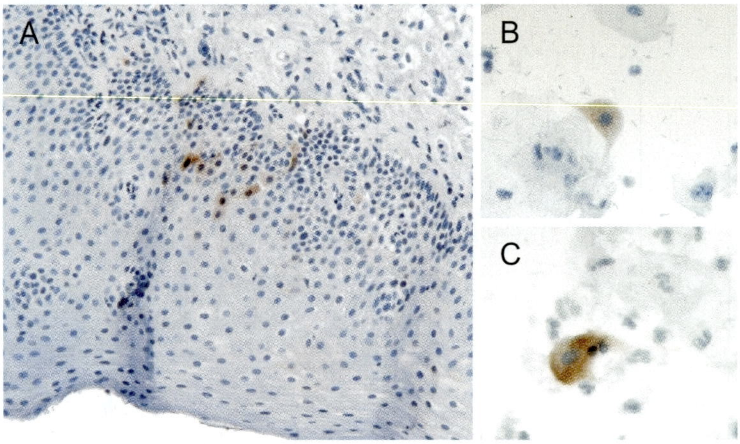

Fig. 3. p16^{INK4a} staining of HPV negative specimens. A: Cervical epithelium with single p16^{INK4a} positive metaplastic cells. B+C: p16^{INK4a} positive metaplastic cell in cytology.

tissues [5]. Expression of p16^{INK4a} in these cells induces immediate irreversible cell cycle arrest and may finally lead to apoptosis. Thus, independent from HPV, expression of p16^{INK4a} is sometimes observed in single cells that undergo modifications of their normal differentiation program due to aging or genomic stress. Particularly in metaplastic or atrophic epithelial changes in older women, p16^{INK4a} positive cells in the differentiated intermediate or superficial parts of the epithelium may be found that are not considered to be related to HPV oncogene expression (Figs 3 A–C). Non-dysplastic epithelia infected with LR- or HR-HPV do not diffusely stain for p16^{INK4a} (Fig. 4A+B).

In sharp contrast to this expression pattern of p16^{INK4a} in resting cells with aberrant differentiation, the pathological expression in HPV transformed cells is indicated by a very strong diffuse staining pattern in the replicating cells of the basal and parabasal cell layer (Fig. 4C–F). Basically all cervical carcinomas, CIN3 lesions, as well as the majority of CIN2 lesions were found to be diffusely positive in immunohistochemistry (IHC) (Fig. 4C–F). In contrast, only a subset of the CIN1 lesions is p16^{INK4a} positive [56,57]. p16^{INK4a} IHC improved the reproducibility of histological assessment of CIN lesions in comparison to the conventional H&E staining [56]. Recent studies have shown that p16^{INK4a} positive low grade lesions have a higher risk of progression than p16^{INK4a} negative lesions [76,109,111], suggesting that p16^{INK4a} could be used as a marker to discriminate lesions with a higher progression risk from those that most likely regress spontaneously. Based on the successful application of p16^{INK4a} in IHC, a cytological assay was developed to investigate the p16^{INK4a} expression in exfoliated cells [104]. Several studies have shown that p16^{INK4a} cytology can detect underlying HGCIN with high sensitivity [40,77,78,128]. Some authors have counted p16^{INK4a} positive cells and have applied cut off levels for the detection of a relevant number of p16^{INK4a} positive cells to detect high grade cervical lesions [87, 88]. In order to improve the specificity of p16^{INK4a} cytology, a nuclear score was defined that facilitates the assessment of p16^{INK4a} positive cells [114]. Using this score, specificity for the detection of relevant lesions was superior to counting p16^{INK4a} positive cells, while sensitivity was not affected. In a direct comparison with Pap cytology, p16^{INK4a} cytology identified 98% of the HSIL cases, while only 1% of the normal cases and 10% of the LSIL cases showed abnormal p16^{INK4a} positive cells (Fig. 4G–I).

Based on these results, p16^{INK4a} immunocytology might be used to highlight potentially abnormal cells in a background of normal, reactive or other non malignant cells (locator function). Positive cells can then in a second step be score according to morphological criteria (Interpreter function). p16^{INK4a} immunostaining has been used to triage ASCUS and LSIL cases for high grade CIN [20]. In an independent ASC-US/ LSIL triage study, p16^{INK4a} cytology applying the above described scoring of nuclear abnormalities had 95% sensitivity and 84% specificity in ASC-US and 100% sensitivity and 82% specificity in LSIL for the detection of biopsy proven HGCIN (Wentzensen in press). Since p16^{INK4a} can be performed from the initial cytology specimen, this application could be a new option for the regular follow up of unclear cytology results. The promising results of this triage study and the high potential for automation of p16^{INK4a} cytology warrant

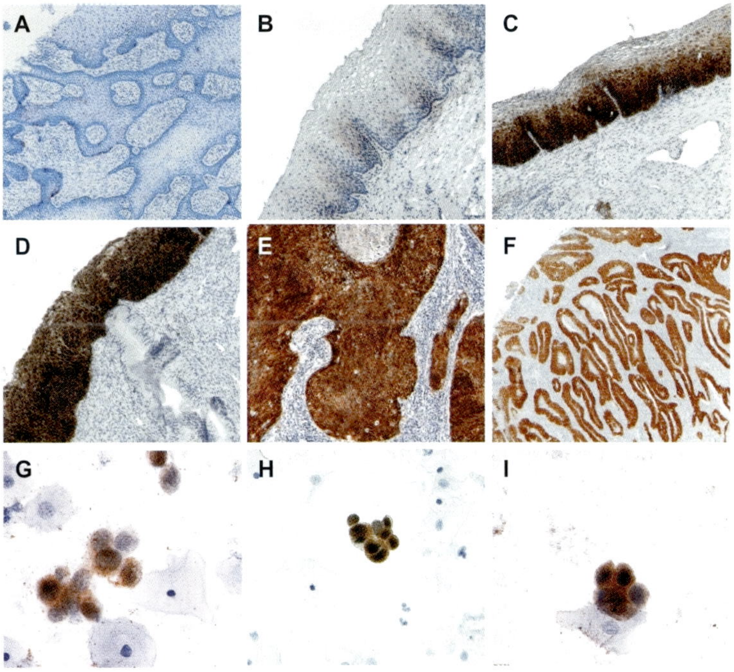

Fig. 4. $p16^{INK4a}$ staining of HPV positive specimens. A: Low risk HPV positive condyloma, no $p16^{INK4a}$ staining. B: High risk HPV positive cervical specimen, no $p16^{INK4a}$ staining C: CIN2 lesion, diffuse $p16^{INK4a}$ staining D: CIN3 lesion, diffuse $p16^{INK4a}$ staining E: Cervical squamous cell carcinoma, diffuse $p16^{INK4a}$ staining F: Cervical adenocarcinoma, diffuse $p16^{INK4a}$ staining G-I: Cytological specimens with $p16^{INK4a}$ positive abnormal cervical cells displaying nuclear abnormalities (H: Seroa Cytoscreen liquid based cytology, G+I: Cytyc Thinprep liquid based cytology).

the evaluation of $p16^{INK4a}$ cytology as a primary cytology screening test along with automated imaging techniques.

A further simplified application of biomarkers in cervical cancer screening is the direct detection of the markers by biochemical techniques in cervical samples. Recently, a biochemical test has been developed that allows to measure $p16^{INK4a}$ levels in solubilized samples obtained from cervical smears. The advantage of this approach is a dichotomous result that is not dependent on the observers' education and experience. Protein based assays are robust and allow for rapid $p16^{INK4a}$ detection procedures that would make a $p16^{INK4a}$ based point of care test possible. An initial study has shown good sensitivity of the assay to detect high grade cervical dysplasia in a disease enriched population [115]. The ELISA based detection of $p16^{INK4a}$ in cervical samples could serve as a quick point of care test in various settings of cervical cancer screening. In countries with cytology screening, it might back up or complement current procedures. In developing countries with no access to screening infrastructure, it could be implemented in visual screening to discriminate lesions with deregulated HPV oncogene expression from non-specific changes that do not require treatment.

5.2. Markers of chromosomal instability

5.2.1. DNA aneuploidy

Duensing et al. [27,28] have shown that disturbances of the mitotic spindle apparatus are induced early by deregulated expression of HPV oncogenes resulting in non-diploid nuclei (aneuploidy). Consequently, aneuploidy is characteristic for HPV transformed lesions even at precancerous stages [8,9,67]. Different techniques exist to measure the DNA content of single cervical cells: Bollmann et al. [8,9] have measured the DNA content of single cells in cytology specimens directly on glass slides using laser scanning microscopy. Melsheimer et al. [67] applied a protocol using minced fresh frozen biopsy specimens followed by flow cytometry DNA content analysis. The studies have shown an association between aneuploidy and increasing dysplasia. Melsheimer and colleagues showed that aneuploidy precedes HPV integration in advanced dysplastic lesions further supporting the notion that integration of viral genomes is the consequence but not the cause of chromosomal instability and transformation [67].

5.2.2. HPV integration

It is believed that HPV DNA is integrated by chance during the cellular repair processes of double strand breaks. As such, HPV integration is an indicator of severe ongoing chromosomal instability and an advanced stage of the transformation process [117]. Several methods exist to detect the integration of HPV DNA into the host genome. A simple approach is the real time PCR-based quantification of the E2 and E6/E7 gene ratio [82]. E2 is frequently lost upon HPV integration and the theoretical ratio of 1:1 between the two genes is expected to be shifted towards E6/E7. However, in many high grade lesions and less advanced cancers, many episomal and few integrated genome copies are found concomitantly, rendering the direct quantification very difficult. Direct proofs of HPV integration are more laborious, since HPV genomes are integrated at random positions in the genome and thus lack a specific sequence that can be amplified. Integration detection assays use primers binding to specific restriction enzyme sites for amplification [103], or perform digestion of the target DNA and ligate either adaptors [63] or use self ligation [52] to construct templates that allow for amplification and sequencing of the unknown cellular sequence.

The RNA-based amplification of viral-cellular fusion transcripts specific for HPV integration [58] is less laborious than the DNA based integration detection assays but requires fresh frozen material with proper RNA quality. Several clinical applications of HPV integration detection exist: HPV integration detection is highly specific for advanced lesions, but lacks sensitivity since all studies measuring HPV integration directly have not shown more than 80–90% integration positive cervical cancers. HPV integration points to advanced lesions with a very high progression potential, i.e. lesions that would clearly require treatment. Although some clustering of HPV integration events has been found most probably related to fragile sites in that region, every HPV integration event is unique with respect to the exact integration site [116,131]. It was shown that all cells are clonally related with respect to the HPV integration site in cervical cancers and in high grade precancer lesions [106,131] allowing to use HPV integration as a very specific tumor marker in post-treatment surveillance.

5.3. Markers of proliferation and host cell genome replication

5.3.1. ki67

The increased proliferation of cervical epithelial cells induced by deregulated HPV oncogene expression is reflected by the activation of proliferation markers such as ki67 (MIB-1). This protein is strongly expressed in CIN lesions, but can also be found expressed in normal basal cells that retain proliferation capacity [38,83]. By analyzing the association between lesion grade and the epithelial location of ki67 positive cell clusters, Kruse et al. have demonstrated that ki67 cell clusters are a good criterion to discriminate low grade CIN lesions from normal and reactive epithelia [60].

5.3.2. MYC

The cellular oncogene MYC is frequently found amplified and overexpressed in cervical cancer. Several studies have shown MYC activation at premalignant stages, indicating that MYC detection might be used to assess dysplastic lesions. Golijow et al. have performed PCR based detection of MYC amplification on histological and cytological specimens and found MYC levels increasing with lesion grade at premalignant stages [39]. In a consecutive study, Abba et al. [1] showed a tight correlation between MYC expression and HPV16 infection at pre-invasive stages, indicating different oncogenic properties of different HR-HPV types.

5.3.3. Cyclins

Cyclins are a large family of regulatory proteins with central functions in the coordination of the cell cycle. The expression of several cyclins has been analyzed in cervical cancer and precancer. Cyclin D1 was found to be overexpressed in low grade lesions induced by LR-HPV, while it was absent in HR-HPV induced lesions [98]. Other cyclins such as A, B, and E were found to be overexpressed in premalignant cervical lesions [31,53]. Weaver et al. have analyzed the expression of Cyclin E in liquid based cytology specimens and found a strong association of Cyclin E with HPV induced cellular abnormalities [113].

5.3.4. Telomerase

Telomerase expression is important to counteract the loss of sequences located at the outermost chromosome endings that naturally occurs during every cell division. To prevent loss of relevant chromosomal sequences, the telomerase complex adds short repetetive DNA stretches to the chromosome endings. Telomerase consists of a protein subunit and an RNA subunit that is template for the repetitive sequences. The gene encoding the RNA subunit, TERC, is located on chromosome 3q, a region that is frequently amplified in cervical cancer and precancer. Since telomerase is necessary to maintain telomere length in proliferating cells, it is found overexpressed in many human cancers. Several groups have used a functional telomerase assay to evaluate telomerase activity on cervical smears. Increased telomerase activity was mainly found in advanced dysplasias with varying sensitivity for the detection of HGCIN [4,49].

5.3.5. Replication complex proteins

MCM5 and CDC6 belong to the DNA pre-replication complex that is usually expressed in replicating, but not in quiescent cells. The replication licensing complex is disassembled during replication to prevent immediate reinitiating of the cell cycle. In dysplastic cervical cells, a continuous activation of the replication complex is found. Williams et al. have analyzed of a modified Pap staining protocol including immunocytochemical detection of the replication complex proteins CDC6 and MCM5. The authors describe good sensitivity and specificity of the assay for the detection of SIL in a series of 92 cervical smears [120]. These results were confirmed by Murphy et al. in an independent study [71]. In frame of the HPV-PathogenISS study, Branca and colleagues found that topoisomerase II alpha (TOP2A) expression was correlated with the progression from CIN2 to CIN3 [15]. The detection of two proliferation associated proteins, MCM2 and TOP2A, has been recently made commercially available. An initial study [92] showed 100% positivity of the marker combination in high grade SIL cytology specimens without staining of normal specimens, while 50% of LSIL and 20% of ASC-US cases were found to be positive.

5.4. Markers of cellular stress and invasion

HSPs are chaperones protecting cellular functions in response to various cellular stresses that were found to be overexpressed in a number of cancers. In cervical precancer, overexpression of HSP40, HSP60 and HSP70 were associated with increasing lesion grade [21]. The Carbonic anhydrase 9 is a transmembrane protein induced by lowered oxygen tension. The CA9/MN antigen has been identified as a marker for all grades of CIN [85]. Liao et al. have analyzed CA9 expression on cervical smears and found expression in all grades of dysplasia as well as some slides exhibiting only atypical cells. For the cytological diagnosis of atypical glandular cells of unknown significance (AGUS), CA9/MN expression pointed to relevant lesions [62]. Laminin 5 is part of cell adhesion complexes and is an important constituent of the extracellular matrix. It was found to be an invasion marker in various epithelial tumors, including cervical cancer [96]. Laminin 5 seems to be a late marker of the cervical transformation process indicating the first steps of invasion [79].

5.5. Epigenetic markers, factors enhancing viral oncogene activity

Methylation of CpG islands is an epigenetic modifier of gene expression. In many cancers, tumor suppressor genes were found to be inactivated by methylation. Likewise, many studies have looked at gene methylation alterations in cervical cancer and precancer. RASSF1 methylation was found in cervical cancer and seems to complement the frequent LOH and CGH losses detected at the 3p21 region [129]. TSLC1 has been described as a cellular tumor suppressor gene involved in cervical cancer development. TSLC1 was found inactivated by methylation in a subset of high grade dysplasias and cervical carcinomas [100]. Recently, methylation studies were performed on cytological and corresponding histological specimens of women with CIN and cervical cancer [33]. Using three target genes, DAPK1, RARB, or TWIST1, the authors found a 60% sensitivity for the detection of CIN3 with a specificity of 95%.

The brn-3a transcription factor is a potent activator of HR-HPV gene expression. A massive overexpression was found in women with CIN3 as compared to women without cervical lesion [74]. Interestingly, the massive overxpression was not only observed in the lesions, but also in the non-diseased tissue surrounding the CIN3 lesions suggesting that high brn-3a expression might be an important risk factor for the development of HR-HPV induced high grade lesions [72]. The group has analyzed the use of brn-3a mRNA quantification from cytology specimens and found a correlation between high brn-3a levels and increased risk of progression to high grade lesions in different populations [73,94,95].

6. Identification of biomarkers for cervical cancer screening by profiling approaches

6.1. Chromosomal abnormalities

Comparative genomic hybridization (CGH) assays can measure altered distributions of genomic DNA on a genome wide basis. The resolution of the CGH mapping has substantially increased during the last years from bacterial artificial chromosomes to array CGH using short DNA clones. In various independent studies, more gains than losses have been observed in CGH studies of cervical cancer [48,127]. Chromosomal aberrations can be identified already in precancerous lesions [45], the frequency of imbalances was found to increase from 19% in CIN1 to over 90% in CIN3 lesions [105,127]. The typical chromosomal losses are 2q, 3p, 4p, 4q, 5q, 6q, 11q, 13q, and 18q, frequently gained regions are 1q, 3q, 5p, and 8q [41,44,45,55,66, 84,105,127].

The most consistently observed alteration seems to be the gain of chromosome 3q, an event that has been associated with the progression from severe dysplasia to invasive cancer [42,43]. The TERC gene coding for the RNA subunit of telomerase is located on 3q. The frequent alterations at this locus together with other functional studies on the role of telomerase in cervical carcinogenesis [130] suggest that TERC amplification might be a necessary step for cervical cancer development. Heselmeyer-Haddad et al. [43] have analyzed the use of a 3q specific probe set on Pap stained cervical smears to detect lesions progressing to CIN3. The authors were able to identify CIN1/2 progressing to CIN3 with a 100% sensitivity, while 70% of the regressing lesions were negative for 3q gain.

Recently, Huang et al. [47] have found a potentially cervical cancer promoting gene, PRKAA1, located on the frequently amplified short arm of chromosome 5 by detailed analysis of gene copy number of several candidate genes in that region.

In a recent paper, Fitzpatrick and colleagues [34] have performed extensive gene expression analysis based on 3 different microarray platforms to compare expression data with chromosomal imbalances. There was a good correlation between chromosomal gains and alterations of genes located on 3q and 12q as well as loss of 6p and 4q.

6.1.1. Alterations of gene expression

Nees et al. [75] have compared gene expression patterns between tumorigenic and non-tumorigenic HPV16 immortalized human foreskin keratinocytes and identified 49 significantly altered genes, among them the proliferation associated gene C4.8 that was found to be overexpressed in high grade cervical lesions [121]. Wong et al. [123] have used microarray expression patterns to discriminate normal cervical tissue from cervical cancers. Using specific gene expression signatures, the authors were able to stratify stage Ib and IIb cancers and to predict the patients response to radiotherapy. Chen et al. [23] have determined global expression patterns of 34 cervical tissues derived from different disease stages and identified 35 candidate biomarkers that were validated on tissue microarrays including a number of cell cycle regulatory genes.

Ahn et al. [2] have analyzed gene expression patterns of primary cancer tissue of 11 patients and found 74 differentially regulated genes. Fujimoto et al. [36] have used gene expression patterns to compare morphologically different cervical cancer cell lines derived from one donor. In a recent analysis, Steinau et al. [101] have compared primary cervical tissue with normal exfoliated cells from 7 donors to evaluate the differences between the two tissue sources. About 50% of the genes present in the primary tissue could also be identified in exfoliated cells indicating that this is only a partial representation probably related to the under-representation of normal basal cells in exfoliated tissue. In addition, the gene expression patterns between 15 CIN3 lesions and 15 normal or CIN1 tissues were compared, 6 commonly altered genes were identified. Santin et al. [90] have performed a microarray analysis comparing gene expression patterns of cervical carcinomas and normal cervical keratinocytes. Among more than 500 differentially regulated genes, the authors identified several biomarkers that have been previously analyzed in functional studies of HPV-induced transformation, including CDKN2A/p16^{INK4a}, topoisomerase 2A, and minichromosome maintenance proteins 2, 4, and 5.

6.1.2. Alteration of protein expression, serum based markers

So far, only few studies exist that have used proteomic tools to identify new cervical cancer biomarkers. Lee et al. [61] have analyzed the proteomic changes induced by transfection of E7 into the HPV negative cell line C33a to identify proteins regulated by E7. Wong et al. [122] have used the SELDI technology to compare protein mass patterns between cervical cancer and non-diseased tissue and achieved a 87% sensitivity and 100% specificity for the classification of tissue using seven specific protein mass patterns.

A number of protein biomarkers have been analyzed in serum to detect cervical cancer, among them the SCC antigen [32], IGF2 and VEGF-C [65,68] and CYFRA 21.1 [69]. Recently, the methylation of CDH1 and CDH2 genes has been analyzed in serum samples [119]. None of these markers has shown a clinical utility superior to the analysis of directly sampled exfoliated cells so far.

The analysis of humoral immune responses against HPV antigens has not been proven to be a valuable tool for cervical cancer screening [93], however, with the introduction of more powerful techniques covering a wide spectrum of HPV antigens [112], new possible fields of application for HPV serology are conceivable, especially considering the forthcoming vaccination against some HPV types.

6.2. Markers analyzed in the HPV-Pathogen ISS study

The HPV-Pathogen ISS study aims at systematically analyzing 13 different biomarkers in defined retrospective, cross-sectional, and prospective cohorts of HIV positive and negative women [12]. The women are followed both with epidemiological surveys and regular colposcopy including sampling for HPV and biomarker analysis. The 13 markers were selected from different sources, mainly including genes known to be involved in the carcinogenesis of other tumor entities, some identified in profiling analysis and some known to be associated with HPV-related transformation. Until now, several markers have been analyzed in retrospective, cross-sectional and prospective analyses, including ERK1 [11], Survivin [19], VEGF-C [18], 67kd-laminin receptor [16], nucleosid diphosphate kinase nm23-h1 [13], MMP2 and TIMP-2 [10], E-cadherin [14], and NF-kappa-B [17]. Two very promising marker candidates analyzed in this series are Survivin and VEGF-C. Survivin is involved both in cell cycle and apoptosis regulation [118]. Survivin gene expression is usually repressed by wild type p53. As such, its overexpression indirectly indicates E6 mediated p53 degradation. Survivin was found to be an early marker of cervical carcinogenesis, expression strength increased with lesion grade [19]. VEGF is upregulated by E6 independent from p53. VEGF overexpression was found to be an early marker of CIN and correlated linearly with lesion grade [18].

7. Summary

Currently, a number of potential biomarkers for cervical screening are being analyzed. The best data are available for HPV DNA based markers, the comprehensive exploration of HPV DNA in the progression from transient infection to cervical cancer raises the bar for the validation of new potential biomarkers. These analyses, however, have also clearly demonstrated that there is a need for new tools that can discriminate lesions with high risk of progression from those that will regress spontaneously. Such markers might be viral markers, like HPV mRNA or HR-HPV single typing. The advantage of cellular markers like $p16^{INK4a}$ is the association with the transformation process independent of the underlying HPV type. This allows to analyze only a single marker, while HPV based assays will always need to target several oncogenic types. In histology applications, $p16^{INK4a}$ has shown excellent results in improving the reproducibility of cervical precancer histology diagnoses. Several approaches to identify high grade lesions using $p16^{INK4a}$ cytology have been published. It is very likely that a combined protocol using $p16^{INK4a}$ staining as a biomarker and nuclear assessment of $p16^{INK4a}$ positive cells might substantially improve the triage of unclear cytology results. The $p16^{INK4a}$ ELISA format may offer a quick and simple assay that can determine the risk of underlying high grade disease independent of the observer's education and a skillful lab environment.

A clear demand in the assessment of novel biomarkers is a standardized approach. Most studies on cervical cancer biomarkers are not comparable and thus do not allow to draw meaningful conclusions at this point. With regard to standardization, the approach of the HPV-PathogenISS study is very helpful and it will be interesting to see more prospective data on different biomarkers. A further step in that direction is the SUCCEED study, a combined epidemiological, pathological, and clinical approach to identify new and validate existing biomarker, conducted by the NCI. The study aims at collecting biological material from more than 1500 women with transient HPV infection, different grades of cervical dysplasia, and cervical cancer and will allow for a thorough comparison of different candidate biomarkers at different steps in the progression to cervical cancer.

Finally, the soon expected introduction of regular vaccination programs against the oncogenic high risk types HPV16 and HPV18 is expected to have an influence on the incidence of HPV infections and HPV associated lesions in the short term and on cervical cancer incidence in the long term. It is assumed that these changes in disease prevalence and a possible shift towards more frequent infections by HPV types not targeted by the vaccine might make cytology based screening more ineffective than it is now and will therefore increase the demand for new biomarkers.

References

[1] M.C. Abba, R.M. Laguens, F.N. Dulout and C.D. Golijow, The c-myc activation in cervical carcinomas and HPV 16 infections, *Mutat Res* **557**(2) (2004), 151–158.

[2] W.S. Ahn, S.M. Bae, J.M. Lee, S.E. Namkoong, S.J. Han, Y.L. Cho YL et al., Searching for pathogenic gene functions to cervical cancer, *Gynecol Oncol* **93**(1) (2004), 41–48.

[3] M. Arbyn, F. Buntinx, M. Van Ranst, E. Paraskevaidis, P. Martin-Hirsch and J. Dillner, Virologic versus cytologic triage of women with equivocal Pap smears: a meta-analysis of the accuracy to detect high-grade intraepithelial neoplasia, *J Natl Cancer Inst* **96**(4) (2004), 280–293.

[4] K.A. Ault, H.K. Allen, S.L. Phillips, M.B. Zimmerman and A.J. Klingelhutz, Telomerase activity as a potential diagnostic marker for triage of abnormal Pap smears, *J Low Genit Tract Dis* **9**(2) (2005), 93–99.

[5] C.M. Beausejour, A. Krtolica, F. Galimi, M. Narita, S.W. Lowe, P. Yaswen et al., Reversal of human cellular senescence: roles of the p53 and p16 pathways, *EMBO J* **22**(16) (2003), 4212–4222.

[6] L. Berdichevsky, R. Karmin and L. Chuang, Treatment of high-grade squamous intraepithelial lesions: a 2- versus 3-step approach, *Am J Obstet Gynecol* **190**(5) (2004), 1424–1426.

[7] B. Bhattacharjee and S. Sengupta, CpG methylation of HPV 16 LCR at E2 binding site proximal to P97 is associated with cervical cancer in presence of intact E2. Virology 2006.

[8] R. Bollmann, M. Bollmann, D.E. Henson and M. Bodo, DNA cytometry confirms the utility of the Bethesda system for the classification of Papanicolaou smears, *Cancer* **93**(3) (2001), 222–228.

[9] R. Bollmann, G. Mehes, R. Torka, N. Speich, C. Schmitt and M. Bollmann, Determination of features indicating progression in atypical squamous cells with undetermined significance: human papillomavirus typing and DNA ploidy analysis from liquid-based cytologic samples, *Cancer* **99**(2) (2003), 113–117.

[10] M. Branca, M. Ciotti, C. Giorgi, D. Santini, L. Di Bonito, S. Costa et al., Matrix metalloproteinase-2 (MMP-2) and its tissue inhibitor (TIMP-2) are prognostic factors in cervical cancer, related to invasive disease but not to high-risk human papillomavirus (HPV) or virus persistence after treatment of CIN, *Anticancer Res* **26**(2B) (2006), 1543–1556.

[11] M. Branca, M. Ciotti, D. Santini, L.D. Bonito, A. Benedetto, C. Giorgi et al., Activation of the ERK/MAP kinase pathway in cervical intraepithelial neoplasia is related to grade of the lesion but not to high-risk human papillomavirus, virus clearance, or prognosis in cervical cancer, *Am J Clin Pathol* **122**(6) (2004), 902–911.

[12] M. Branca, S. Costa, L. Mariani, F. Sesti, A. Agarossi, A. di Carlo et al., Assessment of risk factors and human papillomavirus (HPV) related pathogenetic mechanisms of CIN in HIV-positive and HIV-negative women. Study design and baseline data of the HPV-PathogenISS study, *Eur J Gynaecol Oncol* **25**(6) (2004), 689–698.

[13] M. Branca, C. Giorgi, M. Ciotti, D. Santini, L. Di Bonito, S. Costa et al., Down-regulated nucleoside diphosphate (NDP) kinase nm23-h1 expression is unrelated to high-risk human papillomavirus (HPV) but associated with progression of cin and unfavourable prognosis in cervical cancer, *J Clin Pathol* (2006).

[14] M. Branca, C. Giorgi, M. Ciotti, D. Santini, L. Di Bonito, S. Costa et al., Down-regulation of E-cadherin is closely associated with progression of cervical intraepithelial neoplasia (CIN), but not with high-risk human papillomavirus (HPV) or disease outcome in cervical cancer, *Eur J Gynaecol Oncol* **27**(3) (2006), 215–223.

[15] M. Branca, C. Giorgi, M. Ciotti, D. Santini, L. Di Bonito, S. Costa et al., Over-Expression of Topoisomerase IIalpha is Related to the Grade of Cervical Intraepithelial Neoplasia (CIN) and High-Risk Human Papillomavirus (HPV), but does not Predict Prognosis in Cervical Cancer or HPV Clearance after Cone Treatment, *Int J Gynecol Pathol* **25**(4) (2006), 383–392.

[16] M. Branca, C. Giorgi, M. Ciotti, D. Santini, L. Di Bonito, S. Costa et al., Relationship of up-regulation of 67-kd laminin receptor to grade of cervical intraepithelial neoplasia and to high-risk HPV types and prognosis in cervical cancer, *Acta Cytol* **50**(1) (2006), 6–15.

[17] M. Branca, C. Giorgi, M. Ciotti, D. Santini, L. Di Bonito, S. Costa et al., Upregulation of nuclear factor-kappaB (NF-kappaB) is related to the grade of cervical intraepithelial neoplasia, but is not an independent predictor of high-risk human papillomavirus or disease outcome in cervical cancer, *Diagn Cytopathol* **34**(8) (2006), 555–563.

[18] M. Branca, C. Giorgi, D. Santini, L. Di Bonito, M. Ciotti, A. Benedetto et al., Aberrant expression of VEGF-C is related to grade of cervical intraepithelial neoplasia (CIN) and high risk HPV, but does not predict virus clearance after treatment of CIN or prognosis of cervical cancer, *J Clin Pathol* **59**(1) (2006), 40–47.

[19] M. Branca, C. Giorgi, D. Santini, L. Di Bonito, M. Ciotti, S. Costa et al., Survivin as a marker of cervical intraepithelial neoplasia and high-risk human papillomavirus and a predictor of virus clearance and prognosis in cervical cancer, *Am J Clin Pathol* **124**(1) (2005), 113–121.

[20] F. Carozzi, S. Cecchini, M. Confortini, V. Becattini, M.P. Cariaggi, G. Pontenani et al., Role of P16((INK4a)) expression in identifying CIN2 or more severe lesions among HPV-positive patients referred for colposcopy after abnormal cytology, *Cancer* (2006).

[21] P.E. Castle, R. Ashfaq, F. Ansari and C.Y. Muller, Immunohistochemical evaluation of heat shock proteins in normal and preinvasive lesions of the cervix, *Cancer Lett* **229**(2) (2005), 245–252.

[22] P.E. Castle, D. Solomon, M. Schiffman and C.M. Wheeler, Human papillomavirus type 16 infections and 2-year absolute risk of cervical precancer in women with equivocal or mild cytologic abnormalities, *J Natl Cancer Inst* **97**(14) (2005), 1066–1071.

[23] Y. Chen, C. Miller, R. Mosher, X. Zhao, J. Deeds, M. Morrissey et al., Identification of cervical cancer markers by cDNA and tissue microarrays, *Cancer Res* **63**(8) (2003), 1927–1935.

[24] J. Cuzick, M.H. Mayrand, G. Ronco, P. Snijders and P. Wardle, Chapter 10: New dimensions in cervical cancer screening, *Vaccine* **24**(Suppl 3) (2006), S90–S97.

[25] J. Cuzick, A. Szarewski, H. Cubie, G. Hulman, H. Kitchener, D. Luesley et al., Management of women who test positive for high-risk types of human papillomavirus: the HART study, *Lancet* **362**(9399) (2003), 1871–1876.

[26] L. Denny, L. Kuhn, M. De Souza, A.E. Pollack, W. Dupree and T.C. Wright, Jr., Screen-and-treat approaches for cervical cancer prevention in low-resource settings: a randomized controlled trial, *JAMA* **294**(17) (2005), 2173–2181.

[27] S. Duensing and K. Munger, Centrosome abnormalities, genomic instability and carcinogenic progression, *Biochim Biophys Acta* **1471**(2) (2001), M81–M88.

[28] S. Duensing and K. Munger, The human papillomavirus type 16 E6 and E7 oncoproteins independently induce numerical and structural chromosome instability, *Cancer Res* **62**(23) (2002), 7075–7082.

[29] M. Durst, D. Glitz, A. Schneider and H. zur Hausen, Human papillomavirus type 16 (HPV 16) gene expression and DNA replication in cervical neoplasia: analysis by in situ hybridization, *Virology* **189**(1) (1992), 132–140.

[30] S. Eaker, H.O. Adami, F. Granath, E. Wilander and P. Sparen, A large population-based randomized controlled trial to increase attendance at screening for cervical cancer, *Cancer Epidemiol Biomarkers Prev* **13**(3) (2004), 346–354.

[31] A.A. El Ghobashy, A.M. Shaaban, J. Herod, J. Innes, W. Prime and C.S. Herrington, Overexpression of cyclins A and B as markers of neoplastic glandular lesions of the cervix, *Gynecol Oncol* **92**(2) (2004), 628–634.

[32] M.D. Esajas, J.M. Duk, H.W. de Bruijn, J.G. Aalders, P.H. Willemse, W. Sluiter et al., Clinical value of routine serum squamous cell carcinoma antigen in follow-up of patients with early-stage cervical cancer, *J Clin Oncol* **19**(19) (2001), 3960–3966.

[33] Q. Feng, A. Balasubramanian, S.E. Hawes, P. Toure, P.S. Sow, A. Dem et al., Detection of hypermethylated genes in women with and without cervical neoplasia, *J Natl Cancer Inst* **97**(4) (2005), 273–282.

[34] M.A. Fitzpatrick, M.C. Funk, D. Gius, P.C. Huettner, Z. Zhang, M. Bidder et al., Identification of chromosomal alterations important in the development of cervical intraepithelial neoplasia and invasive carcinoma using alignment of DNA microarray data, *Gynecol Oncol* (2006).

[35] E.L. Franco, J. Cuzick, A. Hildesheim and S. de Sanjose, Chapter 20: Issues in planning cervical cancer screening in the era of HPV vaccination, *Vaccine* **24**(Suppl 3) (2006), S171–S177.

[36] T. Fujimoto, A. Nishikawa, M. Iwasaki, N. Akutagawa, M. Teramoto and R. Kudo, Gene expression profiling in two morphologically different uterine cervical carcinoma cell lines derived from a single donor using a human cancer cDNA array, *Gynecol Oncol* **93**(2) (2004), 446–453.

[37] A. Goel, G. Gandhi, S. Batra, S. Bhambhani, V. Zutshi and P. Sachdeva, Visual inspection of the cervix with acetic acid for cervical intraepithelial lesions, *Int J Gynaecol Obstet* **88**(1) (2005), 25–30.

[38] M.M. Goel, A. Mehrotra, U. Singh, H.P. Gupta and J.S. Misra, MIB-1 and PCNA immunostaining as a diagnostic adjunct to cervical Pap smear, *Diagn Cytopathol* **33**(1) (2005), 15–19.

[39] C.D. Golijow, M.C. Abba, S.A. Mouron, M.A. Gomez and F.N. Dulout, c-myc gene amplification detected in preinvasive intraepithelial cervical lesions, *Int J Gynecol Cancer* **11**(6) (2001), 462–465.

[40] M. Guo, L. Hu, M. Baliga, Z. He and M.D. Hughson, The Predictive Value of p16^(INK4a) and Hybrid Capture 2 Human Papillomavirus Testing for High-Grade Cervical Intraepithelial Neoplasia, *Am J Clin Pathol* **122**(6) (2004), 894–901.

[41] C.P. Harris, X.Y. Lu, G. Narayan, B. Singh, V.V. Murty and P.H. Rao, Comprehensive molecular cytogenetic characterization of cervical cancer cell lines, *Genes Chromosomes Cancer* **36**(3) (2003), 233–241.

[42] K. Heselmeyer, E. Schrock, M.S. du, H. Blegen, K. Shah, R. Steinbeck et al., Gain of chromosome 3q defines the transition from severe dysplasia to invasive carcinoma of the uterine cervix, *Proc Natl Acad Sci USA* **93**(1) (1996), 479–484.

[43] K. Heselmeyer-Haddad, K. Sommerfeld, N.M. White, N. Chaudhri, L.E. Morrison, N. Palanisamy et al., Genomic amplification of the human telomerase gene (TERC) in pap smears predicts the development of cervical cancer, *Am J Pathol* **166**(4) (2005), 1229–1238.

[44] A. Hidalgo, M. Baudis, I. Petersen, H. Arreola, P. Pina, G. Vazquez-Ortiz et al., Microarray comparative genomic hybridization detection of chromosomal imbalances in uterine cervix carcinoma, *BMC Cancer* **5** (2005), 77.

[45] A. Hidalgo, C. Schewe, S. Petersen, M. Salcedo, P. Gariglio, K. Schluns et al., Human papilloma virus status and chromosomal imbalances in primary cervical carcinomas and tumour cell lines, *Eur J Cancer* **36**(4) (2000), 542–548.

[46] A.H. Hopman, M.A. Kamps, F. Smedts, E.J. Speel, C.S. Herrington and F.C. Ramaekers, HPV in situ hybridization: impact of different protocols on the detection of integrated HPV, *Int J Cancer* **115**(3) (2005), 419–428.

[47] F.Y. Huang, P.M. Chiu, K.F. Tam, Y.K. Kwok, E.T. Lau, M.H. Tang et al., Semi-quantitative fluorescent PCR analysis identifies PRKAA1 on chromosome 5 as a potential candidate cancer gene of cervical cancer, *Gynecol Oncol* **103**(1) (2006), 219–225.

[48] F.Y. Huang, Y.K. Kwok, E.T. Lau, M.H. Tang, T.Y. Ng and H.Y. Ngan, Genetic abnormalities and HPV status in cervical and vulvar squamous cell carcinomas, *Cancer Genet Cytogenet* **157**(1) (2005), 42–48.

[49] E.A. Jarboe, L.C. Thompson, D. Heinz, J.A. McGregor and K.R. Shroyer, Telomerase and human papillomavirus as diagnostic adjuncts for cervical dysplasia and carcinoma, *Hum Pathol* **35**(4) (2004), 396–402.

[50] S. Jeon, B.L. Allen-Hoffmann and P.F. Lambert, Integration of human papillomavirus type 16 into the human genome correlates with a selective growth advantage of cells, *J Virol* **69**(5) (1995), 2989–2997.

[51] S. Jeon and P.F. Lambert, Integration of human papillomavirus type 16 DNA into the human genome leads to increased stability of E6 and E7 mRNAs: implications for cervical carcinogenesis, *Proc Natl Acad Sci USA* **92**(5) (1995), 1654–1658.

[52] M. Kalantari, E. Blennow, B. Hagmar and B. Johansson, Physical state of HPV16 and chromosomal mapping of the integrated form in cervical carcinomas, *Diagn Mol Pathol* **10**(1) (2001), 46–54.

[53] J.T. Keating, A. Cviko, S. Riethdorf, L. Riethdorf, B.J. Quade, D. Sun et al., Ki-67, cyclin E, and p16INK4 are complimentary surrogate biomarkers for human papilloma virus-related cervical neoplasia, *Am J Surg Pathol* **25**(7) (2001), 884–891.

[54] S.N. Khleif, J. DeGregori, C.L. Yee, G.A. Otterson, F.J. Kaye, J.R. Nevins et al., Inhibition of cyclin D-CDK4/CDK6 activity is associated with an E2F-mediated induction of cyclin kinase inhibitor activity, *Proc Natl Acad Sci USA* **93**(9) (1996), 4350–4354.

[55] M. Kirchhoff, H. Rose, B.L. Petersen, J. Maahr, T. Gerdes, C. Lundsteen et al., Comparative genomic hybridization reveals a recurrent pattern of chromosomal aberrations in severe dysplasia/carcinoma in situ of the cervix and in advanced-stage cervical carcinoma, *Genes Chromosomes Cancer* **24**(2) (1999), 144–150.

[56] R. Klaes, A. Benner, T. Friedrich, R. Ridder, S. Herrington, D. Jenkins et al., p16INK4a immunohistochemistry improves interobserver agreement in the diagnosis of cervical

intraepithelial neoplasia, *Am J Surg Pathol* **26**(11) (2002), 1389–1399.
[57] R. Klaes, T. Friedrich, D. Spitkovsky, R. Ridder, W. Rudy, U. Petry et al., Overexpression of p16(INK4A) as a specific marker for dysplastic and neoplastic epithelial cells of the cervix uteri, *Int J Cancer* **92**(2) (2001), 276–284.
[58] R. Klaes, S.M. Woerner, R. Ridder, N. Wentzensen, M. Duerst, A. Schneider et al., Detection of high-risk cervical intraepithelial neoplasia and cervical cancer by amplification of transcripts derived from integrated papillomavirus oncogenes, *Cancer Res* **59**(24) (1999), 6132–6136.
[59] L.G. Koss, The Papanicolaou test for cervical cancer detection. A triumph and a tragedy, *JAMA* **261**(5) (1989), 737–743.
[60] A.J. Kruse, J.P. Baak, T. Helliesen, K.H. Kjellevold, M.G. Bol and E.A. Janssen, Evaluation of MIB-1-positive cell clusters as a diagnostic marker for cervical intraepithelial neoplasia, *Am J Surg Pathol* **26**(11) (2002), 1501–1507.
[61] K.A. Lee, J.W. Kang, J.H. Shim, C.W. Kho, S.G. Park, H.G. Lee et al., Protein profiling and identification of modulators regulated by human papillomavirus 16 E7 oncogene in HaCaT keratinocytes by proteomics, *Gynecol Oncol* **99**(1) (2005), 142–152.
[62] S.Y. Liao and E.J. Stanbridge, Expression of MN/CA9 protein in Papanicolaou smears containing atypical glandular cells of undetermined significance is a diagnostic biomarker of cervical dysplasia and neoplasia, *Cancer* **88**(5) (2000), 1108–1121.
[63] F. Luft, R. Klaes, M. Nees, M. Durst, V. Heilmann, P. Melsheimer et al., Detection of integrated papillomavirus sequences by ligation-mediated PCR (DIPS-PCR) and molecular characterization in cervical cancer cells, *Int J Cancer* **92**(1) (2001), 9–17.
[64] F. Mantovani and L. Banks, The human papillomavirus E6 protein and its contribution to malignant progression, *Oncogene* **20**(54) (2001), 7874–7887.
[65] S.P. Mathur, R.S. Mathur, E.A. Gray, D. Lane, P.G. Underwood, M. Kohler et al., Serum vascular endothelial growth factor C (VEGF-C) as a specific biomarker for advanced cervical cancer: Relationship to insulin-like growth factor II (IGF-II), IGF binding protein 3 (IGF-BP3) and VEGF-A [corrected], *Gynecol Oncol* **98**(3) (2005), 467–483.
[66] C.P. Matthews, K.A. Shera and J.K. McDougall, Genomic changes and HPV type in cervical carcinoma, *Proc Soc Exp Biol Med* **223**(3) (2000), 316–321.
[67] P. Melsheimer, S. Vinokurova, N. Wentzensen, G. Bastert and M. von Knebel Doeberitz, DNA aneuploidy and integration of human papillomavirus type 16 e6/e7 oncogenes in intraepithelial neoplasia and invasive squamous cell carcinoma of the cervix uteri, *Clin Cancer Res* **10**(9) (2004), 3059–3063.
[68] A. Mitsuhashi, K. Suzuka, K. Yamazawa, H. Matsui, K. Seki and S. Sekiya, Serum vascular endothelial growth factor (VEGF) and VEGF-C levels as tumor markers in patients with cervical carcinoma, *Cancer* **103**(4) (2005), 724–730.
[69] R. Molina, X. Filella, J.M. Auge, E. Bosch, A. Torne, J. Pahisa et al., CYFRA 21.1 in patients with cervical cancer: comparison with SCC and CEA, *Anticancer Res* **25**(3A) (2005), 1765–1771.
[70] K. Munger, J.R. Basile, S. Duensing, A. Eichten, S.L. Gonzalez, M. Grace et al., Biological activities and molecular targets of the human papillomavirus E7 oncoprotein, *Oncogene* **20**(54) (2001), 7888–7898.
[71] N. Murphy, M. Ring, C.C. Heffron, B. King, A.G. Killalea, C. Hughes et al., p16INK4A, CDC6, and MCM5: predictive biomarkers in cervical preinvasive neoplasia and cervical cancer, *J Clin Pathol* **58**(5) (2005), 525–534.
[72] D. Ndisang, V. Budhram-Mahadeo, A. Singer and D.S. Latchman, Widespread elevated expression of the human papilloma virus (HPV)-activating cellular transcription factor Brn-3a in the cervix of women with CIN3 (cervical intraepithelial neoplasia stage 3), *Clin Sci (Lond)* **98**(5) (2000), 601–602.
[73] D. Ndisang, F. Lorenzato, M. Sindos, A. Singer and D.S. Latchman, Detection of cervical abnormalities in a developing country using measurement of Brn-3a in cervical smears, *Gynecol Oncol* **100**(1) (2006), 89–94.
[74] D. Ndisdang, P.J. Morris, C. Chapman, L. Ho, A. Singer and D.S. Latchman, The HPV-activating cellular transcription factor Brn-3a is overexpressed in CIN3 cervical lesions, *J Clin Invest* **101**(8) (1998), 1687–1692.
[75] M. Nees, E. van Wijngaarden, E. Bakos, A. Schneider and M. Durst, Identification of novel molecular markers which correlate with HPV-induced tumor progression, *Oncogene* **16**(19) (1998), 2447–2458.
[76] G. Negri, F. Vittadello, F. Romano, A. Kasal, F. Rivasi, S. Girlando et al., P16(INK4a) expression and progression risk of low-grade intraepithelial neoplasia of the cervix uteri, *Virchows Arch* (2004).
[77] S. Nieh, S.F. Chen, T.Y. Chu, H.C. Lai and E. Fu, Expression of p16 INK4A in Papanicolaou smears containing atypical squamous cells of undetermined significance from the uterine cervix, *Gynecol Oncol* **91**(1) (2003), 201–208.
[78] S. Nieh, S.F. Chen, T.Y. Chu, H.C. Lai, Y.S. Lin, E. Fu et al., Is p16(INK4A) expression more useful than human papillomavirus test to determine the outcome of atypical squamous cells of undetermined significance-categorized Pap smear? A comparative analysis using abnormal cervical smears with follow-up biopsies, *Gynecol Oncol* **97**(1) (2005), 35–40.
[79] J.C. Noel, S. Fernandez-Aguilar, I. Fayt, F. Buxant, M.H. Ansion, P. Simon et al., Laminin-5 gamma 2 chain expression in cervical intraepithelial neoplasia and invasive cervical carcinoma, *Acta Obstet Gynecol Scand* **84**(11) (2005), 1119–1123.
[80] A.G. Ostor, Natural history of cervical intraepithelial neoplasia: a critical review, *Int J Gynecol Pathol* **12**(2) (1993), 186–192.
[81] J.P. O'Sullivan, R.P. A'Hern, P.A. Chapman, L. Jenkins, R. Smith, A. al Nafussi et al., A case-control study of true-positive versus false-negative cervical smears in women with cervical intraepithelial neoplasia (CIN) III, *Cytopathology* **9**(3) (1998), 155–161.
[82] P. Peitsaro, B. Johansson and S. Syrjanen, Integrated human papillomavirus type 16 is frequently found in cervical cancer precursors as demonstrated by a novel quantitative real-time PCR technique, *J Clin Microbiol* **40**(3) (2002), 886–891.
[83] E.C. Pirog, R.N. Baergen, R.A. Soslow, D. Tam, A.E. DeMattia, Y.T. Chen et al., Diagnostic Accuracy of Cervical Low-Grade Squamous Intraepithelial Lesions Is Improved With MIB-1 Immunostaining, *Am J Surg Pathol* **26**(1) (2002), 70–75.
[84] P.H. Rao, H. Arias-Pulido, X.Y. Lu, C.P. Harris, H. Vargas, F.F. Zhang et al., Chromosomal amplifications, 3q gain and deletions of 2q33-q37 are the frequent genetic changes in cervical carcinoma, *BMC Cancer* **4** (2004), 5.
[85] M. Resnick, S. Lester, J.E. Tate, E.E. Sheets, C. Sparks and C.P. Crum, Viral and histopathologic correlates of MN and

MIB-1 expression in cervical intraepithelial neoplasia, *Hum Pathol* **27**(3) (1996), 234–239.
[86] G. Ronco, N. Segnan, P. Giorgi-Rossi, M. Zappa, G.P. Casadei, F. Carozzi et al., Human papillomavirus testing and liquid-based cytology: results at recruitment from the new technologies for cervical cancer randomized controlled trial, *J Natl Cancer Inst* **98**(11) (2006), 765–774.
[87] S. Sahebali, C.E. Depuydt, G.A. Boulet, M. Arbyn, L.M. Moeneclaey, A.J. Vereecken et al., Immunocytochemistry in liquid-based cervical cytology: Analysis of clinical use following a cross-sectional study, *Int J Cancer* (2005).
[88] S. Sahebali, C.E. Depuydt, K. Segers, L.M. Moeneclaey, A.J. Vereecken, E. Van Marck et al., P16INK4a as an adjunct marker in liquid-based cervical cytology, *Int J Cancer* **108**(6) (2004), 871–876.
[89] T. Sano, T. Oyama, K. Kashiwabara, T. Fukuda and T. Nakajima, Expression status of p16 protein is associated with human papillomavirus oncogenic potential in cervical and genital lesions, *Am J Pathol* **153**(6) (1998), 1741–1748.
[90] A.D. Santin, F. Zhan, E. Bignotti, E.R. Siegel, S. Cane, S. Bellone et al., Gene expression profiles of primary cervical cancers, *Virology* **331**(2) (2005), 269–291.
[91] V. Shanta, S. Krishnamurthi, C.K. Gajalakshmi, R. Swaminathan and K. Ravichandran, Epidemiology of cancer of the cervix: global and national perspective, *J Indian Med Assoc* **98**(2) (2000), 49–52.
[92] K.R. Shroyer, P. Homer, D. Heinz and M. Singh, Validation of a novel immunocytochemical assay for topoisomerase II-alpha and minichromosome maintenance protein 2 expression in cervical cytology, *Cancer* (2006).
[93] I. Silins, E. Avall-Lundqvist, A. Tadesse, K.U. Jansen, U. Stendahl, P. Lenner et al., Evaluation of antibodies to human papillomavirus as prognostic markers in cervical cancer patients, *Gynecol Oncol* **85**(2) (2002), 333–338.
[94] M. Sindos, D. Ndisang, N. Pisal, C. Chow, A. Deery, A. Singer et al., Detection of cervical neoplasia using measurement of Brn-3a in cervical smears with persistent minor abnormality, *Int J Gynecol Cancer* **13**(4) (2003), 515–517.
[95] M. Sindos, D. Ndisang, N. Pisal, C. Chow, A. Singer and D.S. Latchman, Measurement of Brn-3a levels in Pap smears provides a novel diagnostic marker for the detection of cervical neoplasia, *Gynecol Oncol* **90**(2) (2003), 366–371.
[96] B. Skyldberg, S. Salo, E. Eriksson, U. Aspenblad, B. Moberger, K. Tryggvason et al., Laminin-5 as a marker of invasiveness in cervical lesions, *J Natl Cancer Inst* **91**(21) (1999), 1882–1887.
[97] D. Solomon, D. Davey, R. Kurman, A. Moriarty, D. O'Connor, M. Prey et al., The 2001 Bethesda System: terminology for reporting results of cervical cytology, *JAMA* **287**(16) (2002), 2114–2119.
[98] S.A. Southern and C.S. Herrington, Differential cell cycle regulation by low- and high-risk human papillomaviruses in low-grade squamous intraepithelial lesions of the cervix, *Cancer Res* **58**(14) (1998), 2941–2945.
[99] M. Spitzer, B.S. Apgar and G.L. Brotzman, Management of histologic abnormalities of the cervix, *Am Fam Physician* **73**(1) (2006), 105–112.
[100] R.D. Steenbergen, D. Kramer, B.J. Braakhuis, P.L. Stern, R.H. Verheijen, C.J. Meijer et al., TSLC1 gene silencing in cervical cancer cell lines and cervical neoplasia, *J Natl Cancer Inst* **96**(4) (2004), 294–305.
[101] M. Steinau, D.R. Lee, M.S. Rajeevan, S.D. Vernon, M.T. Ruffin and E.R. Unger, Gene expression profile of cervical tissue compared to exfoliated cells: impact on biomarker discovery, *BMC Genomics* **6**(1) (2005), 64.
[102] M.H. Stoler, C.R. Rhodes, A. Whitbeck, S.M. Wolinsky, L.T. Chow and T.R. Broker, Human papillomavirus type 16 and 18 gene expression in cervical neoplasias, *Hum Pathol* **23**(2) (1992), 117–128.
[103] E.C. Thorland, S.L. Myers, D.H. Persing, G. Sarkar, R.M. McGovern, B.S. Gostout et al., Human papillomavirus type 16 integrations in cervical tumors frequently occur in common fragile sites, *Cancer Res* **60**(21) (2000), 5916–5921.
[104] M.J. Trunk, G. Dallenbach-Hellweg, R. Ridder, U. Petry, H. Ikenberg, V. Schneider et al., Morphologic Characteristics of $p16^{INK4a}$-Positive Cells in Cervical Cytology Samples, *Acta Cytol* **48**(6) (2004), 771–782.
[105] K. Umayahara, F. Numa, Y. Suehiro, A. Sakata, S. Nawata, H. Ogata et al., Comparative genomic hybridization detects genetic alterations during early stages of cervical cancer progression, *Genes Chromosomes Cancer* **33**(1) (2002), 98–102.
[106] S. Vinokurova, N. Wentzensen, J. Einenkel, R. Klaes, C. Ziegert, P. Melsheimer et al., Clonal history of papillomavirus-induced dysplasia in the female lower genital tract, *J Natl Cancer Inst* **97**(24) (2005), 1816–1821.
[107] M. von Knebel Doeberitz, T. Bauknecht, D. Bartsch and H. zur Hausen, Influence of chromosomal integration on glucocorticoid-regulated transcription of growth-stimulating papillomavirus genes E6 and E7 in cervical carcinoma cells, *Proc Natl Acad Sci USA* **88**(4) (1991), 1411–1415.
[108] M. von Knebel Doeberitz, New markers for cervical dysplasia to visualise the genomic chaos created by aberrant oncogenic papillomavirus infections, *Eur J Cancer* **38**(17) (2002), 2229–2242.
[109] J.L. Wang, B.Y. Zheng, X.D. Li, T. Angstrom, M.S. Lindstrom and K.L. Wallin, Predictive significance of the alterations of p16INK4A, p14ARF, p53, and proliferating cell nuclear antigen expression in the progression of cervical cancer, *Clin Cancer Res* **10**(7) (2004), 2407–2414.
[110] S.S. Wang, M.E. Sherman, A. Hildesheim, J.V. Lacey, Jr. and S. Devesa, Cervical adenocarcinoma and squamous cell carcinoma incidence trends among white women and black women in the United States for 1976–2000, *Cancer* **100**(5) (2004), 1035–1044.
[111] S.S. Wang, M. Trunk, M. Schiffman, R. Herrero, M.E. Sherman, R.D. Burk et al., Validation of p16INK4a as a marker of oncogenic human papillomavirus infection in cervical biopsies from a population-based cohort in Costa Rica, *Cancer Epidemiol Biomarkers Prev* **13**(8) (2004), 1355–1360.
[112] T. Waterboer, P. Sehr, K.M. Michael, S. Franceschi, J.D. Nieland, T.O. Joos et al., Multiplex human papillomavirus serology based on in situ-purified glutathione s-transferase fusion proteins, *Clin Chem* **51**(10) (2005), 1845–1853.
[113] E.J. Weaver, A.J. Kovatich and M. Bibbo, Cyclin E expression and early cervical neoplasia in ThinPrep specimens. A feasibility study, *Acta Cytol* **44**(3) (2000), 301–304.
[114] N. Wentzensen, C. Bergeron, F. Cas, D. Eschenbach, S. Vinokurova and M. von Knebel Doeberitz, Evaluation of a nuclear score for p16INK4a-stained cervical squamous cells in liquid-based cytology samples, *Cancer* **105**(6) (2005), 461–467.
[115] N. Wentzensen, M. Hampl, M. Herkert, A. Reichert, M.J. Trunk, C. Poremba et al., Identification of high-grade cervical dysplasia by the detection of p16(INK4a) in cell lysates obtained from cervical samples, *Cancer* **107**(9) (2006), 2307–2313.

[116] N. Wentzensen, R. Ridder, R. Klaes, S. Vinokurova, U. Schaefer and M. von Knebel Doeberitz, Characterization of viral-cellular fusion transcripts in a large series of HPV16 and 18 positive anogenital lesions, *Oncogene* **21**(3) (2002), 419–426.

[117] N. Wentzensen, S. Vinokurova and M. von Knebel Doeberitz, Systematic review of genomic integration sites of human papillomavirus genomes in epithelial dysplasia and invasive cancer of the female lower genital tract, *Cancer Res* **64**(11) (2004), 3878–3884.

[118] S.P. Wheatley and I.A. McNeish, Survivin: a protein with dual roles in mitosis and apoptosis, *Int Rev Cytol* **247** (2005), 35–88.

[119] A. Widschwendter, L. Ivarsson, A. Blassnig, H.M. Muller, H. Fiegl, A. Wiedemair et al., CDH1 and CDH13 methylation in serum is an independent prognostic marker in cervical cancer patients, *Int J Cancer* **109**(2) (2004), 163–166.

[120] G.H. Williams, P. Romanowski, L. Morris, M. Madine, A.D. Mills, K. Stoeber et al., Improved cervical smear assessment using antibodies against proteins that regulate DNA replication, *Proc Natl Acad Sci USA* **95**(25) (1998), 14932–14937.

[121] V. Wollscheid, R. Kuhne-Heid, I. Stein, L. Jansen, S. Kollner, A. Schneider et al., Identification of a new proliferation-associated protein NET-1/C4.8 characteristic for a subset of high-grade cervical intraepithelial neoplasia and cervical carcinomas, *Int J Cancer* **99**(6) (2002), 771–775.

[122] Y.F. Wong, T.H. Cheung, K.W. Lo, V.W. Wang, C.S. Chan, T.B. Ng et al., Protein profiling of cervical cancer by protein-biochips: proteomic scoring to discriminate cervical cancer from normal cervix, *Cancer Lett* **211**(2) (2004), 227–234.

[123] Y.F. Wong, Z.E. Selvanayagam, N. Wei, J. Porter, R. Vittal, R. Hu et al., Expression genomics of cervical cancer: molecular classification and prediction of radiotherapy response by DNA microarray, *Clin Cancer Res* **9**(15) (2003), 5486–5492.

[124] T.C. Wright, Jr., J.T. Cox, L.S. Massad, J. Carlson, L.B. Twiggs and E.J. Wilkinson, 2001 consensus guidelines for the management of women with cervical intraepithelial neoplasia, *Am J Obstet Gynecol* **189**(1) (2003), 295–304.

[125] T.C. Wright, Jr., J.T. Cox, L.S. Massad, L.B. Twiggs and E.J. Wilkinson, 2001 Consensus Guidelines for the management of women with cervical cytological abnormalities, *JAMA* **287**(16) (2002), 2120–2129.

[126] T.C. Wright, Jr., M. Schiffman, D. Solomon, J.T. Cox, F. Garcia, S. Goldie et al., Interim guidance for the use of human papillomavirus DNA testing as an adjunct to cervical cytology for screening, *Obstet Gynecol* **103**(2) (2004), 304–309.

[127] Y.C. Yang, W.Y. Shyong, M.S. Chang, Y.J. Chen, C.H. Lin, Z.D. Huang et al., Frequent gain of copy number on the long arm of chromosome 3 in human cervical adenocarcinoma, *Cancer Genet Cytogenet* **131**(1) (2001), 48–53.

[128] T. Yoshida, T. Fukuda, T. Sano, T. Kanuma, N. Owada and T. Nakajima, Usefulness of liquid-based cytology specimens for the immunocytochemical study of p16 expression and human papillomavirus testing: a comparative study using simultaneously sampled histology materials, *Cancer* **102**(2) (2004), 100–108.

[129] M.Y. Yu, J.H. Tong, P.K. Chan, T.L. Lee, M.W. Chan, A.W. Chan et al., Hypermethylation of the tumor suppressor gene RASSFIA and frequent concomitant loss of heterozygosity at 3p21 in cervical cancers, *Int J Cancer* **105**(2) (2003), 204–209.

[130] A. Zhang, J. Wang, B. Zheng, X. Fang, T. Angstrom, C. Liu et al., Telomere attrition predominantly occurs in precursor lesions during *in vivo* carcinogenic process of the uterine cervix, *Oncogene* **23**(44) (2004), 7441–7447.

[131] C. Ziegert, N. Wentzensen, S. Vinokurova, F. Kisseljov, J. Einenkel, M. Hoeckel et al., A comprehensive analysis of HPV integration loci in anogenital lesions combining transcript and genome-based amplification techniques, *Oncogene* **22**(25) (2003), 3977–3984.

[132] H. zur Hausen, Immortalization of human cells and their malignant conversion by high risk human papillomavirus genotypes, *Semin Cancer Biol* **9**(6) (1999), 405–411.

[133] H. zur Hausen, Papillomaviruses and cancer: from basic studies to clinical application, *Nat Rev Cancer* **2**(5) (2002), 342–350.

Disease Markers 23 (2007) 331–336
IOS Press

A long way: History of the prophylactic papillomavirus vaccine

Martin Müller and Lutz Gissmann*
Deutsches Krebsforschungszentrum Heidelberg, Germany

1. History of papillomaviruses as infectious agents in animals and humans

For more than one and a half centuries, papillomaviruses have been recognized as causative agents for benign and malignant disease in humans as well as in a number of animal species [43]. It took more than five decades to provide sufficient evidence for the general acceptance of HPV as necessary cause for the development of anogenital cancer in humans. At the end of this long road of extensive studies on papillomaviruses by countless scientists worldwide there is finally a prophylactic papillomavirus vaccine at hand. Clearly, the scientific progress in vaccine development was hampered by the fact that papillomaviruses cannot be readily cultivated *in vitro*. In this review we will discuss the path that led to the introduction of the prophylactic vaccine to the public.

Earliest reports about a putative infectious agent being involved in the development of cervical cancers came from observations made by the Italian physician Domenico Rigoni-Stern [51]. He noted that cancer of the womb is found most frequently among women in their fourth and fifth decade and he described behavioural risk factors for this cancer that are still being in the focus of modern epidemiology: age at first sexual intercourse and promiscuity. Despite an imprecise baseline of his study (Rigoni-Stern did not differentiate between cancer of the endometrial and cervical cancer) the link to cervical cancer was later confirmed by other investigators in the 1950s eventually linking cervical cancer to sexually transmitted agents [22,62,63]. In the following, a number of known pathogens were suspected to play a role in cervical cancer development. More refined investigations were subsequently able to rule out an involvement of *Treponema pallidum* (Syphilis) or Herpes Simplex Virus 2 and others in anogenital cancer [66].

Another line of evidence for papillomaviruses being responsible for tumor development was established by experimental transmission of warts and condylomas in man. As early as in the 1890s several investigators induced skin warts in volunteers by the inoculation of hand wart extracts [41,64]. In 1907 Ciuffo demonstrated that a filterable agent is able to induce hand warts [10]. Similar experiments were later performed for condylomas by Waelsch [67]. With the introduction of electron microscopy, virus particles were identified in extracts of hand warts and condylomas. Already in the early 1930s Shope described a virus inducing papillomas in cottontail and domestic rabbits [60]. Shope observed that experimentally induced papillomas in domestic rabbits progress to cancer in high frequency providing the first example of a DNA virus as causative agent for cancers in mammals. Later, Ito and Evans demonstrated that papillomas and tumors can be induced solely with naked viral DNA [33].

In 1976 zur Hausen noted that the epidemiological patterns of cervical cancer and condylomas showed striking similarities [72]. As papillomaviruses had been already tracked down for causing condylomas it was postulated that they might also be causatively involved in the development of cervical cancer. With the onset of molecular biology, a number of genital papillo-

*Corresponding author: Lutz Gissmann, DKFZ ATV F020, Im Neuenheimer Feld 242, 69120 Heidelberg, Germany. Tel.: +49 6221 424603; Fax: +49 6221 424932; E-mail: L.Gissmann@dkfz.de.

ISSN 0278-0240/07/$17.00

mavirus types were isolated and cloned into plasmid vectors in the following. HPV 6 DNA was cloned from condylomas, the closely related HPV 11 was isolated from laryngeal papillomas but also detected in genital warts [23,24,59]. With these low-risk papillomavirus genomes at hand, it was possible to prove, for the first time, presence of papillomavirus-related DNA in biopsies of cervical cancer. Shortly after, the two most prevalent high-risk HPV types 16 and 18 were cloned from tumor biopsies [4,15].

2. History of PV vaccination

2.1. Therapeutic approaches

Over the centuries, there have been numerous and sometimes venturesome attempts to treat skin and genital warts which makes it difficult to pinpoint the first therapeutic vaccination against PV. Early observations were made in the course of experimental induction of warts in rabbits and humans. It was noted, that warts develop only in a proportion of the individuals which was interpreted either as inefficiency of the virus to establish infections or 'resistance' of a given individual [26]. Further, it was clear that warts in animals and humans spontaneously regress. During a series of self-inoculations with wart extracts Findlay stated that he became 'immune' to wart induction [21]. It was also observed that local inflammation precedes regression of warts and that warts frequently disappear simultaneously [45]. In the 1930s and 1940s a number of therapeutic vaccination trials were performed based on the injection of autologous and heterologous wart extracts. During his trials, Biberstein inoculated hundreds of patients with filtered extracts from warts and condylomas and was able to record wart regression in the majority of the cases [3]. The likely involvement of the immune system in controlling papillomavirus infections was also underlined by the observation that genital warts but also genital cancer is more frequently found in immuno-suppressed patients [49].

The rabbit papillomavirus model proved to be particular valuable for the study of immune therapy of PV infections. Early studies showed that regression of papillomas and transplanted CRPV-induced tumors can be induced by injection of wart extracts linking papillomas and malignant tumors to the same antigens [18]. In later years, viral antigens responsible for wart regression were identified. The early proteins E1, E2, E6, and E7 protect against virus challenge and induce regression of already existing warts and malignant tumors [28,29]. In recent years a number of efforts have been undertaken to develop therapeutic papillomavirus vaccines some of which have entered clinical trials. It would go beyond the scope of this review to summarize all therapeutic papillomvirus vaccines, most of the approaches are directed to induce cellular immune responses against the E7 tumor antigen (for review see [14,16,61]). Synthetic E7-derived peptides have been analyzed for the treatment of low grade CIN lesion. Anti-E7 immune responses have also been induced by the use of recombinant vaccinia viruses. Interestingly, it was shown that Virus-like particles, the bases for current prophylactic vaccines, are also able to mount strong cellular immune responses likely, because they can directly interact with dendritic, antigen-presenting cells [55,57].

2.2. Prophylactic vaccination

Preventive vaccines are based on the induction of virus-neutralizing antibodies. In case of papillomaviruses this has first been achieved by immunization with formalin-fixed wart extracts and subsequently by inactivated purified viruses [34]. Lacking an appropriate infection model, it was difficult to determine the neutralizing activity of serum antibodies. The first *in vitro* assay for neutralization was the inhibition of focus formation of mouse cells in culture that was, for a long time, limited to BPV virions [53]. Inhibition of hemagluttination, which is based on binding of PV virions to mouse erythrocytes in a receptor-dependent manner, can be achieved by neutralizing antibodies hence this assay is considered a surrogate for measuring inhibition of infectivity [54]. A more complex neutralization assay was introduced by Kreider and coworkers: grafts of normal human tissue infected *in vitro* with HPV 11 or HPV 16 were implanted under the renal capsule of immuno-deficient mice where typical lesions develop [38]. Infection is then monitored by RT-PCR. Only very recently, a potentially high throughput neutralization assay became available which allows detection of neutralizing antibodies in an *in vitro* setting [48].

Neutralizing antibodies are directed against the major structural protein L1 and, to a much lesser degree, also against the minor capsid protein L2. In fact, in an early study *E. coli*-derived L1 protein was used for prophylactic vaccination [50] but was, despite initial promising results not followed up. The reason for the moderate success is that, for induction of neutralizing antibodies, the L1 protein is required to be presented in a correctly folded conformation. This became only possible with the production of L1 in form of virus-like particles. In 1986 it had already been shown that purified VP1 of mouse polyomavirus spontaneously assembles into virus-like particles [56]. This inspired in the early 1990s the production of papillomavirus-like particles by different researchers. Zhou and colleagues used a vaccinia virus expression system to produce HPV 16 L1 VLPs, however the yield of this system was extremely low and did not allow further characterization of the antigen e.g. by immunological studies [70].

Shortly after, it was demonstrated that HPV 1, BPV 1 and HPV 11 VLPs can be produced much more efficiently compared to HPV 16 VLPs leading to the speculation whether this might be due to intrinsic properties of the L1 protein of different PV types [27,54,69]. After a report by Kirnbauer and colleagues it became clear, however, that the HPV 16 L1 gene of the original isolate by Dürst et al. harboured a point mutation rendering its encoded L1 protein virtually assembly defective [36]. The HPV 16 prototype genome, used by numerous researchers worldwide was derived from a tumor biopsy, in which the HPV 16 genome was integrated into the cellular genome and thus had been without any selection pressure for the maintenance of intact structural genes. When HPV 16 genomes obtained from early, virus-producing lesions were analyzed, the respective L1 proteins assembled with much greater efficiency into VLPs. Sequence analysis revealed that this difference was based on a single histidine to aspartic acid exchange at position 202. VLPs were subsequently produced successfully in insect cells, later also in yeast, in plants and even in cell free systems. Meanwhile, VLPs of several animal and human papillomaviruses have been produced, i.e. cottobtail rabbit papillomavirus, rabbit oral papillomavirus, BPV 1 and 4, canine oral papillomavirus and HPV types 1, 2, 6, 8, 11, 13, 16, 18, 31, 33, 39, 45, 58 and 59 [5,9,11–13], for review see [58]. The production of VLPs in larger quantities made structural and immunological studies possible.

The compelling data obtained from several animal models fostered the concept of prophylactic vaccines against HPV infections. Virus-like particles proved to be prime candidates for prophylactic vaccination since they induce high-titer conformational antibodies both in non-human primates and in man [2,8,17,19,20,31, 35,42,47]. Such antibodies proved to have neutralizing capacity [53]. By passive transfer of IgG from immunized animals it was shown that they confer protection against experimental challenge [7].

The first clinical trial with VLPs involving human subjects was initiated in 1996 (for reference see [32]). HPV 11 VLPs were produced in insect cells and at that time laboriously purified by ultracentrifugation, a procedure that is inadequate for large scale production of a human vaccine. Nevertheless, the success of this trial spiked further HPV vaccine development. In several phase I clinical trials safety and immunogenicity of HPV 11, 16 and 18-specific VLPs generated by expression of the L1 protein in yeast or in insect cells infected with recombinant baculovirus were demonstrated [2,17,19,20,31]. Three VLP-based vaccines (HPV 16, HPV 16 + 18, HPV 6 + 11 + 16 + 18) were already brought into clinical efficacy trials. It should be noted that the vaccine provided by Merck & Co (Gardasil^{TM}) contains in addition to the most relevant cancer-associated HPV types 16 and 18 also VLPs of the low-risk HPV types 6 and 11 aiming for protection against genital warts whereas the product developed by GlaxoSmithKline targets only the two high-risk HPVs. The data obtained from immunization of about 25,000 young women receiving either vaccine or placebo demonstrated after 4 years of follow-up protection against incident and persistent infection with HPV 6/11, and/or HPV 16 an 18 and the lesions associated therewith (external genital lesions, high grade CIN, adenocarcinoma in situ) [1,30,37,44, 65]. It is as yet unclear to what extent the protection is HPV type-specific. Obviously it would be beneficial for the overall efficacy if the reactivity is not only restricted to HPV types included in the vaccine. Longer follow-up and large scale population-based efficacy trials will be required to evaluate the potential of these vaccines to reduce the incidence of cervical cancer [6,40]. Based on the existing data, however, the regulatory agencies in different countries have approved the first vaccine, the second product is expected to be licensed soon. It will be more difficult to evaluate the efficacy towards genital warts since the information about the incidence of this disease is rather scarce (http://wrongdiagnosis.com/g/genital_warts).

The question of acceptance of HPV-specific vaccines within different cultures also needs to be addressed [39, 71]. This includes the issue whether the vaccine will be marketed as preventive measures against a sexually transmitted disease or as anti-cancer prophylaxis [46]. Other issues are the duration of immune protection and the participation of vaccinated women in Pap-screening programs HPV 16 and 18 account for about 70% of cervical cancer cases [68] hence the risk for this disease by other high-risk HPV types is far from negligible. Therefore, vaccinated women need to be educated about the necessity to keep up with the screening program although the intervals of the visits can possibly extended [25]. Obviously prophylactic vaccination will be highly desirable in areas where screening programs are not offered to the general population and where cervical cancer is a major public health problem. The high price clearly is prohibitive and joint efforts of scientists (developing more cost effective protocols), providers and politicians (discussing multi-tiered pricing) and public and philanthropic foundations (providing large amounts of money) are needed to make the vaccines available to the populations of highest need.

References

[1] K.A. Ault, Prophylactic use of quadrivalent human papillomavirus (HPV) (types 6, 11, 16, 18) L1 virus-like particle (VLP) vaccine reduces cervical intraepithelial neoplasia (CIN) 2/3 and adenocarcinoma in situ (AIS) risk, *European Journal of Cancer Supplements* **3**(4) (2005), 11.

[2] K.A. Ault, A.R. Giuliano, R.P. Edwards, G. Tamms, L.L. Kim, J.F. Smith, K.U. Jansen, M. Allende, F.J. Taddeo, D. Skulsky and E. Barr, A phase I study to evaluate a human papillomavirus (HPV) type 18 L1 VLP vaccine, *Vaccine* **22**(23–24) (2004), 3004–3007.

[3] Biberstein, Immunization therapy of warts, *Arch Dermatol Syphilol* **50** (1944), 12–22.

[4] M. Boshart, L. Gissmann, H. Ikenberg, A. Kleinheinz, W. Scheurlen and H. zur Hausen, A new type of papillomavirus DNA, its presence in genital cancer biopsies and in cell lines derived from cervical cancer, *Embo J* **3**(5) (1984), 1151–1157.

[5] J.N. Bouwes Bavinck, S. Stark, A.K. Petridis, M.E. Marugg, J. Ter Schegget, R.G. Westendorp, P.G. Fuchs, B.J. Vermeer and H. Pfister, The presence of antibodies against virus-like particles of epidermodysplasia verruciformis-associated humanpapillomavirus type 8 in patients with actinic keratoses, *Br J Dermatol* **142**(1) (2000), 103–109.

[6] M.C. Bratti, A.C. Rodriguez, M. Schiffman, A. Hildesheim, J. Morales, M. Alfaro, D. Guillen, M. Hutchinson, M.E. Sherman, C. Eklund, J. Schussler, J. Buckland, L.A. Morera, F. Cardenas, M. Barrantes, E. Perez, T.J. Cox, R.D. Burk and R. Herrero, Description of a seven-year prospective study of human papillomavirus infection and cervical neoplasia among 10000 women in Guanacaste, Costa Rica, *Rev Panam Salud Publica* **15**(2) (2004), 75–89.

[7] F. Breitburd, R. Kirnbauer, N.L. Hubbert, B. Nonnenmacher, C. Trin-Dinh-Desmarquet, G. Orth, J.T. Schiller and D.R. Lowy, Immunization with viruslike particles from cottontail rabbit papillomavirus (CRPV) can protect against experimental CRPV infection, *J Virol* **69**(6) (1995), 3959–3963.

[8] D.R. Brown, J.T. Bryan, J.M. Schroeder, T.S. Robinson, K.H. Fife, C.M. Wheeler, E. Barr, P.R. Smith, L. Chiacchierini, A. DiCello and K.U. Jansen, Neutralization of human papillomavirus type 11 (HPV-11) by serum from women vaccinated with yeast-derived HPV-11 L1 virus-like particles: correlation with competitive radioimmunoassay titer, *J Infect Dis* **184**(9) (2001), 1183–1186.

[9] N.D. Christensen, N.M. Cladel, C.A. Reed and R. Han, Rabbit oral papillomavirus complete genome sequence and immunity following genital infection, *Virology* **269**(2) (2000), 451–461.

[10] Ciuffo, Innesto positivo con filtrato di verruca volgare, *Giorn Ital Mal Venerol* **48** (1907), 12–17.

[11] A.L. Combita, M.M. Bravo, A. Touze, O. Orozco and P. Coursaget, Serologic response to human oncogenic papillomavirus types 16, 18, 31, 33, 39, 58 and 59 virus-like particles in colombian women with invasive cervical cancer, *Int J Cancer* **97**(6) (2002), 796–803.

[12] V. Cuberos, J. Perez, C.J. Lopez, F. Castro, L.V. Gonzalez, L.A. Correa, G. Sanclemente, A. Gaviria, M. Muller and G.I. Sanchez, Molecular and serological evidence of the epidemiological association of HPV 13 with focal epithelial hyperplasia: a case-control study, *J Clin Virol* **37**(1) (2006), 21–26.

[13] H.A. Cubie, M. Plumstead, W. Zhang, O. de Jesus, L.A. Duncan and M.A. Stanley, Presence of antibodies to human papillomavirus virus-like particles (VLPs) in 11-13-year-old schoolgirls, *J Med Virol* **56**(3) (1998), 210–216.

[14] D.M. Da Silva, G.L. Eiben, S.C. Fausch, M.T. Wakabayashi, M.P. Rudolf, M.P. Velders and W.M. Kast, Cervical cancer vaccines: emerging concepts and developments, *J Cell Physiol* **186**(2) (2001), 169–182.

[15] M. Dürst, L. Gissmann, H. Ikenberg and H. zur Hausen, A papillomavirus DNA from a cervical carcinoma and its prevalence in cancer biopsy samples from different geographic regions, *Proc Natl Acad Sci USA* **80**(12) (1983), 3812–3815.

[16] G.L. Eiben, D.M. da Silva, S.C. Fausch, I.C. Le Poole, M.I. Nishimura and W.M. Kast, Cervical cancer vaccines: recent advances in HPV research, *Viral Immunol* **16**(2) (2003), 111–121.

[17] R.T. Emeny, C.M. Wheeler, K.U. Jansen, W.C. Hunt, T.M. Fu, J.F. Smith, S. MacMullen, M.T. Esser and X. Paliard, Priming of human papillomavirus type 11-specific humoral and cellular immune responses in college-aged women with a virus-like particle vaccine, *J Virol* **76**(15) (2002), 7832–7842.

[18] C.A. Evans, L.R. Gorman, Y. Ito and R.S. Weiser, A vaccination procedure which increases the frequency of regressions of Shope papillomas of rabbits, *Nature* **193** (1962), 288–289.

[19] T.G. Evans, W. Bonnez, R.C. Rose, S. Koenig, L. Demeter, J.A. Suzich, D. O'Brien, M. Campbell, W.I. White, J. Balsley and R.C. Reichman, A Phase 1 study of a recombinant viruslike particle vaccine against human papillomavirus type 11 in healthy adult volunteers, *J Infect Dis* **183**(10) (2001), 1485–1493.

[20] K.H. Fife, C.M. Wheeler, L.A. Koutsky, E. Barr, D.R. Brown, M.A. Schiff, N.B. Kiviat, K.U. Jansen, H. Barber, J.F. Smith, A. Tadesse, K. Giacoletti, P.R. Smith, G. Suhr and D.A. Johnson, Dose-ranging studies of the safety and immunogenicity of human papillomavirus Type 11 and Type 16 virus-like particle candidate vaccines in young healthy women, *Vaccine* **22**(21–22) (2004), 2943–2952.

[21] G. Findlay, Warts, in: *A system of bacteriology in relation to medicine*, (Vol. 7), pp. 252–258. H. M. Stationary Office, London, 1930.

[22] F. Gagnon, Contribution to the study of the etiology and prevention of cancer of the cervix of the uterus, *Am J Obstet Gynecol* **60**(3) (1950), 516–522.

[23] L. Gissmann, V. Diehl, H.J. Schultz-Coulon and H. zur Hausen, Molecular cloning and characterization of human papilloma virus DNA derived from a laryngeal papilloma, *J Virol* **44**(1) (1982), 393–400.

[24] L. Gissmann and H. zur Hausen, Partial characterization of viral DNA from human genital warts (Condylomata acuminata), *Int J Cancer* **25**(5) (1980), 605–609.

[25] S.J. Goldie, M. Kohli, D. Grima, M.C. Weinstein, T.C. Wright, F.X. Bosch and E. Franco, Projected clinical benefits and cost-

effectiveness of a human papillomavirus 16/18 vaccine, *J Natl Cancer Inst* **96**(8) (2004), 604–615.

[26] W. Grigg and G. Wilhelm, Epidemiological study of plantar warts among school children, *Public Health Report US* **68** (1953), 985–988.

[27] M.E. Hagensee, N.H. Olson, T.S. Baker and D.A. Galloway, Three-dimensional structure of vaccinia virus-produced human papillomavirus type 1 capsids, *J Virol* **68**(7) (1994), 4503–4505.

[28] R. Han, N.M. Cladel, C.A. Reed, X. Peng and N.D. Christensen, Protection of rabbits from viral challenge by gene gun-based intracutaneous vaccination with a combination of cottontail rabbit papillomavirus E1, E2, E6, and E7 genes, *J Virol* **73**(8) (1999), 7039–7043.

[29] R. Han, C.A. Reed, N.M. Cladel and N.D. Christensen, Immunization of rabbits with cottontail rabbit papillomavirus E1 and E2 genes: protective immunity induced by gene gun-mediated intracutaneous delivery but not by intramuscular injection, *Vaccine* **18**(26) (2000), 2937–2944.

[30] D.M. Harper, E.L. Franco, C. Wheeler, D.G. Ferris, D. Jenkins, A. Schuind, T. Zahaf, B. Innis, P. Naud and N.S. De Carvalho, Efficacy of a bivalent L1 virus-like particle vaccine in prevention of infection with human papillomavirus types 16 and 18 in young women: a randomised controlled trial, *The Lancet* **364**(9447) (2004), 1757–1765.

[31] C.D. Harro, Y.Y. Pang, R.B. Roden, A. Hildesheim, Z. Wang, M.J. Reynolds, T.C. Mast, R. Robinson, B.R. Murphy, R.A. Karron, J. Dillner, J.T. Schiller and D.R. Lowy, Safety and immunogenicity trial in adult volunteers of a human papillomavirus 16 L1 virus-like particle vaccine, *J Natl Cancer Inst* **93**(4) (2001), 284–292.

[32] S. Inglis, A. Shaw and S. Koenig, Chapter 11: HPV vaccines: Commercial Research & Development, *Vaccine* **24**(Suppl 3) (2006), S99–S105.

[33] Y. Ito and C.A. Evans, Tumorigenic Nucleic Acid Extracts from Tissues of a Transplantable Carcinoma, Vx7, *J Natl Cancer Inst* **34** (1965), 431–437.

[34] W.F. Jarrett, B.W. O'Neil, J.M. Gaukroger, K.T. Smith, H.M. Laird and M.S. Campo, Studies on vaccination against papillomaviruses: the immunity after infection and vaccination with bovine papillomaviruses of different types, *Vet Rec* **126**(19) (1990), 473–475.

[35] R. Kirnbauer, L.M. Chandrachud, B.W. O'Neil, E.R. Wagner, G.J. Grindlay, A. Armstrong, G.M. McGarvie, J.T. Schiller, D.R. Lowy and M.S. Campo, Virus-like particles of bovine papillomavirus type 4 in prophylactic and therapeutic immunization, *Virology* **219**(1) (1996), 37–44.

[36] R. Kirnbauer, J. Taub, H. Greenstone, R. Roden, M. Dürst, L. Gissmann, D.R. Lowy and J.T. Schiller, Efficient self-assembly of human papillomavirus type 16 L1 and L1-L2 into virus-like particles, *J Virol* **67**(12) (1993), 6929–6936.

[37] L.A. Koutsky, K.A. Ault, C.M. Wheeler, D.R. Brown, E. Barr, F.B. Alvarez, L.M. Chiacchierini and K.U. Jansen, A controlled trial of a human papillomavirus type 16 vaccine, *N Engl J Med* **347**(21) (2002), 1645–1651.

[38] J.W. Kreider, M.K. Howett, A.E. Leure-Dupree, R.J. Zaino and J.A. Weber, Laboratory production *in vivo* of infectious human papillomavirus type 11, *J Virol* **61**(2) (1987), 590–593.

[39] E. Lazcano-Ponce, L. Rivera, E. Arillo-Santillan, J. Salmeron, M. Hernandez-Avila and N. Munoz, Acceptability of a human papillomavirus (HPV) trial vaccine among mothers of adolescents in Cuernavaca, Mexico, *Arch Med Res* **32**(3) (2001), 243–247.

[40] M. Lehtinen and J. Paavonen, Effectiveness of preventive human papillomavirus vaccination, *Int J STD AIDS* **14**(12) (2003), 787–792.

[41] W. Licht, Om Vorters Smitsomhed, *Ugeskrift Laeger* **1** (1894), 368–369.

[42] R.S. Lowe, D.R. Brown, J.T. Bryan, J.C. Cook, H.A. George, K.J. Hofmann, W.M. Hurni, J.G. Joyce, E.D. Lehman, H.Z. Markus, M.P. Neeper, L.D. Schultz, A.R. Shaw and K.U. Jansen, Human papillomavirus type 11 (HPV-11) neutralizing antibodies in the serum and genital mucosal secretions of African green monkeys immunized with HPV-11 virus-like particles expressed in yeast, *J Infect Dis* **176**(5) (1997), 1141–1145.

[43] D. Lowy and P. Howley, Papillomaviruses, in: *Fields Virology*, (Vol. 1), D. Knipe and P. Howley, eds, 2001,pp. 2231–2264. 2 vols. Lippincott, Williams and Wilkins, Philadelphia, USA.

[44] C. Mao, L.A. Koutsky, K.A. Ault, C.M. Wheeler, D.R. Brown, D.J. Wiley, F.B. Alvarez, O.M. Bautista, K.U. Jansen and E. Barr, Efficacy of Human Papillomavirus-16 Vaccine to Prevent Cervical Intraepithelial Neoplasia: A Randomized Controlled Trial, *Obstet Gynecol* **107**(1) (2006), 18–27.

[45] A.M. Massing and W.L. Epstein, Natural history of warts. A two-year study, *Arch Dermatol* **87** (1963), 306–310.

[46] R.M. Mays, L.A. Sturm and G.D. Zimet, Parental perspectives on vaccinating children against sexually transmitted infections, *Soc Sci Med* **58**(7) (2004), 1405–1413.

[47] T.J. Palker, J.M. Monteiro, M.M. Martin, C. Kakareka, J.F. Smith, J.C. Cook, J.G. Joyce and K.U. Jansen, Antibody, cytokine and cytotoxic T lymphocyte responses in chimpanzees immunized with human papillomavirus virus-like particles, *Vaccine* **19**(27) (2001), 3733–3743.

[48] D.V. Pastrana, C.B. Buck, Y.Y. Pang, C.D. Thompson, P.E. Castle, P.C. FitzGerald, S. Kruger Kjaer, D.R. Lowy and J.T. Schiller, Reactivity of human sera in a sensitive, high-throughput pseudovirus-based papillomavirus neutralization assay for HPV16 and HPV18, *Virology* **321**(2) (2004), 205–216.

[49] I. Penn, Cancers of the anogenital region in renal transplant recipients. Analysis of 65 cases, *Cancer* **58**(3) (1986), 611–616.

[50] W.P. Pilacinski, D.L. Glassman, K.F. Glassman, D.E. Reed, M.A. Lum, R.F. Marshall, C.C. Muscoplat and A.J. Faras, Immunization against bovine papillomavirus infection, *Ciba Found Symp* **120** (1986), 136–156.

[51] Rigoni-Stern, Fatti statisici relativi alle malatie cancerose, *G Serve Prog Pathol Terap* **2** (1842), 507–517.

[52] R.B. Roden, N.L. Hubbert, R. Kirnbauer, F. Breitburd, D.R. Lowy and J.T. Schiller, Papillomavirus L1 capsids agglutinate mouse erythrocytes through a proteinaceous receptor, *J Virol* **69**(8) (1995), 5147–5151.

[53] R.B. Roden, E.M. Weissinger, D.W. Henderson, F. Booy, R. Kirnbauer, J.F. Mushinski, D.R. Lowy and J.T. Schiller, Neutralization of bovine papillomavirus by antibodies to L1 and L2 capsid proteins, *J Virol* **68**(11) (1994), 7570–7574.

[54] R.C. Rose, R.C. Reichman and W. Bonnez, Human papillomavirus (HPV) type 11 recombinant virus-like particles induce the formation of neutralizing antibodies and detect HPV-specific antibodies in human sera, *J Gen Virol* **75**(Pt 8) (1994), 2075–2079.

[55] M.P. Rudolf, S.C. Fausch, D.M. Da Silva and W.M. Kast, Human dendritic cells are activated by chimeric human papillomavirus type-16 virus-like particles and induce epitope-specific human T cell responses *in vitro*, *J Immunol* **166**(10) (2001), 5917–5924.

[56] D.M. Salunke, D.L. Caspar and R.L. Garcea, Self-assembly of purified polyomavirus capsid protein VP1, *Cell* **46**(6) (1986), 895–904.

[57] K. Schafer, M. Müller, S. Faath, A. Henn, W. Osen, H. Zentgraf, A. Benner, L. Gissmann and I. Jochmus, Immune response to human papillomavirus 16 L1E7 chimeric virus-like particles: induction of cytotoxic T cells and specific tumor protection, *Int J Cancer* **81**(6) (1999), 881–888.

[58] J.T. Schiller and D.R. Lowy, Papillomavirus-like particle vaccines, *J Natl Cancer Inst Monogr* (28) (2001), 50–54.

[59] E. Schwarz, M. Dürst, C. Demankowski, O. Lattermann, R. Zech, E. Wolfsperger, S. Suhai and H. zur Hausen, DNA sequence and genome organization of genital human papillomavirus type 6b, *Embo J* **2**(12) (1983), 2341–2348.

[60] R. Shope, Infectious papillomatosis of rabbits; with a note on histopathology, *J Exp Med* **58** (1933), 607–624.

[61] M.A. Stanley, Progress in prophylactic and therapeutic vaccines for human papillomavirus infection, *Expert Rev Vaccines* **2**(3) (2003), 381–389.

[62] R.S. Taylor, B.E. Carroll and J.W. Lloyd, Mortality among women in 3 Catholic religious orders with special reference to cancer, *Cancer* **12** (1959), 1207–1225.

[63] J.E. Towne, Carcinoma of the cervix in nulliparous and celibate women, *Am J Obstet Gynecol* **69**(3) (1955), 606–613.

[64] G. Variot, Un cas d'inoculation experimentale des verruces de l'enfant a l'homme, *J Clin Therapy Infant* **2** (1894), 529–534.

[65] L.L. Villa, R.L. Costa, C.A. Petta, R.P. Andrade, K.A. Ault, A.R. Giuliano, C.M. Wheeler, L.A. Koutsky, C. Malm, M. Lehtinen, F.E. Skjeldestad, S.E. Olsson, M. Steinwall, D.R. Brown, R.J. Kurman, B.M. Ronnett, M.H. Stoler, A. Ferenczy, D.M. Harper, G.M. Tamms, J. Yu, L. Lupinacci, R. Railkar, F.J. Taddeo, K.U. Jansen, M.T. Esser, H.L. Sings, A.J. Saah and E. Barr, Prophylactic quadrivalent human papillomavirus (types 6, 11, 16, and 18) L1 virus-like particle vaccine in young women: a randomised double-blind placebo-controlled multicentre phase II efficacy trial, *Lancet Oncol* **6**(5) (2005), 271–278.

[66] V. Vonka, J. Kanka, J. Jelinek, I. Subrt, A. Suchanek, A. Havrankova, M. Vachal, I. Hirsch, E. Domorazkova, H. Zavadova et al., Prospective study on the relationship between cervical neoplasia and herpes simplex type-2 virus. I. Epidemiological characteristics, *Int J Cancer* **33**(1) (1984), 49–60.

[67] L. Waelsch, Übertragungsversuche mit spitzen Kondyloma, *Arch Dermatol Syphilis* **124** (1918), 625–646.

[68] J.M. Walboomers, M.V. Jacobs, M.M. Manos, F.X. Bosch, J.A. Kummer, K.V. Shah, P.J. Snijders, J. Peto, C.J. Meijer and N. Munoz, Human papillomavirus is a necessary cause of invasive cervical cancer worldwide, *J Pathol* **189**(1) (1999), 12–19.

[69] J. Zhou, D.J. Stenzel, X.Y. Sun and I.H. Frazer, Synthesis and assembly of infectious bovine papillomavirus particles *in vitro*, *J Gen Virol* **74** (Pt 4) (1993), 763–768.

[70] J. Zhou, X.Y. Sun, H. Davies, L. Crawford, D. Park and I.H. Frazer, Definition of linear antigenic regions of the HPV16 L1 capsid protein using synthetic virion-like particles, *Virology* **189**(2) (1992), 592–599.

[71] G.D. Zimet, R.M. Mays, Y. Winston, R. Kee, J. Dickes and L. Su, Acceptability of human papillomavirus immunization, *J Womens Health Gend Based Med* **9**(1) (2000), 47–50.

[72] H. zur Hausen, Condylomata acuminata and human genital cancer, *Cancer Res* **36**(2 pt 2) (1976), 794.

Disease Markers 23 (2007) 337–352
IOS Press

Therapeutic vaccination for HPV induced cervical cancers

Joeli A. Brinkman[a], Sarah H. Hughes[b], Pamela Stone[b], Angela S. Caffrey[b], Laila I. Muderspach[b], Lynda D. Roman[b], Jeffrey S. Weber[c] and W. Martin Kast[a,d,*]
[a]*Norris Comprehensive Cancer Center, University of Southern California, Keck School of Medicine, Los Angeles, CA, USA*
[b]*Department of Obstetrics and Gynecology, University of Southern California, Keck School of Medicine, Los Angeles, CA, USA*
[c]*Department of Medicine, University of Southern California, Keck School of Medicine, Los Angeles, CA, USA*
[d]*Department of Molecular Microbiology and Imunology, University of Southern California, Keck School of Medicine, Los Angeles, CA, USA*

Abstract. Cervical Cancer is the second leading cause of cancer – related deaths in women worldwide and is associated with Human Papillomavirus (HPV) infection, creating a unique opportunity to treat cervical cancer through anti-viral vaccination. Although a prophylactic vaccine may be available within a year, millions of women, already infected, will continue to suffer from HPV-related disease, emphasizing the need to develop therapeutic vaccination strategies. A majority of clinical trials examining therapeutic vaccination have shown limited efficacy due to examining patients with more advanced-stage cancer who tend to have decreased immune function. Current trends in clinical trials with therapeutic agents examine patients with pre-invasive lesions in order to prevent invasive cervical cancer. However, longer follow-up is necessary to correlate immune responses to lesion regression. Meanwhile, preclinical studies in this field include further exploration of peptide or protein vaccination, and the delivery of HPV antigens in DNA-based vaccines or in viral vectors. As long as pre-clinical studies continue to advance, the prospect of therapeutic vaccination to treat existing lesions seem good in the near future. Positive consequences of therapeutic vaccination would include less disfiguring treatment options and fewer instances of recurrent or progressive lesions leading to a reduction in cervical cancer incidence.

Keywords: Human papillomavirus (HPV), therapeutic vaccination, clinical trials

1. Introduction

Cervical cancer, the second most common cause of cancer-related deaths in women worldwide, is highly associated with Human Papillomaviruses (HPV) infection of the anogenital region. HPV is detected in 99.7% of cervical carcinomas [104]. World-wide approximately 510,000 new cases and 288,000 deaths due to cervical cancer are reported annually [3]. In the United States Papanicicoloau (Pap) smear screening has reduced cervical cancer mortality by 70% in the last 50 years [63]. However, despite the availability of Pap smear screening, approximately 13,000 new cervical cancer cases and 4,500 deaths occur yearly making cervical cancer the tenth most common cancer in women in the US [1,10].

Approximately 30–50% of the general population is positive for HPV DNA in the anogenital region making HPV one of the most common sexually transmitted infections of viral origin. There are over 30 known HPV types that infect the anogenital region [18]. These types are classified as being low, intermediate or high-risk based on their in-vitro ability to interact with cell cycle

*Corresponding author: W. Martin Kast, Ph.D., University of Southern California, 1501 San Pablo Street, ZNI 245, MC 2821, Los Angeles, CA 90089-2821, USA. Tel.: +1 323 442 3870; Fax: +1 323 442 4433; E-mail: mkast@usc.edu.

ISSN 0278-0240/07/$17.00

Table 1
Clinical trial phases

Phase I	Phase II	Phase III	Phase IV
Involve a small number of people (20–80), are the first studies on humans. The goal is to see if the treatment is safe, if it has harmful side effects, and how it is best administered. If the results are positive, researchers move on to phase II	A small number of participants (100–300) are used to determine the effectiveness of a therapeutic agent. The major outcomes can be clinical and/or immunological responses. If benefit is demonstrated, it moves on to phase III	A large number of partipants (1,000–3,000) participants at different hospitals and research centers are utilized to confirm the treatments effectiveness, monitor side effects, and compare it to commonly used treatments, and collect information that will allow the treatment to be used safely. Most phase III studies are randomized and blinded trials	Post marketing studies after the treatment has received FDA approval delineate additional information including the drug's optimal use and cost benefit analysis

Adapted from: [4, 5, 7].

proteins and clinical association with causing cervical cancer. Low risk HPV types like 6 and 11 are associated with causing the sexually transmitted disease of genital warts [40]. High-risk HPV types, like 16, 18, 31, and 45 are closely associated with anogenital malignancies including penile, anal, vaginal and vulva carcinomas and have been implicated in the etiology of most, if not all cervical cancers with high risk types HPV 16 and 18 accounting for nearly 70% of cases [62]. Interestingly, while HPV infection is highly prevalent in the general population, the infection is asymptomatic in most people largely due to host immune system's ability to control the virus and usually does not lead to cancer [62]. In contrast to many other cancers, the fact that cervical cancer is highly associated with a viral infection and that host immune responses control the infection in a majority of infected subjects, opens the possibility of vaccination against HPV viruses as a unique opportunity to either prevent or treat cervical cancer. A prophylactic vaccine for cervical cancer may be available within the next year. However, prophylactic vaccination will have no effect on millions of women already infected with HPV or women who will become infected before the vaccine is available. Additionally, even with conventional treatments mortality from cervical cancer is approximately 40% [22] and conventional treatments for HPV-related pre-malignant lesions can effect female reproduction and cause discomfort. Also HPV associated pre-malignant lesions have a high rate of recurrence, signifying the necessity to develop effective therapeutic vaccines to treat existing disease. The purpose of this article is to discuss therapeutic anti HPV strategies that are currently in clinical trials, a definition of clinical trial stages appears in Table 1, and to indicate innovations in pre-clinical trials of therapeutic vaccines to treat cervical cancers.

1.1. HPV Biology

HPV is a virus with icosahedral symmetry and 72 capsomeres, arranged in a pentameric structure surrounding the genome [15]. The genetic information of HPV viruses is encoded in a double stranded, circular genome that is approximately 8 Kb long. The genome can be divided into three major regions: early genes, late genes, and control genes [91].

The lifecycle of HPV encompasses infection of the basal epithelium and is closely linked to keratinocyte differentiation [108]. The basal epithelial layer is the only layer in the epithelium that is actively dividing [72] and minor trauma to the outer epithelial layer is probably required in order for the virus to reach this layer and initiate infection [67]. Once infection is initiated in the basal cell layer, the viral genome is maintained as a low copy episome. As the keratinocyte undergoes differentiation, viral gene expression and genome amplification both increase until late gene expression of the L1 and L2 capsid forming proteins occurs in terminally differentiated superficial cells [94]. Another form of infection is non-permissive, transformable infection in which viral replication does not occur. In this situation, viral DNA persists as either an extrachromosomal element or becomes integrated into the host cell chromosome at a random site [80]. Viral integration into the host cell DNA is believed to be a necessary step in cellular transformation in mucosal HPV.

E6 and E7 are the major oncogenic proteins involved in HPV carcinogenesis. Both proteins interfere with the normal mechanisms of cell cycle control [97]. HPV types that are low risk for causing cancer have weak interactions with the cell cycle control components, p53 and Rb, whereas high-risk types have stronger binding affinities for these cellular components. The E6 protein of high-risk HPV types forms a complex with the cellular protein E6 associated AP or E6 AP. The E6

AP complex then binds to and degrades p53 through ubiquitin-directed proteolysis [49,71]. P53 is essential for DNA repair as it mediates either G1 growth arrest or apoptosis in response to DNA damage in the cell. Degradation of p53 would result in the lack of cell cycle control leading to the accumulation of mutations and in genetic instability [40]. The E7 protein of high-risk HPV types binds the retinoblastoma tumor suppressor protein (pRb) with higher affinity than low risk types. The binding of the E7 protein to pRb causes Rb to release the transcription factor E2F. This results in activation of certain E2F dependent genes required for DNA synthesis and cell cycle control [49,71]. The effect is deregulated cell cycle control and uncontrolled cellular proliferation. When the virus integrates into the host chromosome, the E1/E2 genes, which regulate E6 and E7 protein production, are interrupted with a resultant increase in both of these oncogenes. Given that expression of E6 and E7 is required for maintenance of the transformed state [103] and expression levels are higher in transformed cells [23,34,40], expression of the oncoproteins and is not likely to be lost due to immunological pressures. This makes the E6 and E7 oncoproteins logical targets for HPV-specific therapeutic vaccine approaches.

1.2. HPV Immunology

In patients having early stage cervical carcinoma and HPV induced CIN lesions, cytotoxic T cell (CTL) responses have been demonstrated against HPV-16 and HPV-18 [36,73,85]. In addition, T helper cell responses directed against HPV-16 E6 and E7 have been detected in patients with abnormal cervical cytology [29, 30,56,68,105,106]. Epidemiological studies involving screening cohorts for the presence of HPV antibodies indicate that neutralizing conformational IgG antibodies directed toward the major capsid antigen (L1) occur in a majority in people having past or current HPV infection. However, these antibody titers are generally low and type specific. Thus antibodies to one HPV type are not protective for other HPV types [42]. These studies may indicate that while effective antiviral immunity is generated in a majority of HPV infected individuals, this immunity may develop too late or be of too low of magnitude to prevent the development of cancer in some individuals. However, these data do indicate that through enhancement of the host's immune response via vaccination, infection with certain high risk types can be prevented or even treated.

Effective eradiation of virally infected cells is generally mediated by a Th1 type immune response characterized by the presence of activated CTL and CD4+ T helper cells. Helper T cells aid in viral eradication and tumor ablation by helping to activate and maintain CTL-mediated responses to tumor antigens through the induction of Th1 cytokines like IFN-gamma. CTL are considered the major eradicators of both tumor and virally infected cells in the adaptive immune response. Target cells are identified by CTL as a result of the presentation of aberrant or "non-self" antigens, typically 8–10 amino acids in length and complexed with Major Histocompatibility Complex (MHC) class I molecules on the cell surface of a majority cells in the body. "Self" proteins are also presented in the context of MHC I molecules and this allows the cells of the immune system to distinguish between "self" and "non-self" antigens. Aberrant, "non-self" and "self" antigens are endogenous proteins that are degraded by the proteasome complex in the cytosol before they are transported by the TAP transporter into the endoplasmic reticulum for complexing with MHC class I molecules and then transported to the cell surface through the Golgi Complex [86]. Helper T cells interact with professional antigen presenting cells (APC), which present viral and tumor antigens through the MHC II pathway [86]. Viral antigens or components of tumor cells that are present in the extracellular spaces can become ingested by APC through endocytosis and subsequently degraded into 12–15 amino acid peptides in endosomal vesicles [88]. Vesicles containing peptides fuse with vesicles containing newly synthesized MHC class II molecules in the cytosol. The MHC class II molecules and the peptide antigen associate and then the bound peptide is transported to the cell surface of the APC [55]. This process is known as exogenous antigen presentation and unlike MHC class I presentation is restricted to professional APC such as B lymphocytes, macrophages, Langerhans cells (LC), and dendritic cells (DC).

Immature LC and DC are professional antigen presenting cells that specialize in antigen capture in the periphery. Immature DC reside in the dermis, whereas immature LC are found in the epidermis of the skin and in the epithelial layers of all mucosa [12,37]. In the genital tract, HPV infection is initiated in basal epithelial cells and LC are believed to pick up HPV particles and cross present these antigens to naïve T cells [99]. In the process, the LC should undergo maturation to initiate an adaptive immune response. However, the local cytokine environment in which LC encounter HPV antigens contributed to by keratinocytes which secrete

TGF-beta, and IL-10 [54] may result in an APC that is polarized to Th-2 type immunity which may result in a relatively ineffective response against solid tumors and HPV infected cells [99]. Conversely, under conditions of inflammation, keratinocytes can produce pro-inflammatory cytokines which can promote a Th1 type immune response leading to presentation of viral antigens by mature LC and the generation of an effective immune response against HPV infection [99]. The effects of the local cytokine environment upon primary introduction of HPV antigens may explain why some women resolve HPV infection while others progress. An interesting study by Fausch et al. demonstrated that while HPV virus-like particles (VLP) can activate DC they do not do not activate Langerhans cells [37, 38] indicating an intriguing immune escape mechanism employed by HPV [39]. DCs have emerged as one of the best stimulators of naïve T cells [37]. DC have a high density of MHC and co-stimulatory molecules and they efficiently process exogenous antigens through the MHC class I pathway in order to stimulate naïve CD8+ T cells through the process of cross presentation [86]. Targeting HPV antigens to DC by vaccination, resulting in activation and a subsequent Th1 response, as opposed to antigen capture by LC in a natural infection may overcome HPV-induced immune escape and lead to lesion regression in HPV infected subjects.

2. Therapeutic vaccines

While prophylactic vaccination strategies aim to prevent initial infection with the HPV virus by inducing a neutralizing antibody response toward the L1 and the L2 capsid antigens, therapeutic vaccination against HPV attempts to induce strong CTL and Helper T cell responses to HPV antigens, such as the E6 and E7 oncoproteins, which unlike the L1 and L2 capsid antigens are expressed in pre-cancerous and cancerous tissue. In particular the E6 and E7 oncoproteins contain epitopes that are processed and presented in association with the HLA-A2 MHC class I molecule [96]. MHC class I restricted peptide epitopes have been generated for the E6 and E7 protein of HPV 16 and 18 [57,87] that have demonstrated immunogenicity in both human and animal models [9,83]. For these reasons peptides generated from the E6 and E7 protein have been used extensively in clinical trials attempting to treat HPV associated cancers.

2.1. Peptide and protein-based vaccines

A phase I clinical trial sought to examine the efficacy of multiple administrations of an HLA-A*0201-restricted HPV-16 E7 lipopeptide vaccine linked to the non-specific helper peptide PADRE in twelve women with refractory cervical or vaginal cancer [96]. Four subcutaneous injections (s.c) of the E7 86-93 lipopeptide were given at three week intervals. Five of seven patients that were evaluable after two vaccinations and 2/3 patients that were evaluable after all four vaccinations demonstrated an E7 peptide specific CTL response as determined by IFN-γ release assay. However, no clinical responses were associated with vaccination in these studies.

Another phase I-II clinical trial utilized two HPV-16 E7 peptides and the PADRE helper peptide delivered in incomplete Freund's adjuvant (IFA) to perform a dose escalation study in 19 HLA-A*0201+ patients with HPV-16+ cervical carcinoma [101]. Successive patient groups received 100 μg, 300 μg, or 1000 μg of each peptide s.c. every three weeks for four vaccinations. Utilizing radiological evaluation, two patients demonstrated stable disease for one year after vaccination and two patients demonstrated tumor regression after vaccination and subsequent chemotherapy treatments. All other patients experienced progressive disease. Immunohistochemical evaluation of skin biopsies taken from the site of vaccination demonstrated an influx of CD8+, CD4+, and CD3+ T cells in three patients analyzed. A large portion of the patients in the study demonstrated lymphopenia both before and after vaccination, indicating that this study population was fairly immunocompromised due to the nature of their disease. Immunological analysis from peripheral blood mononuclear cells measured after vaccination indicated that there was no E7 peptide-specific CTL induction in these patients at any dose [84] perhaps indicating that these patients were too advanced to benefit from peptide immunization.

Another phase I trial was conducted in women with high-grade cervical or vulvar intraepithelial neoplasia who were HLA-A2 and HPV-16 positive [70]. Eighteen patients were treated with four vaccinations given three weeks apart with escalating doses of the E7 peptide 12–20 in incomplete Freund's adjuvant (IFA). Starting with the eleventh patient, the E7 peptide 86–93 linked to the PADRE helper peptide with a covalently linked lipid tail was added to the vaccine regimen. Three out of 17 patients demonstrated complete and 9/17 demonstrated partial regression of dyplastic lesions. Although T cell frequencies remained the same, 6/6 patients tested by immunohistochemical staining demonstrated an increase in DC infiltrates in dysplastic tissue. Although positive delayed type hypersensitivity (DTH) responses were not detected in any patients after vaccination, E7 peptide specific cytotoxic T lymphocytes (CTL) responses were detected from PBMC in 10/16 patients. Lastly, while Pap smears turned out to be negative, *in situ* RNA hybridization revealed that all biopsy specimens were positive for HPV viral RNA after vaccination, although at a much reduced level. Thus, while the therapeutic vaccine in this study was able to effect complete regression in three patients and partial regression in nine others, demonstration of viral RNA in biopsy specimens post vaccination may be an indication of insufficient follow-up time in order to demonstrate complete viral clearance.

Although in a majority of HPV peptide based vaccine trials an HPV specific CTL response has been detected in some patients, tumor regression has been minimal and these CTL responses do not correlate with clinical outcome. An explanation for the lack of correlation between peptide specific T cell responses and clinical outcome may involve the general state of the patients' immune system such that more advanced stage cancer patients tend to have decreased immune function that correlates with stage of disease. Many of the studies discussed above included patients with advanced stage cancers. Obviously, it is necessary to examine peptide or protein based vaccination in patients with early stage cancers or even pre-invasive lesions in order to assess whether in vitro immune reactivity can predict tumor regression or prevent disease progression. One such clinical trial was recently conducted in women having CIN 1-3 lesions [47]. The vaccine agent was a fusion protein (PD-E7) containing mutated HPV-16 E7 protein conjugated to protein D of *Haemophilus influenzae* and delivered intramuscularly with AS02B adjuvant. Five out of seven patients in the study demonstrated significant increases in IFN-γ responses and all vaccinated patients had significant titers of E7 antibodies. However, clinical responses were not correlated with immune responses in this study and the investigators suggested that the efficacy of this agent needs to be further examined in a larger cohort of CIN patients having a high and persistent HPV viral load. Similarly, a recombinant fusion protein consisting of heat shock protein (Hsp 65) from *Mycobacterium Bovis* BCG and the E7 protein of HPV 16 was developed to treat HPV related diseases. A recent Phase II clinical trial utilizing this agent demonstrated high statistical significance for lengthening the interval between de-bulking surgeries for patients with recurrent respiratory papillomatosis (RRP). The results from a separate phase II clinical trial demonstrated that HspE7 is likely active in anal intraepithelial neoplasia (AIN) in converting most patients from high grade to low grade squamous intraepithelial lesions within 3–6 months of starting therapy. An interesting finding in this study was that vaccination with this agent also caused regression of anogenital genital warts in several patients [46]. However, a recent adjunct of this trial involving 133 patients [8], designed to confirm previous results, indicated that the drug exceeded the treatment effect, but the anticipated placebo effect doubled as estimated by experts through studies of natural history, and thus there was no difference between drug and placebo. In this study there was a highly discordant level of interpreted degree of dysplasia between separate pathologists and thus additional measurements of HPV, such as viral load, need to be evaluated in Phase III anal dysplasia trials. The use of this agent to treat 21 women with HPV-related CIN lesions was shown to induce a 40% response rate within 8 weeks. However, Elucidation of the full extent of the clinical benefit will require long-term follow-up [2,8]. Additional pre-clinical studies investigating the use of heat shock protein 70 from *Mycobacterium tuberulosis* fused to HPV-16 E6 and E7 mutated proteins has shown regression of established lung metastases in mice [3] suggesting that the use of heat shock proteins as adjuvants requires further investigation.

Two recent clinical trials have examined therapeutic HPV protein-based vaccine strategies in subjects that do not have HPV related disease. A phase I clinical trial was recently conducted in 40 healthy volunteers [31]. The vaccine agent utilized for these studies, TA-CIN, is a single fusion protein of HPV-16 L2, E6 and E7 proteins and it was administered without adjuvant intramuscularly in three doses. The results indicated that E6 and E7 specific T cell immunity was induced in 8/11 evaluable subjects at the highest dose as well as antibody and T cell proliferative responses. A similar recombinant bacterial fusion protein of HPV-16 E6 and E7 has been made and delivered in ISCOMATRIX® adjuvant intramuscularly to 42 healthy volunteers in a Phase I clinical trial. After three injections of the vaccine agent, measurable T cell responses were detected in 80% of vaccinated subjects and all vaccine recipients demonstrated an HPV-16 E6/E7 antibody response [8, 14]. A follow-up study utilized this agent in 31 patients having CIN lesions and demonstrated good immune responses and a reduction in viral load for patients who were HPV-16+ [43]. The preliminary findings in these trials are indeed encouraging but require further evaluation in order to fully access clinical efficacy.

Pre-clinical research utilizing peptide based vaccines has shifted to the examination of proteins [60] or peptides generated from other early genes of HPV that are expressed in cervical cancers delivered with bacterial adjuvants such as CpG oligodeoxynucleotides [19] and to the administration of long peptides or whole protein vaccines as mentioned above. The trend of utilizing long peptides and whole protein is attributable to the desire to allow presentation of more CTL epitopes and T helper epitopes. As mentioned previously, T helper cells are necessary to enhance CTL mediated tumor killing and for the generation of memory responses. One such strategy was recently employed in a preclinical cottontail rabbit papillomavirus model of recurrent respiratory papillomatosis (RRP). In the study, long over-lapping peptides containing CTL and helper epitopes were able to significantly reduce latent infection and control wart growth in cottontail rabbit papillomavirus infected rabbits [98]. A different preclinical study demonstrated complete tumor regression in mice by utilizing adenylate cyclase (CyaA) of Bordetella pertussis, which is able to target DC through its interaction with the CD11b/CD18 integrin, conjugated to HPV-16 E7 protein [81]. Another preclinical study examined prime-boost vaccination with a 35 amino acid HPV-16 E7 peptide that included both CTL and T helper epitopes administered with oligodeoxynucleotide-CpG as adjuvant to activate DC in C57BL/6 mice and compared their results to mice that were immunized with a minimal E7 CTL epitope [109]. The results demonstrated that a more vigorous CTL response and enhanced tumor eradication was seen when vaccinating with the long peptide as compared to vaccination with the minimal CTL epitope. The results of these studies are encouraging and indicate the need for further investigation into vaccination with long peptides and whole proteins and additional exploration into the use of prime boost strategies to vaccinate with peptide-based agents.

2.2. *Dendritic cell vaccination*

Another approach to therapeutic vaccination in cancer patients has been peptide or protein pulsing of autologous DC and then returning these dendritic cells to the patient. DC are a potent APC type with the ability to stimulate and maintain immune responses when pulsed with antigens [13,95]. A recent clinical trial was conducted in 15 stage IV cervical cancer patients utilizing autologous DC pulsed with recombinant HPV-16 or HPV-18 E7 oncoproteins. Although, a specific cellular immune response was seen in 4/11 patients and a specific antibody response was seen in 3/11 patients, no clinical responses were observed [41]. A similar study conducted in four terminal cervical cancer patients utilized DC pulsed with HPV-16 and HPV-18 E7 proteins in adjunct to rIL-2 treatment. In this study, specific humoral and cellular CD4+ T cell responses to the E7 vaccine were detected in two patients and increased numbers of E7-specific IFN-gamma secreting CD8+ T cells were detected in all patients after vaccination. However, no objective clinical responses were observed [89]. The culmination of both of these reports may indicate that more potent adjuvants or even adjunct vaccination may be necessary to treat cervical cancer patients at such a late state. An advantage to using full length protein over single peptides is the possibility of presenting more CTL epitopes for immune recognition, however, single peptides are cheaper to prepare. To this end, a recent study described a new HPV-16 E6 52–61 B57 HLA class I peptide in which T cell clones specific for this peptide were also able to recognize analogous epitopes from HPV types 35, 39, 45, 51, and 73. However, the efficacy of this peptide delivered in DC, administered to HLA-B57 cancer patients, has yet to be determined [59]. Strategies to enhance the potency of DC based therapeutic vaccine delivery include: DC transfected with a rearranged HPV-16 E7 DNA vaccine [79] and DC loaded with HPV peptides and transfected with HPV small interfering RNA targeting the Bak and Bax anti-apoptotic proteins in order to prolong DC life and thus enhance immunity [77]. Even though delivery of peptide or protein based vaccines by pulsing autologous DC with antigen shows promise in tumor immunotherapy, the technique is cumbersome because of the necessity of stimulating the patient's DC *ex vivo*.

2.3. *DNA vaccines*

Recent efforts in the field of HPV tumor immunotherapy have focused on the delivery of peptides in the form of mini-gene vaccines or naked DNA vaccines. DNA based vaccines are attractive candidates for therapeutic vaccines because of the simplicity of delivery, stability, and overall safety. DNA based vaccines can either stably integrate into the genome or be maintained in an episomal form allowing for extended expression of HPV antigens over a longer period of time than peptide vaccination. Furthermore, administration of DNA based vaccines has been shown to induce both CTL and antibody responses to HPV antigens [35]. To date, two phase I clinical trials, assessing the safety of mini-gene administration in the delivery vehicle have taken place. One study examined this vaccine regimen in 12 patients with HPV-16 associated anal dysplasia [61] and a more recent study examined this vaccination strategy in 15 women with CIN 2 or 3 [92]. The ZYC101 vaccination agent utilized for both of these studies consists of bacterial expression plasmid that expresses a segment of the HPV-16 E7 gene which includes several overlapping CTL epitopes and is fused to a secretory leader sequence derived from the HLA-DRA*0101 locus [61, 92]. The construct was delivered to patients with high grade anal dysplasia on a dose escalating scale either by intramuscular (i.m.) injection [61] or i.m. and s.c. injection [92] encapsulated in poly lactide-co-glyolide particles, which enhances delivery to antigen presenting cells [61]. All of the patients utilized in both studies were HLA-A2 and HPV-16 positive. After four i.m. injections at three week intervals, 3/12 patients demonstrated partial regression of anal dysplasia lesions and 10/12 patients demonstrated increased peptide-specific immune responses as determined by direct ELISPOT assay. All ten of these patients maintained heightened immune responses for at least six months and no serious adverse effects were seen [61]. In the study examining women with CIN, three treatments were given at three week intervals and colposcopy was performed at each treatment and at a four month follow-up period. Eleven of 15 women in the study demonstrated peptide – specific T cell responses as judged by IFN-γ release in ELISA assay and five women demonstrated complete regression of cervical lesions. Four of five of the women who regressed developed cervical IgA responses to the E2 protein of HPV-16, suggesting that HPV infected cells are undergoing lysis as a result of immune stimulation due to vaccination and that this is in effect causing epitope spreading of other HPV antigens that are not included in the vaccine formulation [92]. An improved agent, ZYC101a, was recently utilized in a multi-center study involving 127 women with biopsy confirmed CIN 2/3 lesions. Six months after vaccine administration, a higher proportion of vaccinated subjects resolved their lesions than those in the placebo group. However, this effect was most pronounced in subjects who were less than twenty-five years of age [44]. The preliminary results of this study are slightly encouraging; but the study is still ongoing in order to measure the durability of the agent's effect over a longer follow-up period.

Preclinical studies using DNA based vaccine approaches tend to focus on enhancing presentation of HPV antigens via the MHC class I pathway. Several different approaches have been examined including the attachment of ubiquitin to DNA constructs [66,102], targeting of tumor antigens to centrosomal compartments to enhance MHC class I presentation [52] or the attachment to constructs of calreticulin to target HPV antigens to the MHC I pathway [76,78] optimization of codon usage for enhanced expression and presentation of HPV oncogenes [21,65,66], utilization of modified or duplicated genes to increase the number of available CTL epitopes [16,32,74,75], enhancement of intercellular spreading in order to increase the number of cells expressing antigen [53], or even encoding of a single chain trimer containing b2-microglobulin, MHC class I heavy chain, and an immunodominant HPV-16 E6 epitope in order to bypass antigen processing and cause stable presentation of E6 antigens [51]. All of these approaches have demonstrated increased antigen presentation and superior tumor eradication in mouse models. However, further examination is necessary in order to determine if these effects can be achieved in humans.

2.4. Delivery of HPV antigens through viral vectors

Delivery of HPV antigens, particularly those derived from the E6 and E7 oncogenes, in recombinant viruses poses an attractive approach for therapeutic vaccination. It offers an advantage over peptide immunization in that CTL epitopes can be processed and presented naturally and are delivered more efficiently to target cells and it has an advantage over DNA based vaccines because it increases the efficiency of introducing heterologous genes into target cells [20]. Viruses like vaccinia, the agent utilized to vaccinate against the disease Small Pox, are lytic and extremely immunogenic. The lysis of vaccinia infected cells insures uptake of the HPV antigens and the vaccinia virus acts as an adjuvant to enhance the immune response to the HPV antigens. One vaccine based on this scheme is the TA-HPV vaccine which was recently examined for immunogenicity and safety in 29 patients with stage Ib or IIa cervical cancer [58]. The TA-HPV vaccine is a recombinant vaccinia virus that expresses modified forms of the HPV-16 and 18 E6 and E7 oncoproteins. The vaccination was given in two applications ranging from 4–12 weeks apart by dermal scarification and was thought to deliver approximately 2.5×10^5 pfu. The results indicated that after a single vaccination four patients developed HPV specific CTL responses and eight patients developed HPV-specific serological responses. Currently, the investigators of this study are continuing examination of this agent in patients with vulvar and vaginal intraepithelial neoplasia (VIN) [11, 28]. Similarly, an MVA-HPV-IL-2 vaccine has been developed that is currently being tested in three phase II clinical trials for patients with VIN, CIN, or cervical cancer. The MVA-HPV-IL2 agent is based on the Modified Virus Ankara (MVA), a non-propagative highly attenuated vaccinia virus strain expressing modified E6 and E7 proteins as well as IL-2 to enhance both specific and non-specific cellular immune responses [6]. In the study involving patients with CIN lesions partial clinical and/or histological responses were observed in five out of 15 patients treated with a high dose of the agent while CIN regression was not observed in 12 patients treated with the low dose. In the study involving patients with cervical cancer two out of 27 patients demonstrated stable disease at 6 months when treated with a low dose of the agent.In the clinical trial involving patients with VIN, clinical results showed no difference in the patients treated with the vaccine compared to the controlled placebo group. However, the low dose of the agent that was utilized for this and the cervical cancer study and given the dose-related effect seen in the CIN2/3 trial; these results were probably due to the low dose used and the advanced stage of the disease of these patients [6]. Despite the encouraging results of these studies, there may be problems involved in immunizing with vaccinia virus. One problem may lie in the fact that a majority of women in the US over the age of 35 have been previously vaccinated with vaccinia virus and women in this age group are at the peak age for cervical cancer acquisition. In the present study, nine patients had prior vaccination with vaccinia virus but none of the four women who developed a CTL response to the HPV antigens had been previously vaccinated. Therefore it is possible that childhood vaccination with vaccinia virus, in an effort to eradicate small pox, may induce a strong and early memory response that may supersede the response to HPV antigens. One way to overcome this challenge may be heterologous boosting. In animal models, it was demonstrated that the existence of neutralizing antibodies to chimeric VLP may prevent boosting of the CMI response in subsequent vaccinations [25]. But this effect can be overcome, by utilizing different chimeric or heterologous VLP in prime-boost vaccination strategies [26]. One recent study showed good protection in mice by priming with recombinant adenylate cyclase toxoid from *Bordetella pertussis* conjugated to a modified full length HPV-16 E7 protein and then boosting with MVA virus expressing the E7 protein fused to the lysosome-associated LAMP-1 membrane protein [69]. Enhanced CTL immunity was demonstrated in mice by combining TA-HPV, a vaccinia based vaccine containing HPV 16/18 E6/E7, and TA-CIN containing HPV 16 L2, E6 and E7 as a single fusion protein, in a heterologous prime-boost strategy [100]. Recently, this prime boost regime was utilized in a phase II clinical trial [93]. Twenty-nine women with high grade vaginal intraepithelial neoplasia (VIN) received three intramuscular injections of TA-CIN followed by a single dermal scarification with TA-HPV. After twelve weeks 10/27 patients demonstrated increased T cell proliferation responses to HPV antigens and HPV 16 E6 or E7 specific T cells were identified in 11/25 via IFN-gamma production in ELISPOT assay. However, only five out of twenty-nine and one out of twenty-nine patients demonstrated partial and complete clinical responses, respectively. This perhaps indicates a need for longer term follow-up in these studies in order to determine the temporal relationship between induction of vaccine induced immune responses and the regression of HPV induced lesions.

Similarly, preclinical studies have been conducted in mice using adenovirus vectors that have demonstrated good protection against HPV-16+ tumor challenges [64]. However, given that vaccinia and adenoviruses are DNA viruses, another potential drawback of using these vectors to deliver HPV E6 and E7 oncogenes in therapeutic vaccines is the potential integration of these oncogenes into the host genome. One method to overcome the potential integration of DNA viruses is to utilize (VLP) from hepatitis B virus to deliver an immunodominant CTL epitope from the HPV-16 E7 protein. Hepatitis B virus VLP are good inducers of both T and B cell responses and this strategy prevented the establishment of tumors in mice [33]. Other investigators are attempting to overcome the issues of pre-existing immunity and oncogene integration by using alphavirus vectors in therapeutic vaccine regimens. Alphaviruses such as Sindbis virus, Venezuelan Equine Encephalitis virus (VEE) or Semliki Forest Virus (SFV) are cytopathic RNA viruses that express the RNA of the E6 and E7 oncogenes in the cell's cytosol and thus eliminate the potential integration of these oncogenes into the host cell chromosome. Also there is no pre-existing immunity to these viruses in a vast majority of individuals [27,35]. Additionally, Alpha virus vectors have a very wide host range and can infect a variety of different cell types [45] which makes them attractive candidates for delivering antigenic components of vaccines.

Administration of Sindbis virus replicon particles containing herpes simplex virus type 1 (HSV-1) tegument protein linked to HPV-16 E7 resulted in the spread of E7 antigen to neighboring cells and caused a significant increase in the number of E7-specific CD8+T cell precursors and a strong anti-tumor effect against E7-expressing tumors in C57BL/6 mice [20]. Similarly, immunization with recombinant Semliki Forest virus (SFV) encoding a fusion protein of HPV-16 E6 and E7 resulted in complete elimination of established tumors and induced a long term high level of antigen specific CTL activity in tumor bearing mice [27]. Further advances in using the SFV alpha virus vector may be seen by linking *Mycobacterium tuberculosis* heat shock protein 70 (Hsp70) to HPV-16 E7. In a recent study, SFV vector containing E7/Hsp70 fusion genes generated significantly higher E7-specific T cell-mediated immune responses than SFV vector containing the wild-type E7 gene in vaccinated mice. Furthermore the E7/Hsp70 fusion vaccine demonstrated significant potency against established E7-expressing metastatic tumors in mice [50].

Venezuelan Equine Encephalitis Virus (VEE) replicon particles are unlike other alpha viruses because they have the ability to infect dendritic cells which likely leads to better antigen delivery to naïve T cells present in the lymph nodes [17]. Recent studies utilizing this agent containing mutated, fused E6 and E7 genes of HPV-16 and demonstrated 100% protection from tumor challenge in vaccinated mice. Additionally, eradication of established tumors was observed in 90% of C57/BL6 and HLA-A*0201 transgenic mice during therapeutic vaccination [17]. Although these are preclinical studies, the eradication of tumors in the HLA-A*0201 transgenic mice is significant because these mice bear the most common human leukocyte antigen in the human population. Additionally, this same group of researchers has produced VRP encoding mutated fused E6 and E7 genes of types 18, 45, 31, 33, 52, and 58 and shown in a recent study that administration of a combination of monovalent HPV containing VRP did not diminish the immune response to type 16 indicating that the simultaneous administration of different monovalent VRP could be useful for therapeutic treatment of lesions infected with multiple HPV types [82]. These encouraging results provide incentive for further examination of this agent in pre-clinical and clinical trials.

Taken together, results from pre-clinical studies of tumor eradication with therapeutic alpha virus vaccination strategies are very promising and are likely to be taken into clinical trials in the near future. Ongoing research in delivery of HPV antigens through viral vectors may include other vectors like flavivirus or Kunjin virus replicons which are non-cytopathic and may allow prolonged expression of inserted genes for presentation to the host's immune system and enhancement of T cell memory [48].

2.5. *T cell receptor transfer*

One last approach in HPV related tumor therapy that may be utilized in future vaccine trials is the genetic transfer of antigen specific T cell receptors with high affinity for tumor-associated antigens into patients T cells. Presumably, this approach will confer the appropriate tumor killing specificity and has the potential to generate a bank of TCR genes with specificity to various viral tumor antigens that may be selected for any patient with tumor cells expressing the appropriate antigen [90,107]. An additional benefit would be that genetically transferred TCR could be tracked by non-invasive imaging or PCR based technologies targeting the unique sequence of the T cell's CDR3 region.

3. Conclusion

Because infection with high risk mucosal types of Human Papillomavirus is so closely associated with the development of cervical cancer, several vaccination strategies have been examined in both clinical and preclinical trials for both the prevention of HPV infection and the treatment of pre-existing HPV-related disease. Prophylactic vaccines contain virus-like particles (VLP) that express the HPV viral capsid antigens in a conformational manner and aim to induce neutralizing antibodies to prevent infection with high risk HPV types. Findings from clinical trials with VLP indicate good vaccine efficacy and it is predicted that a prophylactic vaccine for cervical cancer may be available within the next year. However, prophylactic VLP vaccination will have no effect on millions of women already infected with HPV and the millions of women who will become infected before the vaccine is made available. Even after vaccination is implemented it is estimated that a reduction in the incidence of cervical cancer will not be apparent for at least a decade [24]. This stresses the importance of continued therapeutic vaccine development.

Therapeutic vaccination aims to prevent the progression of pre-existing HPV associated lesions or cancers

Table 2

Summary of therapeutic HPV vaccines in clinical trials for CIN, VIN, and Cervical Cancer

Vaccine type	Vaccine composition	Adjuvant/ delivery route	Trial phase	Patient population	Immunological responses	Clinical responses	Reference
Peptide and protein based vaccines	Lipopeptide containing E7 aa 86–93 linked to the non-specific helper peptide PADRE	SC	I	12 women with refractory cervical or vaginal cancer	IFN-γ release in response to the E7 peptide in approximately 66% of patients	none	[96]
	2 HPV-16 E7 peptides and the PADRE helper peptide	IFA SC	I-II	19 HLA-A*0201+ patients with HPV-16+ cervical carcinoma	no E7 peptide-specific CTL induction seen	2/19 SD 2/19 PR	[84,101]
	E7 peptide 12–20 and E7 peptide 86–93 linked to the PADRE helper peptide with a lipid tail	IFA SC	I	17 patients with high-grade cervical or vulvar intraepithelial neoplasia	E7 peptide specific cytotoxic T lymphocytes (CTL) responses were detected from PBMC in 10/16 patients	3/17 CR 9/17 PR	[70]
	Fusion protein containing mutated HPV-16 E7 protein conjugated to protein D of *Haemophilus influenzae*	AS02B IM	I/II	5 patients with CIN III 2 patients with CIN I	5/7 patients showed significantly increased IFN-γ CD8+ cell responses	In CIN III patients, 0/5 had lesion regression. In CIN I patients, 2/2 had lesion regression	[47]
	Fusion protein consisting of (Hsp 65) from *Mycobacterium Bovis* BCG and the E7 protein of HPV 16	SC	II	22 patients with anal HSIL 14/22 patients also had anogenital warts	NR	3/14 CR 10/14 PR of anogential warts	[46]
	Fusion protein of HPV-16 L2, E6 and E7 (TA-CIN)	IM	I	40 healthy volunteers	E6 and E7 specific T cell immunity was induced in 8/11 evaluable subjects	No clinical measures in study	[31]
	Recombinant bacterial fusion protein of HPV-16 E6 and E7	ISCOMATRIX® IM	I	8 CIN I 10 CIN II 13 CIN III	5/15 IFN-γ CD8+ specific T cell responses 18/22 DTH response to E6/E7 antigens	4/31 CR 14 HPV-16+ vaccine recipients showed reduced viral load	[43]
Dendritic cell based vaccines	Autologous dendrtic cells pulsed with recombinant HPV16 E7 or HPV18 E7 proteins	SC	I	15 stage IV cervical cancer patients immune responses were monitored in 11 patients	4/11 cellular immune response 3/11 specific antibody response	No objective clinical response was observed	[41]
	DC pulsed with full-length HPV16 or 18 E7 oncoprotein, followed by subcutaneous (s.c.) low doses of human recombinant interleukin-2 (rIL-2)	SC	I	4 HPV16 or 18 cervical cancer patients who have failed conventional treatment modalities	2/4 Specific humoral and cellular CD4+ T cell responses to 4/4 increased numbers of E7-specific IFN-gamma secreting CD8+ T cells	No objective clinical response was observed	[89]
DNA based vaccines	ZYC101 is composed of Zycos 101 plasmid DNA encapsulated in biodegradable polymer microparticles. The plasmid DNA encodes for multiple HLA-A2-restricted epitopes derived from the HPV-16 E7 protein	IM	I	12 subjects with HPV-16 anal dysplasia	10/12 subjects demonstrated an increased immune response to the peptide epitopes of HPV-16 E7	3/12 PR	[61]
	Zycos 101	SC and/or IM	I	15 patients with CIN 2/3	11/15 HPV specific T-cell responses	5/15 CR	[92]

Table 2, continued

Vaccine type	Vaccine composition	Adjuvant/ delivery route	Trial Phase	Patient population	Immunological responses	Clinical responses	Reference
	ZYC101a contains plasmid-DNA-encoding fragments derived from the E6 and E7 proteins of HPV 16 and 18, and is formulated within small biodegradable microparticles	IM	II	127 patients with CIN 2/3 (86 treated)	80/86 Increased T cell specific immune responses	37/86 CR	[44]
HPV antigens delivered in viral vectors	TA-HPV Recombinant vaccinia virus expressing modified forms of the HPV-16 and 18 E6 and E7 proteins	Dermal scarification	I	29 patients with stage Ib or IIa cervical cancer	HPV-specific CTLs were found in 4 patients. 8 patients developed HPV-specific serological responses	N.R	[58]
	TA-HPV	Dermal scarification	II	12 patients with HPV+ high-grade VIN	6/10 T Helper responses 10/10 antibody responses	5/12 PR 1/12 CR	[11]
	TA-HPV	Dermal scarification	II	18 patients with HPV 16-positive high-grade vaginal intraepithelial neoplasia	8/18 T cell proliferation responses 5/18 INF-γ responses 1/18 antibody responses	7/18 PR 1/18 CR	[28]
	MVA-HPV-IL2 agent is based on the Modified Virus Ankara (MVA), an attenuated vaccinia virus expressing modified E6 and E7 proteins and IL-2	IM	II	31 patients with HPV16-related CIN 2/3	NR	5/16 PR 4/16 viral clearance in high dose group	[6]
Heterologous prime boost vaccinations	TA-CIN (HPV-16 L2/E6/E7 fusion protein and TA-HPV	IM and Dermal scarification	II	29 patients with high-grade CIN	10/29 T cell proliferation responses 11/29 INF-γ responses 14/29 antibody responses	5/29 PR 1/29 CR	[93]

SC = subcutaneous, IM = intramuscular, SD = stable disease, PR = partial regression, CR = Complete regression, HSIL = High grade intraepithelial lesion, NR = not reported, CIN = cervical intraepithelial neoplasia, VIN = vulvar intraepithelial neoplasia.

by targeting the E6 or E7 oncogenes because of their role in cellular transformation and continuous expression in cervical cancers. Treating HPV associated lesions with therapeutic vaccination offers an attractive alternative to current clinical procedures. Current therapies like LEEP and cone biopsy procedures can cause damage to the cervix such as stenosis and cervical incompetence. Additionally, these procedures can result in more painful menstrual cycles, excessive bleeding after surgery, secondary infection as the result of surgery, and increased difficultly in taking future Pap smears [10]. Also because these are surgical procedures, when anesthesia is indicated, patient fatality is a remote outcome and these procedures are far more costly than a vaccination which could be administered in a doctor's office. Lastly, given that there is a high recurrence rate with the procedures utilized to treat HPV-associated pre-malignant lesions and the mortality rate from cervical cancer is approximately 40% [22], elimination of the viral infection via therapeutic vaccination will likely reduce recurrence of HPV-associated pre-malignant lesions causing a reduction in cervical cancers. A summary of current therapeutic vaccination in clinical trials is shown in Table 2.

A majority of clinical trials using therapeutic agents have shown limited efficacy in eradicating established tumors in humans. The lack of clinical outcome seen in these studies may involve the general state of the patients' immune system such that more advanced stage cancer patients tend to have decreased immune function that correlates with stage of disease. Many of the studies examining therapeutic vaccination included patients with advanced stage cancers. Future trends in clinical trials with therapeutic agents will examine patients with early stage cancers and pre-invasive lesions in order to prevent invasive cervical cancer. Meanwhile preclinical studies in this field continue and include the further exploration of peptide or protein vaccination, and the delivery of HPV antigens in DNA-based vaccines or in viral vectors. As long as pre-clinical studies continue to advance in this field, the prospect of therapeutic vaccination to treat existing lesions seem highly likely to be developed in the near future. The result of therapeutic vaccination to treat existing HPV-related disease could include the availability of less invasive and disfiguring treatment options and fewer instances of recurrent or progressive lesions leading to an overall reduction in cervical cancer incidence.

Acknowledgements

Parts of the studies mentioned in this article were supported through grants NCI R01 CA 74397 and NCI P01 CA 97296 and the V and Whittier Foundations. JA Brinkman is an Achievement Rewards for College Scholars (ARCS) Fellow. WM Kast holds the Walter A. Richter Cancer Research Chair.

References

[1] http://www.cancer.org., American Cancer Society Inc., 2004.

[2] http://www.stressgen.com, Stressgen Reports HSPE7 Results From Two clinical Trials, 2004.

[3] http://www.who.int/vaccine_research/documents/new_vaccines/en/index8.html, World health Organization: Human Papillomavirures, 2004.

[4] http://www.centerwatch.com/patient/backgrnd.html, Center Watch Clinical trials listing service, 2006.

[5] http://www.clinicaltrials.gov/ct/info/whatis#phases, Clinical trials.gov, 2006.

[6] http://www.transgene.fr/us/index.php, Transgene, 2006.

[7] http://www.vitaloptions.org, Vital Options International, 2006.

[8] http://www.who.int/vaccine_research/diseases/viral_cancers/en/index3.html, World health Organization: Human Papillomavirures, 2006.

[9] M. Alexander, M.L. Salgaller, E. Celis, A. Sette, W.A. Barnes, S.A. Rosenberg and M.A. Steller, Generation of tumor-specific cytolytic T lymphocytes from peripheral blood of cervical cancer patients by in vitro stimulation with a synthetic human papillomavirus type 16 E7 epitope, *Am J Obstet Gynecol* **175** (1996), 1586–1593.

[10] Association of Professors of Gynecology and Obstetrics. APGO Educational Series on Women's Health Issues. Advances in the Screening, Diagnosis, and Treatment of Cervical Disease, (2002). 409 12th Street SW, Washington, DC 20024.

[11] P.J. Baldwin, S.H. Van der Burg, C.M. Boswell, R. Offringa, J.K. Hickling, J. Dobson, J.S. Roberts, J.A. Latimer, R.P. Moseley, N. Coleman, M.A. Stanley and J.C. Sterling, Vaccinia-expressed human papillomavirus 16 and 18 e6 and e7 as a therapeutic vaccination for vulval and vaginal intraepithelial neoplasia, *Clin Cancer Res* **9** (2003), 5205–5213.

[12] J. Banchereau, F. Briere, C. Caux, J. Davoust, S. Lebecque, Y.J. Liu, B. Pulendran and K. Palucka, Immunobiology of dendritic cells, *Annu Rev Immunol* **18** (2000), 767–811.

[13] J. Banchereau and R.M. Steinman, Dendritic cells and the control of immunity, *Nature* **392** (1998), 245–252.

[14] M. Barnden, L. Papalia, R. Davis, C. Millar, N. Nikolic, K. O'Brien, L. Wang, A. McKenzie, O. White and I. and Frazer, Antigen-Specific CD4+ and CD8+ T Cell Responses to HPV16 E6E7 ISCOMATRIX® Vaccine in Healthy Volunteers, (2004). Presented at the 21st International Papillomavirus Conference, Mexico City, Mexico.

[15] K.R. Beutner and S. Tyring, Human papillomavirus and human disease, *Am J Med* **102** (1997), 9–15.

[16] J. Brinkman, X. Xue, M. d. La. Garcia and W.M. Kast, *The Efficacy of an Insertional Duplication DNA Vaccine for Eradicating Established Tumors in Mice*, Presented at the 21st International Papillomavirus Conference Mexico City, Mexico. 2004.

[17] M.C. Cassetti, S.P. McElhiney, V. Shahabi, J.K. Pullen, I.C. Le Poole, G.L. Eiben, L.R. Smith and W.M. Kast, Antitumor efficacy of Venezuelan equine encephalitis virus replicon particles encoding mutated HPV16 E6 and E7 genes, *Vaccine* **22** (2004), 520–527.

[18] S.Y. Chan, H. Delius, A.L. Halpern and H.U. Bernard, Analysis of genomic sequences of 95 papillomavirus types: uniting typing, phylogeny, and taxonomy, *J Virol* **69** (1995), 3074–3083.

[19] Y.F. Chen, C.W. Lin, Y.P. Tsao and S.L. Chen, Cytotoxic-T-lymphocyte human papillomavirus type 16 E5 peptide with CpG-oligodeoxynucleotide can eliminate tumor growth in C57BL/6 mice, *J Virol* **78** (2004), 1333–1343.

[20] W.F. Cheng, C.F. Hung, K.F. Hsu, C.Y. Chai, L. He, J.M. Polo, L.A. Slater, M. Ling and T.C. Wu, Cancer immunotherapy using Sindbis virus replicon particles encoding a VP22-antigen fusion, *Hum Gene Ther* **13** (2002), 553–568.

[21] A. Cid-Arregui, V. Juarez and H. zur Hausen, A synthetic E7 gene of human papillomavirus type 16 that yields enhanced expression of the protein in mammalian cells and is useful for DNA immunization studies, *J Virol* **77** (2003), 4928–4937.

[22] M.P. Coleman, G. Gatta, A. Verdecchia, J. Esteve, M. Sant, H. Storm, C. Allemani, L. Ciccolallo, M. Santaquilani and F. Berrino, EUROCARE-3 summary: cancer survival in Europe at the end of the 20th century, *Ann Oncol* **14**(Suppl 5) (2003), v128–v149.

[23] J.F. Crish, F. Bone, S. Balasubramanian, T.M. Zaim, T. Wagner, J. Yun, E.A. Rorke and R.L. Eckert, Suprabasal expression of the human papillomavirus type 16 oncoproteins in mouse epidermis alters expression of cell cycle regulatory proteins, *Carcinogenesis* **21** (2000), 1031–1037.

[24] C.P. Crum, The beginning of the end for cervical cancer? *N Engl J Med* **347** (2002), 1703–1705.

[25] D.M. Da Silva, D.V. Pastrana, J.T. Schiller and W.M. Kast, Effect of preexisting neutralizing antibodies on the anti-tumor immune response induced by chimeric human papillomavirus virus-like particle vaccines, *Virology* **290** (2001), 350–360.

[26] D.M. Da Silva, J.T. Schiller and W.M. Kast, Heterologous boosting increases immunogenicity of chimeric papillomavirus virus-like particle vaccines, *Vaccine* **21** (2003), 3219–3227.

[27] T. Daemen, A. Riezebos-Brilman, L. Bungener, J. Regts, B. Dontje and J. Wilschut, Eradication of established HPV16-transformed tumours after immunisation with recombinant Semliki Forest virus expressing a fusion protein of E6 and E7, *Vaccine* **21** (2003), 1082–1088.

[28] E.J. Davidson, C.M. Boswell, P. Sehr, M. Pawlita, A.E. Tomlinson, R.J. McVey, J. Dobson, J.S. Roberts, J. Hickling, H.C. Kitchener and P.L. Stern, Immunological and clinical responses in women with vulval intraepithelial neoplasia vaccinated with a vaccinia virus encoding human papillomavirus 16/18 oncoproteins, *Cancer Res* **63** (2003), 6032–6041.

[29] T.D. de Gruijl, H.J. Bontkes, M.J. Stukart, J.M. Walboomers, A.J. Remmink, R.H. Verheijen, T.J. Helmerhorst, C.J. Meijer and R.J. Scheper, T cell proliferative responses against human papillomavirus type 16 E7 oncoprotein are most prominent in cervical intraepithelial neoplasia patients with a persistent viral infection, *J Gen Virol* **77**(Pt 9), (1996), 2183–2191.

[30] T.D. de Gruijl, H.J. Bontkes, J.M. Walboomers, M.J. Stukart, F.S. Doekhie, A.J. Remmink, T.J. Helmerhorst, R.H. Verheijen, M.F. Duggan-Keen, P.L. Stern, C.J. Meijer and R.J. Scheper, Differential T helper cell responses to human papillomavirus type 16 E7 related to viral clearance or persistence in patients with cervical neoplasia: a longitudinal study, *Cancer Res* **58** (1998), 1700–1706.

[31] A. de Jong, T. O'Neill, A.Y. Khan, K.M. Kwappenberg, S.E. Chisholm, N.R. Whittle, J.A. Dobson, L.C. Jack, J.A. Clair Roberts, R. Offringa, S.H. Van der Burg and J.K. Hickling, Enhancement of human papillomavirus (HPV) type 16 E6 and E7-specific T-cell immunity in healthy volunteers through vaccination with TA-CIN, an HPV16 L2E7E6 fusion protein vaccine, *Vaccine* **20** (2002), 3456–3464.

[32] T. Doan, K. Herd, I. Ramshaw, S. Thomson and R.W. Tindle, A polytope DNA vaccine elicits multiple effector and memory CTL responses and protects against human papillomavirus 16 E7-expressing tumour, *Cancer Immunol Immunother* **54** (2005), 157–171.

[33] T. Doan, K. Herd, Y. Woo, H. Netter and R.W. Tindle, *Recombinant Hepatitis B Surface Antigen Delivers Protective CTL Responses to HPV16-Associated Neoplastic Disease*, Presented at the 22nd International Papillomavirus Conference, Vancouver, Canada. May 2005.

[34] M. Durst, D. Glitz, A. Schneider and H. zur Hausen, Human papillomavirus type 16 (HPV 16) gene expression and DNA replication in cervical neoplasia: analysis by in situ hybridization, *Virology* **189** (1992), 132–140.

[35] G.L. Eiben, D.M. Da Silva, S.C. Fausch, I.C. Le Poole, M.I. Nishimura and W.M. Kast, Cervical cancer vaccines: recent advances in HPV research, *Viral Immunol* **16** (2003), 111–121.

[36] E.M. Evans, S. Man, A.S. Evans and L.K. Borysiewicz, Infiltration of cervical cancer tissue with human papillomavirus-specific cytotoxic T-lymphocytes, *Cancer Res* **57** (1997), 2943–2950.

[37] S.C. Fausch, D.M. Da Silva and W.M. Kast, Differential uptake and cross-presentation of human papillomavirus virus-like particles by dendritic cells and Langerhans cells, *Cancer Res* **63** (2003), 3478–3482.

[38] S.C. Fausch, D.M. Da Silva, M.P. Rudolf and W.M. Kast, Human papillomavirus virus-like particles do not activate Langerhans cells: a possible immune escape mechanism used by human papillomaviruses, *J Immunol* **169** (2002), 3242–3249.

[39] S.C. Fausch, L.M. Fahey, D.M. Da Silva and W.M. Kast, Human Papillomavirus Can Escape Immune Recognition through Langerhans Cell Phosphoinositide 3-Kinase Activation, *J Immunol* **174** (2005), 7172–7178.

[40] M. Favre, N. Ramoz and G. Orth, Human papillomaviruses: general features, *Clin Dermatol* **15** (1997), 181–198.

[41] A. Ferrara, M. Nonn, P. Sehr, C. Schreckenberger, M. Pawlita, M. Durst, A. Schneider and A.M. Kaufmann, Dendritic cell-based tumor vaccine for cervical cancer II: results of a clinical pilot study in 15 individual patients, *J Cancer Res Clin Oncol* **129** (2003), 521–530.

[42] I. Frazer, Vaccines for papillomavirus infection, *Virus Res* **89** (2002), 271–274.

[43] I.H. Frazer, M. Quinn, J.L. Nicklin, J. Tan, L.C. Perrin, P. Ng, V.M. O'Connor, O. White, N. Wendt, J. Martin, J.M. Crowley, S.J. Edwards, A.W. McKenzie, S.V. Mitchell, D.W. Maher, M.J. Pearse and R.L. Basser, Phase 1 study of HPV16-specific immunotherapy with E6E7 fusion protein and ISCOMATRIX adjuvant in women with cervical intraepithelial neoplasia, *Vaccine* **23** (2004), 172–181.

[44] F. Garcia, K.U. Petry, L. Muderspach, M.A. Gold, P. Braly, C.P. Crum, M. Magill, M. Silverman, R.G. Urban, M.L. Hedley and K.J. Beach, ZYC101a for treatment of high-grade cervical intraepithelial neoplasia: a randomized controlled trial, *Obstet Gynecol* **103** (2004), 317–326.

[45] H. Garoff and K.J. Li, Recent advances in gene expression using alphavirus vectors, *Curr Opin Biotechnol* **9** (1998), 464–469.

[46] S.E. Goldstone, J.M. Palefsky, M.T. Winnett and J.R. Neefe, Activity of HspE7, a novel immunotherapy, in patients with anogenital warts, *Dis Colon Rectum* **45** (2002), 502–507.

[47] S. Hallez, P. Simon, F. Maudoux, J. Doyen, J.C. Noel, A. Beliard, X. Capelle, F. Buxant, I. Fayt, A. C. Lagrost, P. Hubert, C. Gerday, A. Burny, J. Boniver, J.M. Foidart, P. Delvenne and N. Jacobs, Phase I/II trial of immunogenicity of a human papillomavirus (HPV) type 16 E7 protein-based vaccine in women with oncogenic HPV-positive cervical intraepithelial neoplasia, *Cancer Immunol Immunother* **53** (2004), 642–650.

[48] K.A. Herd, T. Harvey, A.A. Khromykh and R.W. Tindle, Recombinant Kunjin virus replicon vaccines induce protective T-cell immunity against human papillomavirus 16 E7-expressing tumour, *Virology* **319** (2004), 237–248.

[49] P.M. Howley, Papillomaviruses: The Viruses and Their Replication, in: *Fields Virology*, B.N. Field, D.M. Knipe and P.M. Howley, eds, Lippincott-Raven, Philadelphia, 1996, pp. 2045–2076.

[50] K.F. Hsu, C.F. Hung, W.F. Cheng, L. He, L.A. Slater, M. Ling and T.C. Wu, Enhancement of suicidal DNA vaccine potency by linking Mycobacterium tuberculosis heat shock protein 70 to an antigen, *Gene Ther* **8** (2001), 376–383.

[51] C.H. Huang, S. Peng, L. He, Y.C. Tsai, D.A. Boyd, T.H. Hansen, T.C. Wu and C.F. Hung, Cancer immunotherapy using a DNA vaccine encoding a single-chain trimer of MHC class I linked to an HPV-16 E6 immunodominant CTL epitope, *Gene Ther* **12** (2005), 1180–1186.

[52] C.F. Hung, W.F. Cheng, L. He, M. Ling, J. Juang, C.T. Lin and T.C. Wu, Enhancing major histocompatibility complex class I antigen presentation by targeting antigen to centrosomes, *Cancer Res* **63** (2003), 2393–2398.

[53] C.F. Hung, L. He, J. Juang, T.J. Lin, M. Ling and T.C. Wu, Improving DNA vaccine potency by linking Marek's disease virus type 1 VP22 to an antigen, *J Virol* **76** (2002), 2676–2682.

[54] T. Jakob, J. Ring and M.C. Udey, Multistep navigation of Langerhans/dendritic cells in and out of the skin, *J Allergy Clin Immunol* **108** (2001), 688–696.

[55] C.A. Janeway, P. Travers, M. Walport and M.J. and Shlomchick, Immunobiology: The Immune System in Health and Disease, p. 4:15, Garland publishing company, York and London 2005.

[56] A.S. Kadish, G.Y. Ho, R.D. Burk, Y. Wang, S.L. Romney, R. Ledwidge and R.H. Angeletti, Lymphoproliferative responses to human papillomavirus (HPV) type 16 proteins E6 and E7: outcome of HPV infection and associated neoplasia, *J Natl Cancer Inst* **89** (1997), 1285–1293.

[57] W.M. Kast, R.M. Brandt, J.W. Drijfhout and C.J. Melief, Human leukocyte antigen-A2.1 restricted candidate cytotoxic T lymphocyte epitopes of human papillomavirus type 16 E6 and E7 proteins identified by using the processing-defective human cell line T2, *J Immunother* **14** (1993), 115–120.

[58] A.M. Kaufmann, P.L. Stern, E.M. Rankin, H. Sommer, V. Nuessler, A. Schneider, M. Adams, T.S. Onon, T. Bauknecht, U. Wagner, K. Kroon, J. Hickling, C.M. Boswell, S.N. Stacey, H.C. Kitchener, J. Gillard, J. Wanders, J.S. Roberts and H. Zwierzina, Safety and immunogenicity of TA-HPV, a recombinant vaccinia virus expressing modified human papillomavirus (HPV)-16 and HPV-18 E6 and E7 genes, in women with progressive cervical cancer, *Clin Cancer Res* **8** (2002), 3676–3685.

[59] K.H. Kim, A. Santin, S. Bellone and M. Nakagawa, *The HPV 16 E6 52–61 CD8 T Cell Epitope As a Source of Antigen for Dendritic Cell Immunotherapy for Cervical Cancer*, Presented at the 22nd International Papillomavirus Conference, Vancouver, Canada. May 2005.

[60] S.W. Kim and J.S. Yang, Human papillomavirus type 16 e5 protein as a therapeutic target, *Yonsei Med J* **47** (2006), 1–14.

[61] B. Klencke, M. Matijevic, R.G. Urban, J.L. Lathey, M.L. Hedley, M. Berry, J. Thatcher, V. Weinberg, J. Wilson, T. Darragh, N. Jay, M. Da Costa and J.M. Palefsky, Encapsulated plasmid DNA treatment for human papillomavirus 16-associated anal dysplasia: a Phase I study of ZYC101, *Clin Cancer Res* **8** (2002), 1028–1037.

[62] L.A. Koutsky, D.A. Galloway and K.K. Holmes, Epidemiology of genital human papillomavirus infection, *Epidemiol Rev* **10** (1988), 122–163.

[63] R.J. Kurman, D.E. Henson, A.L. Herbst, K.L. Noller and M.H. Schiffman, Interim guidelines for management of abnormal cervical cytology. The 1992 National Cancer Institute Workshop, *JAMA* **271** (1994), 1866–1869.

[64] J. Li, Y. Sun and A. Garen, Immunization and immunotherapy for cancers involving infection by a human papillomavirus in a mouse model, *Proc Natl Acad Sci USA* **99** (2002), 16232–16236.

[65] W.J. Liu, F. Gao, K.N. Zhao, W. Zhao, G.J. Fernando, R. Thomas and I.H. Frazer, Codon modified human papillomavirus type 16 E7 DNA vaccine enhances cytotoxic T-lymphocyte induction and anti-tumour activity, *Virology* **301** (2002), 43–52.

[66] W.J. Liu, K.N. Zhao, F.G. Gao, G.R. Leggatt, G.J. Fernando and I.H. Frazer, Polynucleotide viral vaccines: codon optimisation and ubiquitin conjugation enhances prophylactic and therapeutic efficacy, *Vaccine* **20** (2001), 862–869.

[67] D.R. Lowy and P.M. Howley, Papillomaviruses, in: *Fields Virology*, D.M. Knipe, P.M. Howley, D.E. Griffin, R.A. Lamb, M.A. Martin, B. Roizman and S.E. Straus, eds, Lippincott Williams & Wilkins, 2001.

[68] J.C. Luxton, A.J. Rowe, J.C. Cridland, T. Coletart, P. Wilson and P.S. Shepherd, Proliferative T cell responses to the human papillomavirus type 16 E7 protein in women with cervical dysplasia and cervical carcinoma and in healthy individuals, *J Gen Virol* **77**(Pt 7), (1996), 1585–1593.

[69] J. Mackova, J. Stasikova, L. Kutinova, J. Masin, P. Hainz, M. Simsova, P. Gabriel, P. Sebo and S. Nemeckova, Prime/boost immunotherapy of HPV16-induced tumors with E7 protein delivered by Bordetella adenylate cyclase and modified vaccinia virus Ankara, *Cancer Immunol Immunother* **55** (2006), 39–46.

[70] L. Muderspach, S. Wilczynski, L. Roman, L. Bade, J. Felix, L.A. Small, W.M. Kast, G. Fascio, V. Marty and J. Weber, A phase I trial of a human papillomavirus (HPV) peptide vaccine for women with high-grade cervical and vulvar intraepithelial neoplasia who are HPV 16 positive, *Clin Cancer Res* **6** (2000), 3406–3416.

[71] K. Munger, The molecular biology of cervical cancer, *J Cell Biochem Suppl* **23** (1995), 55–60.

[72] K. Munger, A. Baldwin, K.M. Edwards, H. Hayakawa, C.L. Nguyen, M. Owens, M. Grace and K. Huh, Mechanisms of human papillomavirus-induced oncogenesis, *J Virol* **78** (2004), 11451–11460.

[73] M. Nimako, A.N. Fiander, G.W. Wilkinson, L.K. Borysiewicz and S. Man, Human papillomavirus-specific cytotoxic T lymphocytes in patients with cervical intraepithelial neoplasia grade III, *Cancer Res* **57** (1997), 4855–4861.

[74] P. Ohlschlager, M. Pes, W. Osen, M. Durst, A. Schneider, L. Gissmann and A.M. Kaufmann, *An improved rearranged Human Papillomavirus Type 16 E7 DNA vaccine candidate (HPV-16 E7SH) induces an E7 wildtype-specific T cell response*, Vaccine, 2006.

[75] W. Osen, T. Peiler, P. Ohlschlager, S. Caldeira, S. Faath, N. Michel, M. Muller, M. Tommasino, I. Jochmus and L. Gissmann, A DNA vaccine based on a shuffled E7 oncogene of the human papillomavirus type 16 (HPV 16) induces E7-specific cytotoxic T cells but lacks transforming activity, *Vaccine* **19** (2001), 4276–4286.

[76] S. Peng, H. Ji, C. Trimble, L. He, Y.C. Tsai, J. Yeatermeyer, D.A. Boyd, C.F. Hung and T.C. Wu, Development of a DNA vaccine targeting human papillomavirus type 16 oncoprotein E6, *J Virol* **78** (2004), 8468–8476.

[77] S. Peng, T.W. Kim, J.H. Lee, M. Yang, L. He, C.F. Hung and T.C. Wu, Vaccination with dendritic cells transfected with BAK and BAX siRNA enhances antigen-specific immune responses by prolonging dendritic cell life, *Hum Gene Ther* **16** (2005), 584–593.

[78] S. Peng, C. Trimble, H. Ji, L. He, Y.C. Tsai, B. Macaes, C.F. Hung and T.C. Wu, Characterization of HPV-16 E6 DNA vaccines employing intracellular targeting and intercellular spreading strategies, *J Biomed Sci* **12** (2005), 689–700.

[79] M. Pes, P. Ohlschlager, L. Gissman, A. Schneider, M. Durst and A.M. Kaufman, Dendritic Cells Transfected by a Rearranged HPV16E7 DNA Vaccine Induce *in Vitro* E7 Wildtype-Specific Human T Cells. Presented at the 22nd International Papillomavirus Conference, Vancouver, Canada. May 2005.

[80] N.C. Popescu and J.A. DiPaolo, Preferential sites for viral integration on mammalian genome, *Cancer Genet Cytogenet* **42** (1989), 157–171.

[81] X. Preville, D. Ladant, B. Timmerman and C. Leclerc, *Eradication of Established Tumors by Vaccination With Recombinant Bordetella Pertussis Adenylate Cyclase Carrying the Human Papillomavirus 16 E7 Oncoprotein*, Presented at the 22nd International Papillomavirus Conference, Vancouver, Canada. May 2005.

[82] J.K. Pullen, S.P. McElhiney, M. Lee, W. Al-Rimawi, J. Li, A. Ota-Setlik, R.J. Natuk, J. Kowalski, D.M. Da Silva and W.M. Kast, *Development of a Multivalent Vaccine for Therapeutic Immunization Against HPV-Associated Diseases*, Presented at the 22nd International Papillomavirus Conference, Vancouver, Canada. 2005.

[83] M.E. Ressing, A. Sette, R.M. Brandt, J. Ruppert, P.A. Wentworth, M. Hartman, C. Oseroff, H.M. Grey, C.J. Melief and W.M. Kast, Human CTL epitopes encoded by human papillomavirus type 16 E6 and E7 identified through *in vivo* and *in vitro* immunogenicity studies of HLA-A*0201-binding peptides, *J Immunol* **154** (1995), 5934–5943.

[84] M.E. Ressing, W.J. van Driel, R.M. Brandt, G.G. Kenter, J.H. de Jong, T. Bauknecht, G.J. Fleuren, P. Hoogerhout, R. Offringa, A. Sette, E. Celis, H. Grey, B.J. Trimbos, W.M. Kast and C.J. Melief, Detection of T helper responses, but not of human papillomavirus-specific cytotoxic T lymphocyte responses, after peptide vaccination of patients with cervical carcinoma, *J Immunother* **23** (2000), 255–266.

[85] M.E. Ressing, W.J. van Driel, E. Celis, A. Sette, M.P. Brandt, M. Hartman, J.D. Anholts, G.M. Schreuder, W.B. ter Harmsel, G.J. Fleuren, B.J. Trimbos, W.M. Kast and C.J. Melief, Occasional memory cytotoxic T-cell responses of patients with human papillomavirus type 16-positive cervical lesions against a human leukocyte antigen-A *0201-restricted E7-encoded epitope, *Cancer Res* **56** (1996), 582–588.

[86] A. Ribas, L.H. Butterfield, J.A. Glaspy and J.S. Economou, Current developments in cancer vaccines and cellular immunotherapy, *J Clin Oncol* **21** (2003), 2415–2432.

[87] M.P. Rudolf, S. Man, C.J. Melief, A. Sette and W.M. Kast, Human T-cell responses to HLA-A-restricted high binding affinity peptides of human papillomavirus type 18 proteins E6 and E7, *Clin Cancer Res* **7** (2001), 788s–795s.

[88] R.B. Salit, W.M. Kast and M.P. Velders, Ins and outs of clinical trials with peptide-based vaccines, *Front Biosci* **7** (2002), e204–e213.

[89] A.D. Santin, S. Bellone, M. Palmieri, A. Ravaggi, C. Romani, R. Tassi, J.J. Roman, A. Burnett, S. Pecorelli and M.J. Cannon, HPV16/18 E7-pulsed dendritic cell vaccination in cervical cancer patients with recurrent disease refractory to standard treatment modalities, *Gynecol Oncol* **100** (2006), 469–478.

[90] K.B. Scholten, M.W. Schreurs, J.J. Ruizendaal, E.W. Kueter, D. Kramer, S. Veenbergen, C.J. Meijer and E. Hooijberg, Preservation and redirection of HPV16E7-specific T cell receptors for immunotherapy of cervical cancer, *Clin Immunol* **114** (2005), 119–129.

[91] K.V. Shah and P.M. and Howley, Papillomaviruses, in: *Fields Virology*, D.M. Knipe, P.M. Howley, D.E. Griffin, R.A. Lamb, M.A. Martin, B. Roizman and S.E. Straus, eds, Lippincott Williams & Wilkins, 1990.

[92] E.E. Sheets, R.G. Urban, C.P. Crum, M.L. Hedley, J.A. Politch, M.A. Gold, L.I. Muderspach, G.A. Cole and P.A. Crowley-Nowick, Immunotherapy of human cervical high-grade cervical intraepithelial neoplasia with microparticle-delivered human papillomavirus 16 E7 plasmid DNA, *Am J Obstet Gynecol* **188** (2003), 916–926.

[93] L.J. Smyth, M.I. Van Poelgeest, E.J. Davidson, K.M. Kwappenberg, D. Burt, P. Sehr, M. Pawlita, S. Man, J.K. Hickling, A.N. Fiander, A. Tristram, H.C. Kitchener, R. Offringa, P.L. Stern and S.H. Van der Burg, Immunological responses in women with human papillomavirus type 16 (HPV-16)-associated anogenital intraepithelial neoplasia induced by heterologous prime-boost HPV-16 oncogene vaccination, *Clin Cancer Res* **10** (2004), 2954–2961.

[94] S.A. Southern and C.S. Herrington, Differential cell cycle regulation by low- and high-risk human papillomaviruses in low-grade squamous intraepithelial lesions of the cervix, *Cancer Res* **58** (1998), 2941–2945.

[95] R.M. Steinman, The dendritic cell system and its role in immunogenicity, *Annu Rev Immunol* **9** (1991), 271–296.

[96] M.A. Steller, K.J. Gurski, M. Murakami, R.W. Daniel, K.V. Shah, E. Celis, A. Sette, E.L. Trimble, R.C. Park and F.M. Marincola, Cell-mediated immunological responses in cervical and vaginal cancer patients immunized with a lipidated epitope of human papillomavirus type 16 E7, *Clin Cancer Res* **4** (1998), 2103–2109.

[97] S.K. Tyring, Human papillomavirus infections: epidemiology, pathogenesis, and host immune response, *J Am Acad Dermatol* **43** (2000), S18–S26.

[98] A. Vambutas, J. Devoti, M. Nouri, J. Drijfhout, G. Lipford, V. Bonagura, S. van der Burg and C.J. Melief. Therapeutic Vaccination With Papillomavirus E6 and E7 Long Peptides Results in the Control of Both Established Virus-Induced Lesions and Latently Infected Sites in a Pre-Clinical Cottontail Rabbit Papillomavirus Model. Presented at the 22nd International Papillomavirus Conference, Vancouver, Canada. May 2005.

[99] S.H. Van der Burg, A. de Jong, M.J. Welters, R. Offringa and C.J. Melief, The status of HPV16-specific T-cell reactivity in

health and disease as a guide to HPV vaccine development, *Virus Res* **89** (2002), 275–284.

[100] S.H. Van der Burg, K.M. Kwappenberg, T. O'Neill, R.M. Brandt, C.J. Melief, J.K. Hickling and R. Offringa, Preclinical safety and efficacy of TA-CIN, a recombinant HPV16 L2E6E7 fusion protein vaccine, in homologous and heterologous prime-boost regimens, *Vaccine* **19** (2001), 3652–3660.

[101] W.J. van Driel, M.E. Ressing, G.G. Kenter, R.M. Brandt, E.J. Krul, A.B. van Rossum, E. Schuuring, R. Offringa, T. Bauknecht, A. Tamm-Hermelink, P.A. van Dam, G.J. Fleuren, W.M. Kast, C.J. Melief and J.B. Trimbos, Vaccination with HPV16 peptides of patients with advanced cervical carcinoma: clinical evaluation of a phase I-II trial, *Eur J Cancer* **35** (1999), 946–952.

[102] M.P. Velders, S. Weijzen, G.L. Eiben, A.G. Elmishad, P.M. Kloetzel, T. Higgins, R.B. Ciccarelli, M. Evans, S. Man, L. Smith and W.M. Kast, Defined flanking spacers and enhanced proteolysis is essential for eradication of established tumors by an epitope string DNA vaccine, *J Immunol* **166** (2001), 5366–5373.

[103] M. von Knebel Doeberitz, C. Rittmuller, F. Aengeneyndt, P. Jansen-Durr and D. Spitkovsky, Reversible repression of papillomavirus oncogene expression in cervical carcinoma cells: consequences for the phenotype and E6-p53 and E7-pRB interactions. J Virol 68, (1994), 2811-2821.

[104] J.M. Walboomers, M.V. Jacobs, M.M. Manos, F.X. Bosch, J.A. Kummer, K.V. Shah, P.J. Snijders, J. Peto, C.J. Meijer and N. Munoz, Human papillomavirus is a necessary cause of invasive cervical cancer worldwide, *J Pathol* **189** (1999), 12–19.

[105] D.E. Warrino, W.C. Olson, W.T. Knapp, M.I. Scarrow, L.J. D'Ambrosio-Brennan, R.S. Guido, R.P. Edwards, W.M. Kast and W.J. Storkus, Disease-stage variance in functional CD4(+) T-cell responses against novel pan-human leukocyte antigen-D region presented human papillomavirus-16 E7 epitopes, *Clin Cancer Res* **10** (2004), 3301–3308.

[106] D.E. Warrino, W.C. Olson, M.I. Scarrow, L.J. D'Ambrosio-Brennan, R.S. Guido, D.M. Da Silva, W.M. Kast and W.J. Storkus, Human papillomavirus L1L2-E7 virus-like particles partially mature human dendritic cells and elicit E7-specific T-helper responses from patients with cervical intraepithelial neoplasia or cervical cancer *in vitro*, *Hum Immunol* **66** (2005), 762–772.

[107] S. Xue, R. Gillmore, A. Downs, A. Tsallios, A. Holler, L. Gao, V. Wong, E. Morris and H.J. Stauss, Exploiting T cell receptor genes for cancer immunotherapy, *Clin Exp Immunol* **139** (2005), 167–172.

[108] H. zur Hausen, Papillomaviruses and cancer: from basic studies to clinical application, *Nat Rev Cancer* **2** (2002), 342–350.

[109] S. Zwaveling, S.C. Ferreira Mota, J. Nouta, M. Johnson, G.B. Lipford, R. Offringa, S.H. Van der Burg and C.J. Melief, Established human papillomavirus type 16-expressing tumors are effectively eradicated following vaccination with long peptides, *J Immunol* **169** (2002), 350–358.